Sustainable Ageing

Nestor Asiamah • Hafiz T. A. Khan
Whitney Nesser • Frank Frimpong Opuni
Alex Siu Wing Chan
Editors

Sustainable Ageing

Reimagining Healthy Ageing Through the Lens of Flagship Campaigns

Springer

Editors
Nestor Asiamah
Division of Interdisciplinary Research and Practice
University of Essex
Colchester, Essex, UK

Whitney Nesser
Department of Applied Clinical and Educational Sciences
Indiana State University
Terre Haute, IN, USA

Alex Siu Wing Chan
Hong Kong Polytechnic University
Hung Hom, Kowloon, Hong Kong

Hafiz T. A. Khan
University of West London
London, Middlesex, UK

Frank Frimpong Opuni
Department of Marketing
Accra Technical University
Accra, Ghana

ISBN 978-3-031-69474-5 ISBN 978-3-031-69475-2 (eBook)
https://doi.org/10.1007/978-3-031-69475-2

This Springer imprint is published by the registered company Springer Nature Switzerland AG
The registered company address is: Gewerbestrasse 11, 6330 Cham, Switzerland

Preface

Ageing is a gradual decline in the physiological functions necessary for well-being and survival. Its intensity and frequency determine population ageing, a shift in the distribution of a population towards older ages. The world's population is rapidly ageing owing to improving life expectancy and declining fertility rate. Consequently, the burden of disease and health care will continue to increase, putting pressure on governments and the limited resources available. Many individuals are living with chronic conditions such as diabetes and cancer and are unable to maintain jobs, economic productivity, and autonomy in older age due to limited functional capacity. In response to this development of demographic change, the Decade of Healthy Ageing 2021–2030 initiative and other campaigns were launched by the United Nations.

The foregoing campaign is a flagship initiative championed by the United Nations to support older adults, their families, and communities. Its key action plans include combating ageism, providing age-friendly neighbourhoods, and improving access to long-term and integrated care for those in need of it. These action plans enable the United Nations to streamline interdisciplinary efforts fostering well-being for older adults worldwide. The campaign is undoubtedly timely and provides an opportunity for empowering individuals and communities to maintain well-being across the lifespan. Even so, emerging crises can make its desired outcomes an illusion.

Climate change, outbreak of infectious diseases, extreme industrialization, and war or violence are entrenched health threats. Neighbourhood resources such as parks, social networks, and services facilitating health-seeking behaviour are disoriented by these crises. Climate change events such as heat waves increase disease risk, especially respiratory disorders. Neighbourhood resources necessary for healthy lifestyles and healthy ageing are obliterated by war, violence, and natural disasters. Arguably, the goals of the Decade of Healthy Ageing 2020–2030 and related campaigns may not be realized since efforts against crises are not integrated into the campaigns' action plans. Hence, an interdisciplinary dialogue towards a strategy for manoeuvring or overcoming the crises to achieve the goals of the foregoing campaigns is imperative.

This book provides a forum for re-imagining healthy ageing through the Decade of Healthy Ageing 2020–2030 and other campaigns. It compiles ideas, models, and postulates for manoeuvring crises and realizing healthy longevity in contexts experiencing crises. Most of its chapters draw on action plans of the Decade of Healthy Ageing and related campaigns to create an imaginary path along which healthy ageing can be made more realistic amidst the crises. This book is the first to initiate a debate for rethinking approaches to healthy ageing in response to crises. Its key themes are: (1) age-friendly neighbourhoods, (2) innovation and planning, (3) the use of data and research evidence, and (4) human development.

Chapters of the book were written by a team of scholars from 13 countries and a wide spectrum of disciplines, including public health, architecture, engineering, human resources management, psychology, education, marketing, and finance. The interdisciplinary nature of its authorship makes it an invaluable resource for students, researchers, educators, and stakeholders in different disciplines. Review questions at the end of each chapter maximize the didactic potential of the volume. Enjoy your reading!

Colchester, Essex, UK — Nestor Asiamah
London, Middlesex, UK — Hafiz T. A. Khan
Terre Haute, IN, USA — Whitney Nesser
Accra, Ghana — Frank Frimpong Opuni
Hung Hom, Kowloon, Hong Kong — Alex Siu Wing Chan

Contents

1 Re-imagining Healthy Ageing Through the Lens of Flagship Campaigns: An Introduction 1
Nestor Asiamah, Hafiz T. A. Khan, Whitney Nesser, Frank Frimpong Opuni, and Alex Siu Wing Chan

Part I Age-Friendly Neighbourhoods and Ageing in Place

2 Psychology of "Ageing in Place" Amidst Health and Social Threats: Perspectives on the Decade of Healthy Ageing 13
Nestor Asiamah, Hafiz T. A. Khan, JohnBosco Chika Chukwuorji, Alex Siu Wing Chan, and Happy Griffiths Njoekpume

3 Making the "Smart Cities" Agenda a Reality: The Role of a Proposed Integrated Model 35
Mariana Flores-García

4 A Systematic-Narrative Review of the Determinants of Green Purchasing Capabilities in Developing Countries: Healthy Aging Perspective 45
James Peprah Adu and John Amoah

Part II Innovation, Planning, and Change

5 The Future of Healthy Ageing Amidst Threats: The Role of Innovation for Nigerian Older Adults 75
Jacinta C. Ene, Henry T. Ajibo, and Uzoma O. Okoye

6 Global Social Policy Reform of Healthy Ageing: A Comparison of China and India 93
Jamie P. Halsall, Liping Mei, James Stockton, Kalim Siddiqui, Chloe Holland, Michael Sarfo, and Michael Snowden

7 A Health Promotion Perspective on the "Decade of Healthy Ageing" Initiative 109
Nestor Asiamah, Amar Kanekar, Peter Hjorth, Kyriakos Kouveliotis, and Thomas Rieger

8 Climate Change Adaptation for Healthy Ageing 127
Faith Hope Muhonja, Simon Mawulorm Agyemang, Reginald Arthur-Mensah, and Sarra Sghaier

Part III Data and Research for Healthy Ageing

9 Research-Practice Gap: Impact on Campaigns and Mitigation Strategies 143
Evelyn N. Alvarez, Alexys Garcia, Patricia Amoroto, and Marlene Huerta

10 An Evaluation of the Financing of Healthy Aging Through the Lens of Social Welfare: Healthy Aging Index 159
Özge Kutlu and Mehmet Öçal

11 GIS Objective Measures of Walkability Are Not Always Superior to Psychometric Measures 179
Nestor Asiamah and Hafiz T. A. Khan

12 The Role of PROMs in Mitigating Infectious Disease Crises: A Healthy Ageing Perspective 189
Kasturi Shukla and Asiya Attar

Part IV Human Development for Healthy Ageing

13 Human Development Pathways for Empowering Older Adults: A Decade of Healthy Ageing Perspective 213
Md. Emaj Uddin

14 Empowering Older Adults to Utilise Neighbourhoods: A Healthy Ageing Perspective 227
Simon Mawulorm Agyemang, Faith Hope Muhonja, Sarra Sghaier, Richmond Stephen Sorkpor, and Seyram Kafui Akude

Part V Interventions Against Ageism

15 Combating Ageism and Elderly Abuse: The Roles of Physical Activity Participation, Social Services Utilization, and Legal Interventions 247
Oluwasogo Ruth Ogunleye, Bala Kwata Waziri, and Ferdinand Onwe Agama

16 Initiatives to Fight Ageism, Neglect, and Elderly Abuse During Crises: A Healthy Ageing Perspective 263
Clotilde Dudley-Smith

Index 275

About the Editors

Nestor Asiamah, PhD, FHEA, is a Lecturer (Assistant Professor) and Deputy Director of Postgraduate Research in the School of Health and Social Care at the University of Essex, United Kingdom. He is also a Lecturer at the University of Europe for Applied Sciences and Berlin School of Business and Innovation, which are both in Germany. He is Executive Director and Founding Fellow at the Africa Centre for Epidemiology and leads several international research groups. He reviews for several top journals such as *The Lancet* and serves as an academic editor for several journals (e.g., *BMC Public Health* and *PLoS ONE*). He is a Medical Research Council grant reviewer and has served as a research consultant to the NHS in the United Kingdom.

Hafiz T. A. Khan, PhD, is a Professor of Public Health and Statistics at the University of West London, UK. He is also an Associate Professorial Fellow in the Oxford Institute of Population Ageing at the University of Oxford. Prof Khan has published several articles in top-tier journals and has played editorial roles in Health Sciences journals.

Whitney Nesser, PhD, is a Professor and Gerontology Program Director in the Department of Applied Clinical and Educational Sciences at Indiana State University, USA. Her primary focus is on research and teaching about quality of life, ageing, and intergenerationology. Her PhD is in Health Education and Promotion from the University of Alabama at Birmingham.

Frank Frimpong Opuni, PhD, is an Associate Professor in Marketing at Accra Technical University, Ghana, and has a PhD in Marketing from the University of Bolton, UK. He serves as Director of Business Development and Founding Fellow at the Africa Centre for Epidemiology. His research interests are social marketing, green marketing, and health marketing. He serves on the editorial board of *Social Sciences and Humanities Open* (Elsevier) and reviews for *Journal of Social Marketing*, *Transportation Planning and Technology*, and *BMC Psychology*.

Alex Siu Wing Chan, PhD, is a Chartered Psychologist with the British Psychological Society and a full member of the American Psychological Association. Dr Chan is also a Registered Social Worker. His research focuses on promoting social equality and mental health for the LGBTQ community, including areas such as ageing, homosexuality, psychological well-being, HIV/AIDS, and social inclusion/exclusion among LGBTQ individuals. He serves as an associate editor for *Frontiers in Public Health* and *Frontiers in Urology*. He is a review editor for *Clinical Research in Nephrology* and an editorial board member for *BMC Public Health.*

Contributors

James Peprah Adu, PhD, is a Senior Lecturer at Takoradi Technical University, Ghana, specializing in procurement, logistics, operations management, and supply chain management. He has taught at prestigious institutions such as the Chartered Institute of Logistics and Transport (CILT) and the Ghana Institute of Management and Public Administration (GIMPA). Adu holds a PhD in Supply Chain Management from Durban University of Technology and an MPhil in Business Administration with a focus on Logistics and Supply Chain Management from Kwame Nkrumah University of Science and Technology. He is a Chartered Member of the Chartered Institute of Supply Chain Management, the Chartered Institute of Logistics and Transport, and the Chartered Institute of Procurement and Supply.

Ferdinand Onwe Agama, PhD, is a Lecturer in the Faculty of Law, at the National Open University of Nigeria. He obtained his Doctorate in International Law and Jurisprudence from Nnamdi Azikiwe University, Awka. He is the current Deputy Dean of the Faculty of Law. He is adventurous and has a flair for research.

Simon Mawulorm Agyemang, MPhil, is a Senior Tutor at Abetifi Presbyterian College of Education, Ghana. He is equipped with skills in physical fitness, exercise, and first aid. His research interests are in safety in schools, sustainable green environment, physical activity, sports development, healthy ageing, and climate change.

Henry T. Ajibo, PhD, has a PhD in Public Health Social Work and is Lecturer 1 in the Department of Social Work, University of Nigeria, Nsukka, Enugu state. His research interest is in social work and public health.

Seyram Kafui Akude, MPhil, is a Tutor at Peki College of Education, Ghana, specialized in health, physical education, and sports. He has expertise in physical fitness, exercise, first aid, and teacher development. He is currently a PhD scholar at Ignatius Ajuru University of Education, Port Harcourt, River State, Nigeria. His research interests include health, inclusive education, physical activity, sports management and administration, as well as sports marketing.

Evelyn N. Alvarez, PhD, MPH, is an environmental health scientist and Professor at California State University, Los Angeles (Cal State LA), USA. Her research agenda largely focuses on environmental smartphone applications and wearable technology to promote environmental justice. Her research interests also include examining underrepresented narratives in the climate change dialogue and demystifying sustainable living.

John Amoah, PhD, is a Lecturer in the Department of Marketing and HRM at KAAF University College, Kasoa, Ghana. He holds a PhD in Marketing Management from the Tomas Bata University, Zlin, Czech Republic. Currently, he is the Master's Coordinator of the MBA Program at the Faculty of Business School. He serves on the editorial boards of several journals, including *Cogent Business & Management*. John is an Associate member of the Chartered Institute of Marketing, Ghana. His main research areas are the development of small- and medium-size enterprises, technology adoption, and service marketing.

Patricia Amoroto, MPH, specializes in policy, systems, and environmental change for issues at the intersection of public health and environmental sustainability. Her work revolves around energy equity, particularly focusing on heat mitigation, weatherization, and clean mobility options.

Reginald Arthur-Mensah, MPhil, is a specialist in clinical nursing and a Senior Lecturer at Pentecost University, Ghana. He is currently a PhD scholar at the University of Ghana. His research interests include physical activity, gerontology, and geriatrics.

Asiya Attar is a PhD Scholar with a Junior Research Fellowship at Symbiosis International University, Pune, India. She is a Dental Surgeon with a master's degree in Healthcare and Pharmaceutical Management. Her research interests include patient-centred care, oral health-related quality of life, and dental patient-reported outcomes and experiences.

JohnBosco Chika Chukwuorji, PhD, is currently a Research Associate (Postdoc) in the CS Mott Department of Public Health of the College of Human Medicine at Michigan State University, USA, and was a visiting Fulbright Scholar at Cleveland State University, Cleveland, Ohio, USA (2019–2020). He also holds a Senior Lecturer position in Psychology and a Senior Research Fellow at the IVAN Research Institute. He is a recipient of the Developing Country Fellowship Award (2022) of the International Society for the Study of Behavioural Development (ISSBD). In addition to being guest editor of a special issue on Aging in sub-Saharan Africa for *Innovation in Aging* and Editor of the *Nigerian Journal of Psychological Research*, he holds editorial positions in two developmental science journals—*Journal of Child & Adolescent Trauma*, as well as *Adversity and Resilience Science: Journal of Research and Practice*.

Clotilde Dudley-Smith, EdD, MPA, RDH, HEC-C, is Director and Assistant Professor of Health Sciences at Quinnipiac University in Hamden, CT, USA. She earned her Doctorate in Educational Leadership, a Master's in Public/Healthcare Management, and a Bachelor's in Health Science/Dental Hygiene and certificate in Healthcare Ethics Consulting. Dr Dudley-Smith has presented nationally and internationally. She has numerous publications, book chapters, and grants on healthcare ethics.

Jacinta C. Ene, PhD, holds a PhD in Social Gerontology and is Lecturer 1 in the Department of Social Work at the University of Nigeria, Nsukka, Enugu state. Her research interest is in public health and social gerontology.

Mariana Flores-García, PhD, is a Professor in the Faculty of Architecture at the University La Salle Bajío, León, Guanajuato, Mexico. She holds a PhD in architecture, housing, and contemporary habitat from the University of Seville and serves as Director at the National Institute of Architecture and Urbanism (INAU)—FCARM MÉXICO—UIA.

Alexys Garcia, MPH, CHES®, is a Health Educator for the Los Angeles County Department of Health Services (LADHS), where she provides sexual and reproductive health classes and resources to individuals in substance use disorder (SUD) recovery. Her research interests include the built environment and its health impacts on marginalized communities.

Jamie P. Halsall, PhD, is a Reader in Social Sciences in the Department of Behavioural and Social Sciences at the University of Huddersfield, UK. Jamie's research interests are encompassed within three distinct areas: (1) civil society, social enterprise, and public policy; (2) sustainability and globalization, and (3) coaching and mentorship.

Peter Hjorth, PhD, is a renowned researcher and clinician in psychiatry, focusing on the physical health of individuals with severe mental illness. He earned his PhD from Aarhus University, Denmark, in 2013, and in 2019 became an Associate Professor specializing in the prevention and treatment of physical health problems in people with mental illness.

Chloe Holland has just completed her Master's degree in Public Health and has a keen interest in global health and well-being. Chloe's research focuses on health inequalities and how United Kingdom's policy can be adapted to better support population health.

Marlene Huerta, MPH, has served as a Research Assistant at George Washington University's (GW) i-CHARM Lab. She is currently a Case Manager at Molina Healthcare, where she focuses on ovarian cancer, reproductive and sexual health, and the impact of environmental health on marginalized communities, aiming to enhance overall health outcomes.

Amar Kanekar, PhD, is a Professor and Graduate Program Coordinator for Health Education and Health Promotion at the University of Arkansas at Little Rock. His research areas of interest focus on adolescent health, measurement in health education, global health, online and hybrid pedagogy, and health behaviour interventions.

Kyriakos Kouveliotis, PhD FRSA, is a Professor and the Provost and Chief Academic Officer of the Berlin School of Business and Innovation in Germany. He also serves as a Professor at the Uninettuno University of Rome, Italy, and President at Atheneum Liberal Studies. In the last 20 years, he has guided and taught in many universities and educational organizations globally. He is an expert in developing new curricula, programmes, syllabi, and on e-learning and virtual learning. Professor Kouveliotis has published 12 books and dozens of original scientific articles. Recently, he received a fellowship in the Royal Society of Arts and created in the Hague his own not-for-profit organization, the "Global Degree Foundation".

Özge Kutlu graduated from Social Work and Social Policy Master's Program in 2022. Kutlu, who worked as a Social Worker at Burdur Provincial Health Directorate between 2019 and 2023, has been working as a Lecturer in Burdur Mehmet Akif Ersoy University Elderly Care programme since February 2023. She works on the provision of rights-based social work practices for the elderly and their families.

Liping Mei, PhD, is an Associate Professor at Beijing Youth Politics College, China. Liping is a member of the Chinese Psychological Society and the Vice President of China Pharmaceutical Culture Society Health Science Popularization Branch. Her research interests are encompassed within two areas: (1) ageing and elderly care and (2) comparative study of social welfare policies.

Faith Hope Muhonja, PhD, is a Lecturer and Research Consultant of Public Health at Amref International University, Kenya. Her research interests include the effect of climate change on health, one health, ageing, physical activity, food hygiene and security, adolescent sexual health, and mHealth technology.

Happy Griffiths Njoekpume's academic journey began with a Bachelor of Science in Human Physiology, focusing on the human body's intricate mechanisms. He further pursued a Master of Science in Psychology, which has enhanced his understanding of mind, body, and spirit. As an independent researcher, he explores bidirectional relationship between psychological factors and physical health outcomes.

Mehmet Öçal, PhD, completed his Doctorate education in the Department of Labor Economics and Industrial Relations at Pamukkale University in 2022. He has been working as an Assistant Professor in the Social Work Department of Burdur Mehmet Akif Ersoy University, Turkey. In 2022, he was deemed worthy of the Outstanding Achievement Award from Türkiye Council of Higher Education.

Oluwasogo Ruth Ogunleye, PhD, is a Nigerian health advocate and scholar at the National Open University of Nigeria. She is dedicated to promoting physical fitness, wellness, and healthy living. As the lead author of *Interdisciplinary Approaches to Combating Ageism and Elderly Abuse*, shepromotes holistic well-being through research and teachings.

Uzoma O. Okoye, PhD, is a Professor of Social Gerontology. She is a Lecturer in the Department of Social Work at the University of Nigeria, Nsukka, Enugu state. Her research interests include social gerontology, youth, and family social work.

Thomas Rieger, PhD, is Professor and Programme Director of the MSc in International Public Health Management at the University of Europe for Applied Science, Germany. He is the Founding Dean of the Faculty of Sports, Media and Event. Between 2012 and 2015, he served as Chairman of the Standards Council of the European Health and Fitness Association.

Michael Sarfo is a dedicated Doctoral Researcher at the University of Huddersfield, UK. He also serves as a Tutor in Health at Coventry University's Scarborough campus and is an experienced medical practitioner from Ghana. Michael has a profound research interest in vaccinations, both communicable and non-communicable diseases, and the integration of social enterprise into health initiatives. His current PhD research focuses on exploring the role of social enterprise in the implementation and effectiveness of malaria vaccination programs in Ghana.

Sarra Sghaier, PhD, is a Lecturer and Researcher in Marketing. Her research is interdisciplinary and concentrates on marketing, psychology, sociology, anthropology, and gerontology. She received her first and second degrees as well as PhD in Marketing from the Faculty of Economics Sciences and Management of the University of Tunis, Tunisia. Her PhD was on the impact of subjective age on innovativeness.

Kasturi Shukla, PhD, is an Associate Professor at Symbiosis International (Deemed University), Pune, India. She is a trained Hospital Administrator and an awardee of the Gold Medal for Best Ph.D. Thesis 2012. With more than 18 years of research and industry experience, she has published more than 30 original research articles, 3 books, and 3 registered patents. Her research interests include quality of life, climate change, and sustainability. She is a life member of reputed bodies and on the review board of many journals.

Kalim Siddiqui, PhD, is an economist, specializing in International Political Economy, Development Economics, and Economic Policy. He is a Senior Lecturer in the Department of Accounting, Finance and Economics at the University of Huddersfield, UK. He has a wide range of research interests, and they can be classified into four broad domains: (1) political economy, (2) development economics, (3) economic policy, and (4) international trade.

Michael Snowden, PhD, is a Senior Lecturer of Public Health at the University of Huddersfield, UK. He has a special interest in social enterprise, coaching and mentoring, and how they can be used to promote equality and inclusivity in learning and society. During Mike's long and established career in Higher Education, he has contributed to, led, and developed numerous funded innovative projects, distinct pedagogical innovations, and conceptual models that influence and enhance learning and practice. His expertise is widely recognised as instrumental in developing curricula that support learning enhancement. Mike has published his work widely and is a regular speaker at national and international conferences.

Richmond Stephen Sorkpor, PhD, is a Lecturer and Researcher at the University of Education, Winneba, Ghana. His research interests are in teacher development, curriculum development, mentoring, physical activity engagement for lifelong living, physical fitness, and climate issues.

James Stockton, PhD, is a Post-graduate Researcher in the School of Human and Health Sciences at the University of Huddersfield, UK. His research interests cover four main areas: Health Impacts of Loneliness Isolation and Alienation, Global Development, Pedagogy of Higher Education, and Statistical Research Methods.

Md. Emaj Uddin, PhD, is a Professor in the Department of Social Work at Rajshahi University, Bangladesh. He is interested in family studies, health, and child development. He has written 50 articles and 20 book chapters on socioeconomic status, health, child development, and education in abstracted journals and edited books.

Bala Kwata Waziri, PhD, is a distinguished scholar in Health Education. He brings a deep understanding of community health issues and a passion for education to his work. With a commitment to improving public health and promoting wellness, he has made significant contributions to the broader field of health education.

List of Figures

Fig. 2.1 Authors' conceptualisation of the relationship between contextual and personal factors, outcomes of action plans, and healthy ageing. Note: + represents positive influence; − represents negative influence; ***resilience is analogous to the ability to adapt to biological, environmental, and social changes experienced in ageing; **the influence of a semi-haven or out-of-neighbourhood psychological distance on healthy ageing and Decade of Healthy Ageing outcomes can be negative, positive, or non-significant depending on the intensity and duration of the threats and personal coping ability; *factors listed are not exhaustive; other factors such as social network size and employment may apply 24

Fig. 3.1 Author's conceptualisation of a smart age-friendly context according to Pinheiro (2021) and the Age-Friendly Conceptual Model (PAHO, 2023) 38

Fig. 3.2 Author's conceptualisation of the Age-Friendly Model (second model adapted) 39

Fig. 3.3 Author's conceptualisation of the Smart City Model (third model adapted) 40

Fig. 3.4 The proposed Integrated Model of Smart and Age-Friendly Cities 40

Fig. 4.1 Flow diagram of the search strategy 50

Fig. 7.1 Authors' conceptual framework of the potential influence of health promotion efforts on four societal layers 116

Fig. 8.1 Authors' conceptualisation of the link between adaptation to climate change and healthy ageing. Note: Adaptive capacity (AC), structural adaptation (STA), physiological adaptation (PA), behavioural adaptation (BA), healthy ageing (HA) 135

Fig. 9.1 Chart depicting themes and frequency found in the 23 articles. 148

Fig. 9.2 The author's proposed emphasis of older adults as a priority population in Cooling Center planning 149
Fig. 9.3 The author's proposed application of the Cornell RTP Consensus Workshop Model to the Cooling Centers campaign case study 150
Fig. 10.1 Authors' construction of the parameters affecting healthy aging . . . 165
Fig. 10.2 Authors' ranking of age-friendly countries according to healthy aging index (The age-friendly country ranking was reached as a result of the classification of the HAI according to percentile analysis. Countries in red are called low age-friendly countries, countries in yellow are called moderately age-friendly countries, and countries in green are called age-friendly countries) 168
Fig. 12.1 Authors' multi-level framework for attaining sustainable ageing . . . 203
Fig. 13.1 The author's conceptualisation of the nexus between neighbourhood resources, HD pathways, healthy ageing, and crises. (Note: Not all potential covariates are in the fig. HD, human development; COVID-19, coronavirus disease 2019. Broken arrows and rectangles show the types of variables) 216

List of Tables

Table 2.1 The authors' mapping of psychological distance types onto healthy "ageing in place" implications 23

Table 4.1 Descriptive Statistics 52

Table 4.2 Details of journal sources 53

Table 4.3 The most cited publications, including year, authors, sources, and total citations.... 54

Table 5.1 Summary of the socio-demographic characteristics of the participants of the study 79

Table 7.1 Authors' mapping of health-promoting activities onto action plans of the Decade of Healthy Ageing and the four societal layers 118

Table 8.1 Authors' summary of key attributes of the four levels of adaptation 132

Table 9.1 Overview of the search term combinations utilized regarding Cooling Centers in Los Angeles County.... 146

Table 9.2 Overview of the search term combinations utilized regarding Cooling Centers around the United States and globally 146

Table 9.3 The authors' compilation of primary topics of Cooling Centers in Los Angeles as depicted in the literature 147

Table 9.4 The authors' compilation of categories of Cooling Center types.... 147

Table 9.5 Article coverage of Cooling Centers and healthy aging (by common themes).... 147

Table 10.1 Percentage of population aged 65 years or over for the World and SDG regions.... 162

Table 10.2 Analysis of social policies implemented by selected countries for older people according to the Healthy Aging Index 169

Table 16.1 Authors' suggested actions for realizing the Decade of Healthy Ageing initiative.... 269

Chapter 1
Re-imagining Healthy Ageing Through the Lens of Flagship Campaigns: An Introduction

Nestor Asiamah, Hafiz T. A. Khan, Whitney Nesser, Frank Frimpong Opuni, and Alex Siu Wing Chan

Acronyms and Abbreviations

HD	Human Development
WHO	World Health Organization

1.1 Introduction

The world's population is rapidly ageing and, consequently, experiencing a demographic shift. This phenomenon is characterised by declining fertility and improved life expectancy on a global scale (Dudel, 2021; Nagarajan et al., 2021; Van Der Cammen et al., 2017). Population ageing offers organisations and governments an

N. Asiamah (✉)
School of Health and Social Care, Colchester, Essex, UK

International Public Health Management Programme, University of Europe for Applied Sciences, Iserlohn, Germany

Department of Health Management, Berlin School of Business and Innovation, Berlin, Germany

Department of Gerontology and Geriatrics, Africa Centre for Epidemiology, Accra North, Accra, Ghana
e-mail: n.asiamah@essex.ac.uk

H. T. A. Khan
Public Health Group, College of Nursing, Midwifery, and Healthcare, University of West London, Brentford, UK

Oxford Institute of Population Ageing, University of Oxford, Oxford, UK
e-mail: hafiz.khan@uwl.ac.uk; hafiz.khan@ageing.ox.ac.uk

N. Asiamah et al. (eds.), *Sustainable Ageing*,
https://doi.org/10.1007/978-3-031-69475-2_1

opportunity to savour human capital for an extended period and leverage the unique skills of older adults in volunteering and community engagement programmes. These opportunities can ultimately be realised if people remain healthy and avoid functional limitations as they age. An undesirable global situation is that people are living longer in poor health or disability (Dudel, 2021; Nagarajan et al., 2021), implying that the burden of disease and the cost of healthcare associated with the older adult population would be high. Interventions fostering healthy ageing or enabling people to maintain their health and avoid disability in later life are needed to overcome this situation.

A notable intervention is the Decade of Healthy Ageing 2021–2030, championed by the United Nations through the World Health Organization (WHO) (Rudnicka et al., 2020). This initiative aims to support older adults, their families, and the communities where they live, providing them with opportunities for healthy longevity. Arguably, the Decade of Healthy Ageing 2021–2030 is a timely initiative, not only because the world's population is rapidly ageing but also because several unexpected threats (e.g. climate change, earthquake, infectious disease outbreaks, extreme industrialisation, and war as well as violence) are now making ageing more daunting than ever. The combined influences of these threats exert a powerful force against the ageing process and require more resilience and fortitude for healthy ageing. It is understandable why several scholars have critically analysed and contextualised the joint impact of these threats on health and healthy ageing (Asiamah et al., 2023b; Barchielli et al., 2022).

Healthy ageing is the maintenance of the functional capacity needed for wellbeing in old age (Menassa et al., 2023). Being able to independently make decisions and perform daily social, recreational, and economic tasks is implicit in this ability. Through its Decade of Healthy Ageing 2021–2030 campaign, the WHO advocates healthy ageing efforts and a future where people can live healthy and productive lives in older age. While this initiative is promising and has gained momentum in its implementation (Dixon, 2021; Rudnicka et al., 2020), its action plans were not based on sufficient consideration of the joint influences of the aforesaid health and natural threats. This shortcoming of the initiative is worth addressing because the

W. Nesser
Department of Applied Clinical and Educational Sciences, Indiana State University, Terre Haute, IN, USA
e-mail: whitney.nesser@indstate.edu

F. F. Opuni
Department of Gerontology and Geriatrics, Africa Centre for Epidemiology, Accra North, Accra, Ghana

Department of Marketing, Accra Technical University, Accra Metro, Accra, Ghana
e-mail: fofrimpong@atu.edu.gh

A. S. W. Chan
Department of Applied Social Sciences, The Hong Kong Polytechnic University, Hung Hom, Hong Kong
e-mail: chansw.alex@gmail.com

threats may thwart campaign-related efforts and make healthy ageing unrealistic if not considered in designing interventions.

This book provides a forum for reimagining healthy ageing through the lens of the Decade of Healthy Ageing 2021–2030 and other campaigns fostering healthy ageing. By re-imagining healthy ageing through these campaigns, this book offers ideas, models, and postulates for realising healthy longevity in contexts experiencing health and social threats. It leverages current action plans of the Decade of Healthy Ageing 2021–2030 and related campaigns to create an imaginary path along which healthy ageing can be made more realistic amidst health and social threats. It advances an ongoing debate on 'sustainable ageing', which is the maintenance of the functional abilities necessary for optimal health in contexts experiencing health and social threats (Asiamah, 2023). Sustainable ageing concerns the maintenance of functional capacity and well-being in later life despite living in uncertain socio-environmental conditions (e.g. extreme weather, unsafety, war/violence, and fear) caused by threats.

This chapter is organised into five sections, including an introductory section where the significance of the book is demonstrated. In the second section, the aim and objectives of the book are identified, setting a foundation for formulating the book's focus and contents in the third section. The significance and limitations of the book are outlined in the fourth section whereas concluding remarks are provided in the fifth section.

1.2 Aim and Objectives

Sustainable ageing refers to healthy ageing in contexts where crises or humanitarian situations require extraordinary abilities, including resilience, endurance, and ability to cope (Asiamah, 2023). Life in contexts experiencing crises may be fraught with injury, death, fear, and anxiety, but access to social support and neighbourhood attributes (e.g. services, parks) can enable individuals to achieve resilience and endurance until normalcy is re-established in such contexts. Sustainable ageing ultimately fosters a socio-physical environment where individuals can manage their health through health-seeking behaviours (e.g. healthcare utilisation and engagement in social and physical activities) over the life course without fear of the unexpected. Sustainable ageing from this viewpoint will sustain economic agility and pave the way for people to protect their productivity in later life when experiencing crises.

Interventions should, therefore, aim to (1) provide social support and environments where people can maintain functional capacity and well-being by achieving resilience, coping ability, and endurance against crises, or (2) prevent crises from occurring and empower individuals to maintain functional ability and well-being over the life course. While the latter aim is superior to the former, it is unrealistic in settings where natural disasters cannot be predicted and avoided. Action plans of the Decade of Healthy Ageing 2021–2030 campaign are a potential instrument for realising sustainable ageing with the former aim above for two reasons. First, the initiative targets older adults, families, and communities (Keating, 2022; Rudnicka et al., 2020), thereby setting a foundation for providing inclusive support. Second, the campaign advocates the creation of a convivial socio-physical (age-friendly) environment (Rudnicka et al., 2020) where older adults can enjoy life without ageism, abuse, and unnecessary barriers to healthcare and other community resources.

This notwithstanding, the Decade of Healthy Ageing 2021–2030 and related initiatives could undermine most members of the population if focused on older adults. The campaign may fail to achieve its goals if the stakeholders undermine current crises and their joint impacts on ageing people. Thus, it is imperative amidst crises to employ a life course approach to empower people to maintain functional ability and well-being over the life course. A life course approach in this context refers to interventions that provide social support and age-friendly neighbourhoods for all to maintain well-being and avoid disease and disability across the lifespan. This is a disease prevention pathway that is more likely to empower individuals to live in optimal health in older age (Asiamah, 2023; Duplaga et al., 2016; Menassa et al., 2023).

This book aims to advance emerging schools of thought (Asiamah, 2023; Asiamah et al., 2023b; Baird et al., 2017; Kuruvilla et al., 2018) on how to realise the above life course approach. It compiles models, ideas, and empirical evidence where a multidisciplinary team of scholars re-imagine healthy ageing, with key global campaigns used as a lens. This book initiates a debate on approaches to "sustainable ageing', which is analogous to healthy ageing in contexts experiencing crises. This is the first book to address the crisis as a threat to healthy ageing and its realisation through influential campaigns such as the Decade of Healthy Ageing 2021–2030.

1.3 Scope and Contents

The chapters included in this book were selected as topics consistent with healthy ageing campaigns such as the Decade of Healthy Ageing 2021–2030. The selected titles enable the authors to mirror their ideas in contemporary initiatives that seek to foster healthy ageing globally. The chapters represent significant outcomes from desk research, qualitative synthesis, or statistical analyses of secondary data. The contents of the book build upon recent advances regarding uncertain events in gerontology (Asiamah, 2023; Asiamah et al., 2023b) but initiate a unique interdisciplinary dialogue about realising healthy ageing through campaigns in an era of worsening crisis.

The compilation of chapters into this book was informed by our recognition of the need for (1) global perspectives commensurate with the geographical scope of crises, (2) interdisciplinary perspectives needed for reframing healthy ageing through campaigns, and (3) actionable measures for policymakers and researchers. Based on these needs, an international call for abstracts was published and followed by a double-blind peer review of chapters, resulting in 15 chapters. In total, 43 authors from 5 continents (i.e. Africa, Europe, North America, Asia, and South America) and 13 countries (e.g. Bangladesh, China, Denmark, Germany, Ghana, India, Kenya, Mexico, Nigeria, Turkey, United States of America, and United Kingdom) contributed to the book. Disciplines included are sociology, geography, gerontology, psychology, architecture, finance, human resources management, social marketing, and social work.

Chapter 1 provides insight into the rationale, significance, and aim of the book, including what readers can expect. The other chapters are organised into five themes of varying lengths. Chapter 2 opens the discussion on Theme 1, which comprises four chapters and concerns age-friendly neighbourhoods and ageing in place. In Chap. 2, Asiamah et al. (2024b) elaborates upon the Diminishing Life Space Concept (Asiamah et al., 2023b) to propose the psychology for ageing in place in contexts experiencing crises. Asiamah and colleagues recognise *abridged psychological distance* as the ideal mental state for ageing in place amidst crises.

Chapter 3 by Flores-García (2024) recalls the smart cities campaign that emphasises widening the global network of age-friendly cities. It proposes strategies for progressing the foregoing campaign for healthy ageing in contexts experiencing crises. In Chap. 4, Adu and Amoah (2024) round up the discourse with a narrative review of factors influencing green purchasing capabilities in developing countries. From a social marketing perspective, Adu and Amoah delineate the implications of green purchasing capabilities for creating age-friendly neighbourhoods.

The first chapter under Theme II (Innovation, planning, and change) is Chap. 5, where Ene et al. (2024) draw on findings from a qualitative study conducted in Nigeria to analyse the role of innovation in healthy ageing during crises for Nigerian older adults. The study reveals a need to create institutions or centres where older adults can meet to build friendships and access social support for healthy ageing. Halsall et al. (2024), in Chap. 6, provide a narrative about global social policy reform regarding ageing and analyse the role of entrepreneurship and innovation in healthy ageing reforms. Their ideas were enriched with a parallel analysis of reforms in China and India, emphasising the uniqueness and similarities between the two countries.

To advocate for a change in the approach to healthy ageing, Asiamah et al. (2024a), in Chap. 7, propose a model for health promotion that encapsulates health literacy-enhancing programmes targeted at every segment of the population rather than older adults alone. The model suggests that health education programmes should enable everyone to maintain health-seeking behaviours and well-being across the lifespan. Complementing ideas in Chap. 7 is Chap. 8, where Muhonja et al. (2024) put forth a framework for understanding the role of adaptative behaviour in healthy ageing in contexts experiencing crises. Muhonja and colleagues posit that adaptation amidst crises is necessary for healthy longevity and successful adaptive behaviour, which depends on life experiences and resources available to the individual.

Theme III touches upon the role of data and research in healthy ageing and is introduced in Chap. 9 by Alvarez et al. (2024). This chapter provides a framework for qualifying the threats contributing to a research-practice gap and proposes an adapted model for bridging this gap to promote ageing in place. The authors recommend a need for an evidence-based approach to be employed in the provision and management of cooling systems in California and possibly other contexts. In Chap. 10, Kutlu and Öçal (2024) demonstrate how to fill the research–practice gap with secondary data analysis. The authors analyse pooled data on multiple European countries to compare healthy ageing indexes and delineate how differences in the indexes may be influenced by variations in the macroeconomic standings of countries.

Chapter 11 advances the discourse on Theme III with an experience-based comparative analysis of objective and subjective measures of walkability. With this chapter, Asiamah and Khan (2024) question the prioritisation of objective measures of walkability by researchers and editors over subjective or psychometric measures. They explain why this attitude may widen the research–practice gap and should, therefore, be eschewed. Shukla and Attar (2024) contributed Chap. 12, which concerns the role of health systems in healthy ageing. This chapter provides insights into how the use of patient-reported outcome measures can facilitate healthy ageing and precedes Theme IV, a section comprising two chapters.

Chapter 13, the first chapter under Theme IV, comes from Uddin (2024), who elucidates Human Development (HD) pathways for empowering older adults to utilise neighbourhoods. Uddin emphasise some principles (referred to as HD pathways) and their role in utilising neighbourhood resources for healthy ageing in crisis situations. These principles were discussed in the context of the Decade of Healthy Ageing 2021–2030 initiative. Adding to Uddin's thoughts are Agyemang et al. (2024) who identify different ways to enable older adults to savour neighbourhood resources for healthy ageing in Chap. 14. Training individuals to use technologies, implementation of age-friendly policies, and improving access to services are key strategies proposed for healthy ageing by Agyemang and colleagues.

Theme V focuses on interventions against ageism and comprises two chapters. Ogunleye et al. (2024), in Chap. 15, analyse physical activity participation, social services utilisation, and legal interventions as pathways to combatting ageism and abuse of older adults. This chapter clarifies how these pathways may be relished to empower older adults to voice their experiences with ageism and abuse. In Chap. 16, Dudley-Smith (2024) recognise ageism and abuse as antecedents to social isolation and threats to healthy ageing. They contend that efforts against ageism can improve the inclusiveness of neighbourhoods and provide easy access to community resources (e.g. social support) necessary for healthy ageing.

Despite presenting useful evidence and models, the above chapters do not provide exhaustive information for reimagining healthy ageing through campaigns amidst crises. This shortcoming has implications for practice, as discussed in the following section.

1.4 Limitations, Significance, and Directions for Future Research

The Decade of Healthy Ageing 2021–2030 is undoubtedly a promising initiative spearheaded by WHO, a well-resourced organisation with a global influence. As such, it can facilitate the needed impetus among multidisciplinary stakeholders and champion collective advocacy and actions for healthy ageing. However, the crises are increasingly felt globally (Asiamah et al. 2023b) and are frequent and impactful enough to offset any positive outcome of healthy ageing interventions. This book is significant and timely because it, for the first time, identifies the risk of campaign-related efforts not being realised owing to the crises and initiates an interdisciplinary discourse about how healthy ageing can be achieved with flagship campaigns amidst the crises. By utilising dominant healthy ageing campaigns to elucidate strategies for manoeuvring crises and fostering healthy ageing, this book provides a unique precedence for productive academic debate regarding healthy longevity.

This book, nonetheless, is inexhaustive of all necessary topics and considerations. First, it does not provide a detailed analysis of some topics related to the action plans of the Decade of Healthy Ageing 2021–2030 campaign and similar initiatives. An example of such topics is the use of assistive technologies in older populations and the empowerment of individuals to use such technologies (Asiamah et al., 2023a; Rodeschini, 2011; Rudnicka et al., 2020). Contemporary healthy ageing campaigns recognise the role of context or where people live in healthy longevity, which implies that emerging debates should consider how urban and rural neighbourhoods differently influence health across the lifespan. This consideration is necessitated by the unique disadvantages and advantages offered by rural and urban settings for healthy ageing. Access to services is often higher in urban settings (Cattaneo et al., 2021) but violence and infectious diseases are more likely to break out and spread in them owing to their relatively high population densities.

Given the above limitations of the book, research and future debates are needed on relevant topics this book could not consider. Topics and issues incompletely discussed should be advanced in transdisciplinary debate. Healthy ageing is a product of efforts from stakeholders in many sectors (e.g. education, public health, human resources development, government, healthcare, sociology, social marketing, finance, architecture, and engineering) (Asiamah, 2023; Rudnicka et al., 2020), suggesting that debates towards healthy longevity should be interdisciplinary. Additionally, most of the models proposed in this book have not been empirically tested. Practitioners should, therefore, be circumspect when applying them. Finally, future researchers are encouraged to test these models with data from robustly designed studies.

1.5 Conclusion

The Decade of Healthy Ageing 2021–2030 and related campaigns are timely initiatives aimed at supporting older adults, their families, and communities. Their action plans may, however, be abortive if not designed to foster well-being across the lifespan and against global crises that are disorienting the lives of individuals, especially older adults. This edited book offers an interdisciplinary discourse on how healthy ageing can be made more realistic amidst the crises. It integrates empirical evidence and theoretical perspectives on healthy ageing, using action plans of the above campaigns as a lens. The contents of the book offer thoughtful strategies for realising the goals of the campaigns and span multiple disciplines such as gerontology, architecture, health promotion, healthcare management, engineering, psychology, human resources development, marketing, finance, and environmental science. This book, nevertheless, only initiates a debate for reimagining healthy ageing given worsening crises. Hence, we encourage researchers to advance our work by testing proposed models and extending the scope of topics considered.

References

Adu, J. P., & Amoah, J. (2024). A systematic-narrative review of the determinants of green purchasing capabilities in developing countries: Healthy ageing perspective. In N. Asiamah, H. T. A. Khan, W. Nesser, F. F. Opuni, & A. S. W. Chan (Eds.), *Sustainable ageing: Reimagining healthy ageing through the lens of flagship campaigns*. Springer Nature.

Agyemang, S. M., Muhonja, F., Sghaier, S., Sorkpor, S. S., & Akude, S. K. (2024). Empowering older adults to utilize neighbourhoods: A healthy ageing perspective. In N. Asiamah, H. T. A. Khan, W. Nesser, F. F. Opuni, & A. S. W. Chan (Eds.), *Sustainable ageing: Reimagining healthy ageing through the lens of flagship campaigns*. Springer Nature.

Alvarez, E. N., Garcia, A., Amoroto, P., & Huerta, M. (2024). Research-practice gap: Impact on campaigns and mitigation strategies. In N. Asiamah, H. T. A. Khan, W. Nesser, F. F. Opuni, & A. S. W. Chan (Eds.), *Sustainable ageing: Reimagining healthy ageing through the lens of flagship campaigns*. Springer Nature.

Asiamah, N. (2023). 'Sustainable ageing' in a world of crises. In *Sustainable neighbourhoods for ageing in place* (pp. 217–236). Springer. https://doi.org/10.1007/978-3-031-41594-4_12

Asiamah, N., & Khan, H. T. A. (2024). GIS objective measures of walkability are not always superior to psychometric measures. In N. Asiamah, H. T. A. Khan, W. Nesser, F. F. Opuni, & A. S. W. Chan (Eds.), *Sustainable ageing: Reimagining healthy ageing through the lens of flagship campaigns*. Springer Nature.

Asiamah, N., Danquah, E., Sghaier, S., Mensah, H. K., & Kouveliotis, K. (2023a). Assistive technologies for ageing in place: A theoretical proposition of human development postulates. In *Sustainable neighbourhoods for ageing in place* (pp. 161–178). Springer. https://doi.org/10.1007/978-3-031-41594-4_9

Asiamah, N., Koohsari, M. J., & Lowry, R. (2023b). Ageing in place: The present and future social and health threats. In N. Asiamah, H. T. A. Khan, P. Villalobos Dintrans, M. J. Koohsari, E. Mogaji, E. R. Vieira, R. Lowry, & H. K. Mensah (Eds.), *Sustainable neighbourhoods for ageing in place* (pp. 161–178). Springer Nature, . 15–35. https://doi.org/10.1007/978-3-031-41594-4_2

Asiamah, N., Kanekar, A., Hjorth, P., Kouveliotis, K., & Rieger, T. (2024a). A health promotion perspective on the "decade of healthy ageing" initiative. In N. Asiamah, H. T. A. Khan,

W. Nesser, F. F. Opuni, & A. S. W. Chan (Eds.), *Sustainable ageing: Reimagining healthy ageing through the lens of flagship campaigns*. Springer Nature.

Asiamah, N., Khan, H. T. A., Chukwuorji, J. C., Chan, A. S. W., & Njoekpume, H. G. (2024b). Psychology of "ageing in place" amidst health and social threats: Perspectives on the decade of healthy ageing. In N. Asiamah, H. T. A. Khan, W. Nesser, F. F. Opuni, & A. S. W. Chan (Eds.), *Sustainable ageing: Reimagining healthy ageing through the lens of flagship campaigns*. Springer Nature.

Baird, J., Jacob, C., Barker, M., Fall, C. H. D., Hanson, M., Harvey, N. C., Inskip, H. M., Kumaran, K., & Cooper, C. (2017). Developmental origins of health and disease: A lifecourse approach to the prevention of non-communicable diseases. *Healthcare (Switzerland), 5*(1). https://doi.org/10.3390/healthcare5010014

Barchielli, B., Cricenti, C., Gallè, F., Sabella, E. A., Liguori, F., Da Molin, G., Liguori, G., Orsi, G. B., Giannini, A. M., Ferracuti, S., & Napoli, C. (2022). Climate changes, natural resources depletion, COVID-19 pandemic, and Russian-Ukrainian war: What is the impact on habits change and mental health? *International Journal of Environmental Research and Public Health, 19*(19). https://doi.org/10.3390/ijerph191911929

Cattaneo, A., Nelson, A., & McMenomy, T. (2021). Global mapping of urban-rural catchment areas reveals unequal access to services. *Proceedings of the National Academy of Sciences of the United States of America, 118*(2). https://doi.org/10.1073/PNAS.2011990118

Dixon, A. (2021). The United Nations decade of healthy ageing requires concerted global action. *Nature Aging, 1*(1), 2. https://doi.org/10.1038/s43587-020-00011-5

Dudel, C. (2021). Healthy and unhealthy working-life expectancy: Opportunities and challenges. *The Lancet Healthy Longevity, 2*(10), e604–e605. https://doi.org/10.1016/S2666-7568(21)00211-7

Dudley-Smith, C. (2024). Initiatives to fight ageism, neglect, and elderly abuse during crises: A healthy ageing perspective. In N. Asiamah, H. T. A. Khan, W. Nesser, F. F. Opuni, & A. S. W. Chan (Eds.), *Sustainable ageing: Reimagining healthy ageing through the lens of flagship campaigns*. Springer Nature.

Duplaga, M., Grysztar, M., Rodzinka, M., & Kopec, A. (2016). Scoping review of health promotion and disease prevention interventions addressed to elderly people. *BMC Health Services Research, 16*(Suppl 5), 278. https://doi.org/10.1186/s12913-016-1521-4

Ene, J. C., Ajibo, H. T., & Okoye, U. O. (2024). The future of healthy ageing amidst threats: The role of innovation for Nigerian older adults. In N. Asiamah, H. T. A. Khan, W. Nesser, F. F. Opuni, & A. S. W. Chan (Eds.), *Sustainable ageing: Reimagining healthy ageing through the lens of flagship campaigns*. Springer Nature.

Flores-García, M. (2024). *Making the "smart cities" agenda a reality: The role of a proposed integrated model*. In N. Asiamah, H. T. A. Khan, W. Nesser, F. F. Opuni, & A. S. W. Chan (Eds.), *Sustainable ageing: Reimagining healthy ageing through the lens of flagship campaigns*. Springer Nature.

Halsall, J. P., Mei, L., Stockton, J., Siddiqui, K., Holland, C., Sarfo, M., & Snowden, M. (2024). *Global social policy reform of healthy ageing: A comparison of China and India*. In N. Asiamah, H. T. A. Khan, W. Nesser, F. F. Opuni, & A. S. W. Chan (Eds.), *Sustainable ageing: Reimagining healthy ageing through the lens of flagship campaigns*. Springer Nature.

Keating, N. (2022). A research framework for the United Nations decade of healthy ageing (2021–2030). *European Journal of Ageing, 19*(3), 775–787. https://doi.org/10.1007/s10433-021-00679-7

Kuruvilla, S., Sadana, R., Montesinos, E. V., Beard, J., Vasdeki, J. F., De Carvalho, I. A., Thomas, R. B., Drisse, M. N. B., Daelmans, B., Goodman, T., Koller, T., Officer, A., Vogel, J., Valentine, N., Wootton, E., Banerjee, A., Magar, V., Neira, M., Bele, J. M. O., et al. (2018). A life-course approach to health: Synergy with sustainable development goals. *Bulletin of the World Health Organization, 96*(1), 42–50. https://doi.org/10.2471/BLT.17.198358

Kutlu, O., & Öçal, M. (2024). An evaluation of the financing of healthy ageing through the lens of social welfare: Healthy ageing index. In N. Asiamah, H. T. A. Khan, W. Nesser, F. F. Opuni,

& A. S. W. Chan (Eds.), *Sustainable ageing: Reimagining healthy ageing through the lens of flagship campaigns*. Springer Nature.

Menassa, M., Stronks, K., Khatmi, F., Roa Díaz, Z. M., Espinola, O. P., Gamba, M., Itodo, O. A., Buttia, C., Wehrli, F., Minder, B., Velarde, M. R., & Franco, O. H. (2023). Concepts and definitions of healthy ageing: A systematic review and synthesis of theoretical models. *EClinicalMedicine, 56*, 101821. https://doi.org/10.1016/j.eclinm.2022.101821

Muhonja, F. H., Agyemang, S., Arthur-Mensah, R., & Sghaier, S. (2024). Climate change adaptation for healthy ageing. In N. Asiamah, H. T. A. Khan, W. Nesser, F. F. Opuni, & A. S. W. Chan (Eds.), *Sustainable ageing: Reimagining healthy ageing through the lens of flagship campaigns*. Springer Nature.

Nagarajan, N. R., Teixeira, A. A. C., & Silva, S. T. (2021). Ageing population: Identifying the determinants of ageing in the least developed countries. *Population Research and Policy Review, 40*(2), 187–210. https://doi.org/10.1007/s11113-020-09571-1

Ogunleye, O. R., Waziri, B. K., & Agama, F. O. (2024). Combating ageism and elderly abuse: The roles of physical activity participation, social services utilisation, and legal interventions. In N. Asiamah, H. T. A. Khan, W. Nesser, F. F. Opuni, & A. S. W. Chan (Eds.), *Sustainable ageing: Reimagining healthy ageing through the lens of flagship campaigns*. Springer Nature.

Rodeschini, G. (2011). Gerotechnology: A new kind of care for aging? An analysis of the relationship between older people and technology. *Nursing and Health Sciences, 13*(4), 521–528. https://doi.org/10.1111/j.1442-2018.2011.00634.x

Rudnicka, E., Napierała, P., Podfigurna, A., Męczekalski, B., Smolarczyk, R., & Grymowicz, M. (2020). The World Health Organization (WHO) approach to healthy ageing. *Maturitas, 139*(February), 6–11. https://doi.org/10.1016/j.maturitas.2020.05.018

Shukla, K., & Attar, A. (2024). The role of PROMs in mitigating infectious disease crises: A healthy ageing perspective. In N. Asiamah, H. T. A. Khan, W. Nesser, F. F. Opuni, & A. S. W. Chan (Eds.), *Sustainable ageing: Reimagining healthy ageing through the lens of flagship campaigns*. Springer Nature.

Uddin, M. E. (2024). Human development pathways for empowering older adults: A decade of healthy ageing perspective. In N. Asiamah, H. T. A. Khan, W. Nesser, F. F. Opuni, & A. S. W. Chan (Eds.), *Sustainable ageing: Reimagining healthy ageing through the lens of flagship campaigns*. Springer Nature.

Van Der Cammen, T. J. M., Albayrak, A., VoûTe, E., & Molenbroek, J. F. M. (2017). New horizons in design for autonomous ageing. *Age and Ageing, 46*(1), 11–17. https://doi.org/10.1093/ageing/afw181

Part I
Age-Friendly Neighbourhoods and Ageing in Place

Chapter 2
Psychology of "Ageing in Place" Amidst Health and Social Threats: Perspectives on the Decade of Healthy Ageing

Nestor Asiamah, Hafiz T. A. Khan, JohnBosco Chika Chukwuorji, Alex Siu Wing Chan, and Happy Griffiths Njoekpume

Acronyms and Abbreviations

CODA	Context dynamics in ageing
COVID-19	Coronavirus disease 2019
P–E	Person–environment
SAN	Socially active neighbourhoods
UN	United Nations
WHO	World Health Organization

N. Asiamah (✉)
School of Health and Social Care, Colchester, Essex, UK

International Public Health Management Programme, University of Europe for Applied Sciences, Iserlohn, Germany

Department of Health Management, Berlin School of Business and Innovation, Berlin, Germany

Department of Gerontology and Geriatrics, Africa Centre for Epidemiology, Accra North, Accra, Ghana
e-mail: n.asiamah@essex.ac.uk

H. T. A. Khan
Public Health Group, College of Nursing, Midwifery, and Healthcare, University of West London, Brentford, UK

Oxford Institute of Population Ageing, University of Oxford, Oxford, UK
e-mail: hafiz.khan@uwl.ac.uk; hafiz.khan@ageing.ox.ac.uk

N. Asiamah et al. (eds.), *Sustainable Ageing*,
https://doi.org/10.1007/978-3-031-69475-2_2

2.1 Introduction

The ageing of the world's population is an opportunity for countries to relish human capital for economic growth for a longer period. Citizens may spend more productive years in employment and pay taxes if they live longer. Conversely, the burden of disease and its associated healthcare expenditure are likely to grow with population ageing if individuals do not maintain optimal health. For population ageing to positively influence economies, people must live longer without disease and disability. Researchers (Khan, 2019; Béjot et al., 2019; Chang et al., 2019) have observed that though people are living longer, they are not necessarily living in good health. Moreover, longevity is undesirable if it is accompanied by terminal disease and a progressive decline in functional abilities, while there is a huge economic cost attached to this unhealthy life expectancy.

A way forward, therefore, is by enabling individuals to avoid disease and disability as they age. Stakeholders such as the World Health Organization (WHO) have been remarkable in leading flagship ageing initiatives in this direction. A well-known initiative is the Decade of Healthy Ageing 2021–2030 (Keating, 2022; Rudnicka et al., 2020), which we elaborate upon later in this chapter. Although this and similar campaigns provide strategies for enabling individuals to maintain health as they age, they may not yield desired outcomes in contexts facing crises recently identified as "health and social threats" (Asiamah et al., 2023a, b, c). These threats are climate change incidences, extreme industrialisation, outbreak of infectious diseases, and war and violence. They can prevent stakeholders from realising the goals of the Decade of Healthy Ageing initiative.

The threats have a long history, and their intensity and frequency are increasing. This assertion is echoed by several scholars (Anderberg et al., 2022; Asiamah et al., 2023c; Khojasteh et al., 2022) who have alluded to the future of humankind being more turbulent and uncertain due to these emergencies. Worth noting is the vulnerability of older adults, especially those with physical and cognitive health limitations, to the threats. Researchers (Carnes et al., 2014; Gamble et al., 2013) have

J. C. Chukwuorji
Charles Stewart Mott Department of Public Health, College of Human Medicine, Michigan State University, Flint, MI, USA

Department of Psychology, University of Nigeria, Nsukka, Enugu State, Nigeria

IVAN Research Institute, Enugu, Nigeria
e-mail: johnbosco.chukwuorji@unn.edu.ng

A. S. W. Chan
Department of Applied Social Sciences, The Hong Kong Polytechnic University, Hung Hom, Hong Kong
e-mail: chansw.alex@gmail.com

H. G. Njoekpume
Independent Researcher, Colchester, Essex, UK
e-mail: griffithchannels@yahoo.com

reported adverse impacts of climate change incidences on the physical and mental health of older adults. Their immunity is also susceptible to infectious diseases (Díaz et al., 2020), and spikes in social isolation, depression, and anxiety due to unexpected outbreaks of wars, infectious diseases, and climate change incidences are more likely in older populations. The chance of people maintaining health and avoiding disability while ageing is being reduced by these threats.

Healthy ageing refers to developing and maintaining the functional capacity necessary for well-being in later life and is less possible where the threats are experienced by residents (Rudnicka et al., 2020). This definition implies that well-being in later life depends on "functional ability" or the physical and cognitive capacity to engage in social, physical, and economic activities independently in ways that result in a sense of fulfilment and satisfaction. A number of researchers (Asiamah et al., 2023b, c); Gamble et al., 2013) have reasoned that this ability is endangered by threats, especially among frail older adults living in disadvantaged neighbourhoods. This assertion recalls the concept of "ageing in place" and the effect of the neighbourhood on it.

"Ageing in place" is the ability of individuals to live in their neighbourhoods and homes independently, safely, and comfortably, irrespective of their age, income, or ability (Asiamah et al., 2023a, b, c; Bigonnesse et al., 2018). Since this concept depends on psychosocial factors such as a sense of safety, place attachment, and familiarity with one's community, we contend that ageing in socially unstable places affects the state of mind and psychology, which we define as human behaviour informed by beliefs and feelings (Henriques, 2004). In this chapter, we use the diminishing life space concept (Asiamah et al., 2023c) in analysing this psychology, with the Decade of Healthy Ageing used as a lens. The foregoing psychology plays a role in how individuals respond to humanitarian events and whether their response would support healthy ageing or need stakeholder support. We provide an analysis to draw out implications for improved approaches to healthy ageing in a world where the worst of the threats can be expected.

This chapter comprises nine sections, including the Sect. 2.1 that provides a background of our narrative. Following the introduction, the Sect. 2.2 summarises the Decade of Healthy Ageing initiative and provides a basis for the Sect. 2.3 where the psychology of "ageing in place" is framed. In the Sect. 2.4, relevant tenets of the diminishing life space concept are introduced, and a framework to demonstrate the influence of diminishing life space on healthy ageing is formulated in Sect. 2.5. An analysis of the role of psychological distance in "ageing in place" appears in Sect. 2.6 with implications of our framework for healthy ageing set out in Sect. 2.7. The limitations of our framework appear in Sect. 2.8 with concluding remarks presented in Sect. 2.9.

2.2 Decade of Healthy Ageing and Age-Friendly Contexts

The Decade of Healthy Ageing was developed in 2016 by the United Nations (UN) through the WHO to support older adults, their families, and the communities where they live (Rudnicka et al., 2020). It is a strategic framework of the UN's action plan towards supporting older adults to live independent and happy lives and was tagged "Decade of Healthy Ageing 2016–2020" in its initial implementation. Recently, the UN renewed it to become the "Decade of Healthy Ageing 2021–2030" that comprises four major action plans.

The first action plan aims to change how individuals and communities think, feel, and act towards older adults and ageing (Keating, 2022; Rudnicka et al., 2020). It advocates zero tolerance for ageism and discrimination against older people. The second action plan seeks to provide opportunities through which older adults' abilities are preserved and used. It is based on the principle that people should be enabled to live, grow, work, and age in good economic and social environments. Older people should be able to live healthy autonomous lives in such environments. The third action plan aims to foster quality person-centred, integrated, and primary care targeted at older adults and the fourth action plan seeks to provide access to long-term care for older adults in need of it. Thus, the third and fourth action plans focus on the provision of health services that either preserve health or alleviate disease or disability.

Arguably, the realisation of the first, third, and fourth action plans is implicit in the ability of stakeholders to foster age-friendly environments via the second action plan. Environmental gerontologists (Asiamah et al., 2023a, b, c; Gan et al., 2022; Wahl & Gerstorf, 2020) agree that the physical, social, and economic environment where individuals age is characterised by the built environment (i.e. street connectivity, mixed land use, and a high residential density) and psychosocial factors (i.e. safety, social cohesion, and social support) that jointly influence health-seeking behaviours (e.g. healthcare utilisation and physical activity). Environments where these attributes positively influence health and ageing are generally referred to as age-friendly neighbourhoods (Rudnicka et al., 2020; Wahl & Gerstorf, 2018). A neighbourhood is an area within a 10–15 minutes walk away from home (Sallis et al., 2010), and the terms neighbourhood, context, life space, and community are used interchangeably in this chapter.

Integrated models such as the context dynamics in ageing (CODA) and socially active neighbourhood (SAN) frameworks depict age-friendly neighbourhoods as secure contexts without factors such as ageism, which can undermine safety (Asiamah et al., 2023c; Wahl & Gerstorf, 2018). These models also recognise that age-friendly neighbourhoods can provide sustained access to services, including person-centred, integrated, and long-term care. This being the case, efforts outlined in the Decade of Healthy Ageing 2021–2030 plan to foster the "abilities" of older people through the provision of age-friendly environments will accomplish the other action plans.

Our reasoning suggests that initiatives within neighbourhoods to improve access to services, in fulfilment of action plans 3 and 4, and to eliminate ageist stereotypes in fulfilment of action plan 1, are of utmost relevance to the realisation of the Decade of Healthy Ageing. It also endorses efforts to increase the number of cities and communities taking part in WHO's Global Network of Age-Friendly Cities and Communities (Rudnicka et al., 2020).

Transforming as many communities as possible into age-friendly ecosystems is rooted in research evidence suggesting that the neighbourhood provides resources for maintaining health (Schulz et al., 2018; Yen et al., 2009). Prominent works that paved the way for generating this evidence include Cantor's survey in New York (Cantor, 1975) and the first person–environment (P–E) fit model developed in 1951 (Asiamah et al., 2023a, c). Undoubtedly, understanding how ageing people view or relate with their environment while facing the threats is necessary for realising the aim of the Decade of Healthy Ageing 2021–2030. We provide this understanding with the "psychology" of "ageing in place."

2.3 Psychology of "Ageing in Place": A Contextual Proposition

Some researchers (Bigonnesse et al., 2018) have attempted to enhance the definition of "ageing in place" by extending the scope of the earlier definition. To them, "ageing in place" is an ongoing balance that enables people to develop and maintain independence, have place integration and attachment, mobility, and social participation. This process occurs in an age-friendly environment within which the individual's accessible, functional, adaptable, and affordable home is found. Place integration and attachment are the most important facilitators of "ageing in place" and refer to the active process that links people and the place where they live and transforms them and their relationships (Bigonnesse et al., 2018). The integration process is characterised by four factors: (1) safety, (2) daily activities, (3) familiarity, and (4) habits and routines. Thus, for people to feel integrated into their neighbourhoods and develop familiarity with their communities, they need to be able to perform daily activities, habits, and routines independently.

Place attachment is people's love for their neighbourhood (Bigonnesse et al., 2018; Pitas et al., 2021) or their fondness for their place. People are more likely to enjoy their neighbourhoods and remain in them if they are fond of their psychosocial (e.g. social cohesion, reciprocity, and trust), economic (e.g. employment, shops, and services), and physical environmental attributes (e.g. pavements, traffic lights, parks, and interconnected streets). Place integration and attachment are linked in the sense that the latter is high in socially cohesive contexts where people feel attracted to each other. We refer to place integration and attachment as *affective factors* of neighbourhoods necessary for "ageing in place." These factors determine residents' attitudes and feelings about where they live and represent the bond between people and their communities. They shape feelings about how the social and physical environment supports daily activities and routines.

If older adults' feelings about their neighbourhoods are positive, they are more likely to stay put while ageing in optimal health. A neighbourhood with economic and physical factors (e.g. jobs, services, parks, and streets) influences feelings about life space (Asiamah et al., 2023c; Bigonnesse et al., 2018; Lowen et al., 2015), but these attributes alone cannot encourage or support "ageing in place," especially in contexts experiencing the threats. Assuming a context is characterised by these physical attributes but lacks safety and security owing to entrenched violence and industrial hazards, its older residents will not feel positive about it. The most beautiful and expertly engineered cities and communities cannot support or encourage "ageing in place" without psychosocial factors (e.g. safety, security, and reciprocity) that maximise the positive feelings of residents about their community. Hence, safety is the foundation of the affective factors, without which "ageing in place" is less likely. We refer to safety and the affective factors as the *affective advantage*, a feeling of strong attachment to one's neighbourhood and the people in it. It originates from feelings (e.g. safety, familiarity with the neighbourhood, and tranquillity) that influence how older adults react to threats. A reaction to threats can take different forms, including social isolation or unwanted relocation to another community.

The literature reports other domains of the affective advantage, and a notable example is the "sense of community" (Francis et al., 2012) that encapsulates psychosocial factors (i.e. social cohesion, trust, and reciprocity) and their influence on a sense of belonging felt by residents in the community. A discussion of all components of the affective advantage is beyond the scope of this chapter, but it is worth noting that our framing of this type of psychology is supported by seminal works in environmental gerontology. The earliest of these works is a 1951 P–E fit model which argues that the reaction of residents (in the form of social isolation) can be the consequence of bad feelings about contextual factors such as insecurity and the absence of services (Asiamah et al., 2023a; Wahl & Gerstorf, 2020). Cantor's survey in New York suggests that activities (reactions) like shopping and social engagement are encouraged by the availability of community factors such as service destinations, safety, and related factors (Cantor, 1975). Residents are ideally encouraged and more likely to perform physical and social activities in their neighbourhoods if they feel positive about the environmental circumstances.

The CODA and SAN frameworks also recently recognised safety and other psychosocial factors as determinants of the feelings that older adults have about their neighbourhoods and their pro-health behaviours (Asiamah et al., 2023a; Wahl & Gerstorf, 2018). A growing body of empirical evidence suggests that these behaviours are primary determinants of wellbeing and longevity (Guthold et al., 2020; Hajek et al., 2017; Mäkinen et al., 2012; Wunsch et al., 2017; Yeung et al., 2017), and the WHO's Decade of Healthy Ageing aims to support older adults to maintain wellbeing and achieve healthy longevity. It can, therefore, be inferred that the affective advantage (which is our proposed psychology of "ageing in place") can positively influence healthy reactions in contexts facing threats. These reactions are the individual's positive response to diminishing life space.

2.4 The Diminishing Life Space Concept: A Crisis Perspective

The concept of diminishing life space recognises "social status" as an outcome of a neighbourhood's response to threats (Asiamah et al., 2023c). The social status of a neighbourhood is the situation of peace (i.e. absence of violence and events causing insecurity), economic agility, and congeniality needed to live safely with others in a neighbourhood. In a community with a satisfactory social status, residents safely engage in activities to maintain access to services as well as social and emotional support. If this social status is sustained, residents retain services and psychosocial resources (e.g. social support, trust, and companionship) over the life course, which makes healthy longevity possible. In such contexts, the built environment encourages residents to engage in social, economic, and physical activities (Asiamah et al., 2020; Chudyk et al., 2017; Gan et al., 2022). Crimes, violence, and the adverse effects of extreme industrial practices (e.g. pollution) are absent or rare.

Conversely, some neighbourhoods may experience threats at different levels of intensity. The social climate in these communities can be bleak and terrifying and may compel residents to live in fear and panic. For instance, residents in Syria experienced intense bombardment and lived in extreme fear and panic that resulted in a decline in their mental health and unplanned relocation (Kivlahan et al., 2024). Community life involving participation in social and economic activities was an illusion to victims of the war. Diminishing life space in such contexts means a lack of affective advantage that bars residents from accessing social (e.g. social networks and support), economic (e.g. jobs and markets), and physical (e.g. parks and shops) resources of a neighbourhood. It triggers a decline in the affective advantage because conviviality, safety, and tranquillity are depleted or at least disturbed by threats. For this reason, it sets the community in motion towards a poor health profile, which means residents in such contexts may lose the services and resources necessary for a healthy happy life. Consequently, residents leave the community, become homebound, or crave relocation to another context. Diminishing life space, therefore, refers to (1) leaving a neighbourhood, (2) seeking social isolation at home, and/or (3) yearning to relocate to another context due to a loss of the affective advantage caused by the threats. Any of these three behaviours results in a loss of one's space or a partial use of spatial resources.

A recent piece of research highlights the scope and nature of diminishing life space (Asiamah et al., 2023c. It states that the life space or the neighbourhood is fixed in the sense that nothing can change its size. As such, diminishing life space is not about a literal loss of space or land, but rather, it is about a loss of affective advantage and access to community resources necessary for a healthy happy life. The uncertain situation caused by threats compels people to relocate or seek social isolation and to live in fear. From this viewpoint, diminishing life space occurs "affectively" or in the way the feelings of residents and their attitudes are changed by a lack of safety. For instance, communities in Syria, Ukraine, and Gaza have experienced short supplies of necessities and a cut in access to services (Kivlahan et al., 2024; Oleksiyenko et al., 2021; Quinn et al., 2022; Shreim, 2014). Some residents in these contexts have fled to safer places with high social cohesion, trust, and economic stability. A lack of safety has also been perceived in places experiencing unsafe industrial practices (Asiamah et al. 2023b; Li et al., 2018) and climate change incidences such as extreme weather and landslides (Carnes et al., 2014; Chang et al., 2022).

Diminishing life space can also occur when the structure and distribution of neighbourhood resources, such as services and social networks, are adversely affected, giving rise to a situation where residents lack amenities and necessities. Residents are compelled to either (1) seek isolation away from channels like shops and markets where necessities can be accessed or (2) leave their communities for places where they can access those necessities. In this context, diminishing life space is due to fear and a lack of access to supplies that would ensure survival. In the United States, most of the agelong citizens of the city of Flint, Michigan, left the city following the water crisis of 2014 (Felton, 2016). To save money, the city changed its water supply and started using a nearby river in April of that year, which was when the issues started. Residents complained about the foul-smelling, discoloured, and revolting fluid that was now entering their homes very instantly. Many residents relocated, which has left the city with half of its 1960 population. In most countries in the world, many residents during the outbreak of the Coronavirus pandemic (COVID-19), for example, lost access to services and basic supplies because they were socially isolated (Asiamah et al., 2021; Asiamah et al., 2023c). In some places, residents relocated to less affected places for safety or to maintain access to services and necessities. Diminishing life space, therefore, occurred through the obliteration of resources in the social, physical, and economic environment or through a loss of affective advantage due to fear and panic. Some neighbourhoods experienced diminishing life space through a loss of affective advantage only, whereas others experienced it through a loss of both resources and affective advantage. What is lost depends on the threat and its intensity.

At the outbreak of an infectious disease when only a few cases have been recorded, residents would maintain their affective advantage. As the outbreak becomes more intense, people are expected to worry about their safety, especially if case fatality is high. Residents may begin to seek isolation or leave the neighbourhood for safer places, not because community resources had been obliterated but because it was difficult to access them. In this context, a factor more likely to initiate diminishing life space is a loss of affective advantage emanating from fear and uncertainty. Assuming a natural disaster such as an earthquake occurs in this community, neighbourhood resources would be destroyed, and residents would lose vital necessities in an atmosphere of heightened fear and panic. Diminishing life space in this context would be due to a loss of both affective advantage (linked to fear) and physical resources. During the COVID-19 pandemic, for instance, Ukraine alternated between an atmosphere in which only safety was lost to a bleak social climate where both safety and physical resources were lost at the outbreak of war (Lim et al., 2022; Quinn et al., 2022). Diminishing life space can worsen over time as multiple threats are experienced, a fact that affirms the link between diminishing life space and people's "psychological distance."

2.5 Diminishing Life Space as a Driver of Psychological Distance

Diminishing life space can be a continuum of spatial change over a period of time (Asiamah et al., 2023c). Within this continuum, there are three types of contexts: an infernal, a semi-haven, and a haven. An infernal is where older adults are extremely exposed and vulnerable to threats. Residents live in fear and panic amidst an extended period of social distress. Arguably, Gaza is infernal since Israeli occupation and bombardment of this city has a long history, and the intensity of suffering from war in this space has been high. The opposite of an infernal is a haven, typified by the absence or rare occurrence of any threat. Safety, social cohesion, tranquillity, and affective advantage are high in havens, which is why they offer the best ecological resources for healthy longevity.

A semi-haven is a community where the intensity and frequency of the threats are relatively low (compared to an infernal), but threats occur periodically (Asiamah et al., 2023c). Residents in this space alternate between safe and unsafe social climates and, therefore, live in uncertainty and fear of what may happen next. A semi-haven is typical of communities that experience short episodes of tribal or civil conflicts that are the consequence of periodic resurgence of the conflicts. It is worth noting that the three types of neighbourhoods support "ageing in place" differently in the way they shape the affective advantage and attitudes of older and ageing people. These contexts influence "ageing in place" by creating a sense of "psychological distance" in individuals.

Psychological distance refers to residents' thoughts and feelings about remaining at home (indoors) or leaving their homes for places unexposed or less exposed to threats (Asiamah et al., 2023c). With a psychological distance, residents contemplate remaining indoors or relocating for safety and protection due to fear and anxiety. Two types of psychological distance are *neighbourhood psychological distance* and *out-of-home psychological distance* (Asiamah et al., 2023c).

Neighbourhood psychological distance occurs when people think about remaining at home or leaving their homes to go to other places, such as the home of a relative living in the same neighbourhood, to seek safety or protection. Out-of-home psychological distance, which we prefer to call *out-of-neighbourhood psychological distance*, occurs when people contemplate leaving their homes to places outside their neighbourhoods, such as neighbouring communities or another country, to find safety and protection. Adapting the framework of Asiamah et al. (2023c), we propose a third type of psychological distance called *abridged psychological distance*.

Threats are being felt globally, given that every country and community is experiencing an economic downturn due to war, COVID-19 or other risks (Asiamah et al., 2023b, c). Even though nowhere is completely unaffected by the threats, some countries, such as Iceland and Denmark, are safer and more supportive of healthy ageing than others like Gaza and Yemen. We define abridged psychological distance as positive feelings and thoughts about maintaining a normal life at home and in the neighbourhood without any, or only a negligible, sense of unsafety. Life may not be perfect with this type of psychological distance, but it satisfactorily characterises daily activities and access to spatial resources that people value and use over the life course. The affective advantage associated with abridged psychological distance is sufficient to sustain lifelong utilisation of services, social networks, and other contextual resources to maintain health-seeking behaviours and health. It is worth understanding, going forward, whether the three contexts (i.e. infernal, semi-haven, and haven) are related to the three types of psychological distance. We see a relationship between the two typologies and attempt to conceptualise it with a hypothetical model in the next section.

2.6 The Role of Psychological Distance in "Ageing in Place"

Psychological distance is a mental state that can be triggered by relocation or loss of a preferred home environment. The likelihood of residents leaving their communities for unfamiliar places increases with psychological distance (Asiamah et al., 2023c), so an abridged psychological distance, compared to the other two types, would better support "ageing in place." This section compares the implications of the three types of psychological distance for "ageing in place." This comparison provides a lens for understanding how the threats may affect the implementation of the Decade of Healthy Ageing. These implications are summarised in Table 2.1, with emphasis on the "space retention" and "implications for healthy ageing" columns. Space retention refers to a situation where the residents continue to live in their preferred homes and neighbourhoods, which offer contextual attributes (e.g. services, parks, social cohesion, and social support) needed for health-seeking behaviours.

As Table 2.1 suggests, residents with an abridged psychological distance who live in a haven are more likely to retain their homes. Older residents enjoying life in a safe and resourceful community would not relocate, especially if there is no other neighbourhood as homely as theirs. Such individuals may, nevertheless, temporarily leave their communities to explore life elsewhere in pursuit of hobbies and interests. Though older people with an abridged psychological distance may be mildly anxious about life and threats in other communities or countries, they are better resourced to maintain the physical abilities necessary for autonomy and healthy longevity. The Decade of Healthy Ageing initiative and gerontologists advocate the autonomy of older adults (Bigonnesse et al., 2018; Rudnicka et al., 2020), which signifies the important role of an abridged psychological distance in healthy ageing.

Residents with a neighbourhood psychological distance may maintain a sense of community since they are less inclined to leave their neighbourhood. These individuals may return home, especially when supported to do so because the intensity and geographical spread of the threats they are experiencing are limited (Asiamah et al., 2023c). Their homes may be relatively far from the spot in the neighbourhood where a threat has occurred. Hence, older adults with a neighbourhood psychological distance may maintain the affective advantage. Even so, this type of

Table 2.1 The authors' mapping of psychological distance types onto healthy "ageing in place" implications

Type	Description	What is lost, gained, or maintained	Space retention	Implication(s) for healthy ageing
Abridged psychological distance	One maintains a sense of safety, familiarity, and tranquillity with no or little fear and anxiety	Familiarity, place attachment, safety, and access to resources are maintained	Residents are more likely to retain their space or continue to live in their community	Residents maintain health and physical abilities through the utilisation of services and other resources
Neighbourhood psychological distance	Loss of personal dignity, a sense of attachment to one's home, and contextual resources near the individual's home	Familiarity with the neighbourhood may be maintained but residents would be afraid of losing their dignity and self-worth outside their homes	Residents may remain in their neighbourhood or return home if the threat does not persist	Residents may savour the familiarity of the neighbourhood to use services and other resources to maintain physical abilities, but they may experience mental health declines from living outside their homes
Out-of-neighbourhood psychological distance	A sense of detachment from community and a loss of personal dignity as well as a loss of familiarity	Familiarity, sense of dignity, and place attachment are lost	Residents are likely to lose their home and may not return without support or if the threat persists	Residents may be unable to use resources in the new context to maintain physical abilities and health since they are less familiar with the context

psychological distance may evolve into an out-of-neighbourhood psychological distance if threats persist or escalate. It may also be associated with feelings about the possibility of losing self-worth and dignity in an unfamiliar environment. Therefore, the ultimate neighbourhood for healthy ageing must foster an abridged psychological distance or a better mental state with which access to contextual resources such as services can be maintained across the lifespan.

An out-of-neighbourhood psychological distance is the consequence of intense fear of the unexpected, so it can translate into relocation to places outside the individual's neighbourhood. Space retention and the efficient use of neighbourhood resources to maintain prohealth behaviours and abilities are least likely with this type of psychological distance. This assertion is supported by researchers (Asiamah et al., 2021; Barchielli et al., 2022; Kohrt et al., 2012; Panter-Brick et al., 2018) who have alluded that disability and a decline in mental health are more likely in an infernal or in contexts experiencing extreme threats. The likelihood of experiencing

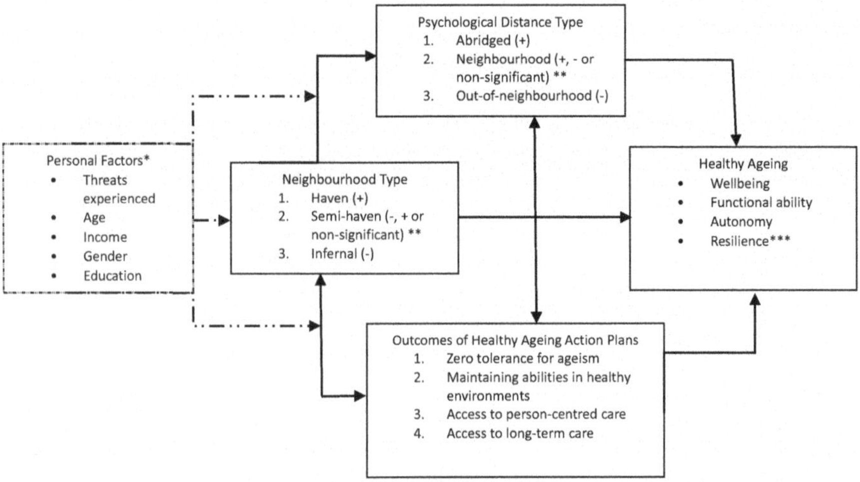

Fig. 2.1 Authors' conceptualisation of the relationship between contextual and personal factors, outcomes of action plans, and healthy ageing. Note: $^{+}$ represents positive influence; $^{-}$ represents negative influence; ***resilience is analogous to the ability to adapt to biological, environmental, and social changes experienced in ageing; **the influence of a semi-haven or out-of-neighbourhood psychological distance on healthy ageing and Decade of Healthy Ageing outcomes can be negative, positive, or non-significant depending on the intensity and duration of the threats and personal coping ability; *factors listed are not exhaustive; other factors such as social network size and employment may apply

an out-of-neighbourhood psychological distance is highest in an infernal (Asiamah et al., 2023c), affirming that healthy ageing and the realisation of the goals of the Decade of Healthy Ageing campaign are more feasible in a haven.

Figure 2.1 illustrates the potential relationship between the three types of neighbourhoods and psychological distance, as well as healthy ageing. In the figure, neighbourhood type would have a direct effect and an indirect effect (through the types of psychological distance) on healthy ageing. A haven, for example, embodies pro-health attributes such as healthcare, parks, supportive social networks, and trust and would, therefore, provide opportunities for maintaining functional abilities and health over the life course. The opposite is true of an infernal, which lacks resources for maintaining health and functional abilities (Asiamah et al., 2023c). The link between neighbourhood type and psychological distance forms the basis of the foregoing indirect effect. Ultimately, a haven maps on to abridged psychological distance, a semi-haven on to neighbourhood psychological distance, and an infernal on to out-of-neighbourhood psychological distance. This mapping is consistent with the diminishing life space continuum (Asiamah et al., 2023c), which assumes that psychological distance is inversely proportional to safety and other attributes that make a context age-friendly.

The bidirectional link between neighbourhood type and healthy ageing action plans is remarkable as it sets the foundation of how contexts experiencing the threats may influence outcomes of the Decade of Healthy Ageing campaign. Ageism and abuse of older adults are implicit in an infernal because these have been reported in the literature as community factors likely to increase worry and fear among older adults along with place detachment (Jacobson, 2006; Vale et al., 2020). Also, residents living in an infernal environment and overwhelmed by threats may lose their sense of altruism, become self-centred and may compete for dwindling resources. This attitudinal change of residents in response to the threats may exacerbate the abuse and discrimination of older adults. If so, efforts made in the context of the Decade of Healthy Ageing to create or improve age-friendly communities must be cognizant of the mental health consequences of threats. The bidirectional link implies that neighbourhood types can be influenced by the outcomes of the action plans. Interventions aimed at providing safe age-friendly contexts, for instance, may transform an infernal into a semi-haven or haven.

The link between psychological distance and the action plans indicates that the lowest incidence of ageism and discrimination would be in havens. Similarly, the highest level of access to services would be in havens where service delivery channels and their accessibility are best preserved (Asiamah et al., 2023c). With the reversible link between the action plans and psychological distance, we contend that residents would experience little or no psychological distance if they lived in neighbourhoods with maximum access to services but without ageist stereotypes. Thus, we recognise two scenarios with this reversible relationship: (1) implementation of the action plans could influence people's psychological distance by changing the social status of a neighbourhood and (2) people's psychological distance could inform where the action plans should be implemented or the impact these plans have on residents.

As illustrated in Fig. 2.1, personal factors play a role in healthy ageing as confounding or moderating variables. Income, for instance, can influence where a person lives (i.e. haven, semi-haven, or infernal), and people with higher incomes live in havens or the most age-friendly communities (Asiamah et al., 2023c). From this perspective, personal factors act as potential confounders of the relationship between neighbourhood type, psychological distance and healthy ageing. The arrows linking the personal factors to the paths between neighbourhood type and psychological distance as well as neighbourhood type and action plans depict a potential moderation of these paths, which stem from the direct link between neighbourhood type and personal factors. "Threats experienced" is treated in the model as a personal factor because the intensity and impact of the threats are perceived differently based on personal circumstances, implying that people would respond to a threat in different ways when equally exposed to it. Understandably, the implementation of healthy ageing initiatives such as the Decade of Healthy Ageing must be cognisant of differences in how people may respond to threats.

2.7 Implications for Healthy Ageing

A key inference that can be drawn from our model (Fig. 2.1) is that healthy ageing efforts may prove futile if stakeholders undermine the impact of threats on older adults. In this section, we delineate pathways to healthy ageing, emphasising threats as a challenge that stakeholders must navigate in their effort to realise the Decade of Healthy Ageing 2021–2030.

2.7.1 Interventions Against Ageism

To recall, the first action plan of the Decade of Healthy Ageing is to change the way people think, feel and act toward older adults in a bid to provide a society free of ageism (Keating, 2022). This plan is important because ageism can weaken or threaten affective advantage and worsen psychological distance among older people. In contexts experiencing the threats, the impact of ageism on older adults and ageing would be more enormous for some reasons. Life in such communities would be more daunting for everyone, including social networks (e.g. kinsmen, friends, and workmates) serving as a source of social support. The difficulty of life in such places may encourage a self-centred lifestyle in a social climate of extreme competition for diminishing resources. Consequently, vulnerable segments of the population, such as older adults, would be marginalised, neglected or abused, "leaving them behind" in defiance of the UN's sustainable development goals.

Consequently, the elimination of ageism in contexts experiencing threats may be difficult or even impossible. In their implementation of the Decade of Healthy Ageing, therefore, stakeholders must recognise the threats as an impediment and incorporate them into their strategies for avoiding the incremental impact of the threats on ageism. Interventions should be developed to monitor and maintain the support that older adults receive from their relatives and caregivers during threats, ensuring that groups responsible for the welfare of older adults are not overwhelmed. Geriatric caregivers would need support and encouragement to maintain their allegiance to older adults and maintain quality of life for themselves during threats. Given the enormity and omnipresence of threats such as climate change, the above considerations ought to be infused into policies that favour the preservation of affective advantage and the prevention of out-of-neighbourhood psychological distance.

2.7.2 Interventions for Age-Friendly Neighbourhoods

Another action plan of the Decade of Healthy Ageing is to provide age-friendly physical and social environments where older and ageing people can maintain physical ability and health over the life course (Keating, 2022; Rudnicka et al., 2020).

Built environment attributes (e.g. street connectivity, a high residential density, and mixed land use) and psychosocial factors (e.g. safety, trust, social cohesion) are the facilitators of health-seeking behaviours in such environments. As the discussion above suggests, access to these resources can be reduced or terminated by threats, even in the most age-friendly contexts. Efforts to provide age-friendly communities without interventions against the threats may consequently prove abortive, which is why programmes designed as part of the Decade of Healthy Ageing campaign must consider the potential impact of the threats on the lives of older adults. This consideration is the basis of a holistic approach to the provision of age-friendly neighbourhoods that support healthy ageing amidst the threats.

We hereby propose two pathways to the realisation of the second action plan of the Decade of Healthy Ageing. The superior pathway involves preventing the occurrence of threats that are within the control of humans (e.g. war, extreme industrialisation and disease outbreaks). In compliance with recommended strategies (Asiamah et al., 2023c; Hao et al., 2021; Rutherford et al., 2007), governments and other stakeholders can roll out policies to prevent systematic violence and conflicts, regulate industrial practices, and provide surveillance systems that prevent or control the outbreak of infectious diseases.

The second pathway is providing welfare systems intended to support victims of the threats or alleviate the impact of the threats on older populations. This approach is suited for threats out of the full control of humans such as climate change. Stakeholders, for example, can provide evacuation centres or villages where older adults can seek refuge at the outbreak of a threat. Victims relocating to evacuation centres may lose their preferred homes, but these centres can shield them from serious injuries or death if designed and equipped to meet the needs of older people. Further to this, a policy aimed at providing special support for older adults may be adopted to ensure that the care and assistance received by them from their families and communities are preserved during threats. This policy must prevent other populations from competing with older adults for services and social support.

2.7.3 Provision of Person-Centred and Long-Term Care

The third and fourth action plans of the Decade of Healthy Ageing aim to provide and improve access to person-centred and long-term care. While this is a laudable plan, it may not be realised in contexts where older adults are experiencing threats. In Gaza, for instance, residents were unable to access healthcare owing to the disruption of the healthcare system by Israeli bombardment (Klin & Clin, 2024; Shreim, 2014). During the COVID-19 pandemic, many individuals lost access to health and social care around the world (Orakani et al., 2024). Casualties, mental health decline, and disabilities sustained by older victims during a threat would increase the demand for person-centred and long-term care. Without an initial consideration of the threat in proposing the Decade of Healthy Ageing campaign, stakeholders possibly underestimated the work required to realise the third and fourth action plans in contexts experiencing the threats.

Prevalence of the threats, therefore, requires concerted efforts toward meeting increased demand for person-centred and long-term care during the threats. Apart from the burden of disease and disability increasing following the threats, health and social care infrastructure is also destroyed or disoriented, as was the case during the outbreak of COVID-19 (Orakani et al., 2024) and the wars in Gaza, Ukraine, and Syria (Jagtap et al., 2022; Klin & Clin, 2024; Strong et al., 2015). There are instances when health and social care facilities have been disrupted or disorientated by climate change incidences such as earthquakes and flooding (Barchielli et al., 2022; Chang et al., 2022; Saulnier et al., 2017). Plans for enhancing access to person-centred and long-term care without consideration of the potential impact of threats on the healthcare infrastructure may, therefore, not yield the expected results. Governments and other stakeholders must think about ways to improve current health systems, ensuring that social care infrastructure is resilient against threats and can meet the highest possible level of demand for person-centred and long-term care.

2.8 Limitations and Future Research

There are limitations to the thoughts and framework set out in this chapter. Firstly, some residents may leave their homes and neighbourhoods not because they are experiencing threats but because they wish to change their environment as their life goals change. Our framework does not apply to this group and focuses on a situation where people contemplate leaving their communities in response to threats. Secondly, the three types of psychological distance have not been empirically confirmed to exist. They are only a proposed typology comprising potential outcomes of residents' exposure to threats. This limitation creates a need for future researchers to develop psychometric tools for measuring the three types of psychological distance, assessing their prevalence in different contexts (e.g. haven, semi-haven, and infernal), and exploring how they influence health and "ageing in place." Future researchers may investigate whether the likelihood of older adults leaving their communities differs across the three mental states. This kind of work would help to consolidate the evidence for the development of policies against the threats.

2.9 Conclusions

The Decade of Healthy Ageing is a timely framework of action plans for supporting older adults to age in optimal health. Yet, this campaign may not yield the desired outcomes in contexts experiencing the threats, which necessitates the incorporation of interventions against the threats into the campaign's action plans. Stakeholders ought to develop and roll out policies to eradicate extreme industrial practices, protect older adults from violence and conflicts, and avoid outbreaks and the spread of infectious diseases, ensuring that the threats do not thwart efforts made through the Decade of Healthy Ageing towards a better life for older people. This policy pathway would contribute to the provision of age-friendly neighbourhoods (i.e. havens) thereby fostering an abridged psychological distance, the ideal mental state for utilising services and other age-friendly contextual resources. A welfare system should be developed to support older adults during threats (e.g. climate change incidences) that are not always in the control of humans. This system may facilitate the safe evacuation of older adults experiencing threats and the preservation of geriatric health and social services, including person-centred and long-term care. Demand for these services would be higher in communities experiencing threats and stakeholders must be prepared to improve the care system to meet this demand.

Review Questions

1. Define diminishing life space and explain how it is affected by the threats.
2. Discuss the differences among the three types of psychological distance. Which of them best supports "ageing in place"?
3. What is an affective advantage? Explain how it influences "ageing in place."
4. Why should stakeholders consider the threats in determining and implementing healthy ageing strategies through the Decade of Healthy Ageing?
5. Discuss three implications of diminishing life space for "ageing in place."

References

Anderberg, D., Rainer, H., & Siuda, F. (2022). Quantifying domestic violence in times of crisis: An internet search activity-based measure for the COVID-19 pandemic. *Journal of the Royal Statistical Society. Series A: Statistics in Society, 185*(2), 498–518. https://doi.org/10.1111/rssa.12780

Asiamah, N., Kouveliotis, K., Eduafo, R., & Borkey, R. (2020). The influence of community-level built environment factors on active social network size in older adults: Social activity as a moderator. *International Quarterly of Community Health Education, 41*(1), 77–87. https://doi.org/10.1177/0272684X20915379

Asiamah, N., Opuni, F. F., Mends-Brew, E., Mensah, S. W., Mensah, H. K., & Quansah, F. (2021). Short-term changes in behaviors resulting from COVID-19-related social isolation and their influences on mental health in Ghana. *Community Mental Health Journal, 57*(1), 79–92. https://doi.org/10.1007/s10597-020-00722-4

Asiamah, N., Bateman, A., Hjorth, P., Khan, H. T. A., & Danquah, E. (2023a). Socially active neighborhoods: Construct operationalization for aging in place, health promotion and psychometric testing. *Health Promotion International, 38*(1), 1–10.

Asiamah, N., Kanekar, A., Khan, H. T. A., & Dintrans, P. V. (2023b). Neighbourhood services and ageing in place: An extreme industrialisation perspective. In N. Asiamah, H. T. A. Khan, P. Villalobos Dintrans, M. J. Koohsari, E. Mogaji, E. R. Vieira, R. Lowry, & H. K. Mensah (Eds.), *Sustainable neighbourhoods for ageing in place* (pp. 91–110). Springer Nature Switzerland. https://doi.org/10.1007/978-3-031-41594-4_6

Asiamah, N., Koohsari, M. J., & Lowry, R. (2023c). Ageing in place: The present and future social and health threats. In N. Asiamah, H. T. A. Khan, P. Villalobos Dintrans, M. J. Koohsari, E. Mogaji,

E. R. Vieira, R. Lowry, & H. K. Mensah (Eds.), *Sustainable neighbourhoods for ageing in place* (pp. 15–35). Springer Nature Switzerland. https://doi.org/10.1007/978-3-031-41594-4_2

Barchielli, B., Cricenti, C., Gallè, F., Sabella, E. A., Liguori, F., Da Molin, G., Liguori, G., Orsi, G. B., Giannini, A. M., Ferracuti, S., & Napoli, C. (2022). Climate changes, natural resources depletion, COVID-19 pandemic, and Russian-Ukrainian war: What is the impact on habits change and mental health? *International Journal of Environmental Research and Public Health, 19*(19). https://doi.org/10.3390/ijerph191911929

Béjot, Y., Bailly, H., Graber, M., Garnier, L., Laville, A., Dubourget, L., Mielle, N., Chevalier, C., Durier, J., & Giroud, M. (2019). Impact of the ageing population on the burden of stroke: The Dijon stroke registry. *Neuroepidemiology, 52*(1–2), 78–85. https://doi.org/10.1159/000492820

Bigonnesse, C., Mahmood, A., Chaudhury, H., Mortenson, W. B., Miller, W. C., & Martin Ginis, K. A. (2018). The role of neighborhood physical environment on mobility and social participation among people using mobility assistive technology. *Disability and Society, 33*(6), 866–893. https://doi.org/10.1080/09687599.2018.1453783

Cantor, M. H. (1975). Life space and the social support system of the inner city elderly of New York. *Gerontologist, 15*(1), 23–27. https://doi.org/10.1093/geront/15.1_Part_1.23

Carnes, B. A., Staats, D., & Willcox, B. J. (2014). Impact of climate change on elder health. *Journals of Gerontology – Series A Biological Sciences and Medical Sciences, 69*(9), 1087–1091. https://doi.org/10.1093/gerona/glt159

Chang, A. Y., Skirbekk, V. F., Tyrovolas, S., Kassebaum, N. J., & Dieleman, J. L. (2019). Measuring population ageing: An analysis of the Global Burden of Disease Study 2017. *The Lancet Public Health, 4*(3), e159–e167. https://doi.org/10.1016/S2468-2667(19)30019-2

Chang, A. Y., Tan, A. X., Nadeau, K. C., & Odden, M. C. (2022). Aging hearts in a hotter, more turbulent world: The impacts of climate change on the cardiovascular health of older adults. *Current Cardiology Reports, 0123456789*. https://doi.org/10.1007/s11886-022-01693-6

Chudyk, A. M., McKay, H. A., Winters, M., Sims-Gould, J., & Ashe, M. C. (2017). Neighborhood walkability, physical activity, and walking for transportation: A cross-sectional study of older adults living on low income. *BMC Geriatrics, 17*(1), 1–14. https://doi.org/10.1186/s12877-017-0469-5

Díaz, A., Beleña, Á., & Zueco, J. (2020). The role of age and gender in perceived vulnerability to infectious diseases. *International Journal of Environmental Research and Public Health, 17*(2). https://doi.org/10.3390/ijerph17020485

Felton, R. (2016, January 16). *Flint's water crisis: What went wrong*. Retrieved on February 17, 2024, from https://www.theguardian.com/environment/2016/jan/16/flints-water-crisis-what-went-wrong

Francis, J., Giles-Corti, B., Wood, L., & Knuiman, M. (2012). Creating sense of community: The role of public space. *Journal of Environmental Psychology, 32*(4), 401–409. https://doi.org/10.1016/j.jenvp.2012.07.002

Gamble, J. L., Hurley, B. J., Schultz, P. A., Jaglom, W. S., Krishnan, N., & Harris, M. (2013). Climate change and older Americans: State of the science. *Environmental Health Perspectives, 121*(1), 15–22. https://doi.org/10.1289/ehp.1205223

Gan, D. R. Y., Mahmood, A., Routhier, F., & Mortenson, W. B. (2022). Walk/wheelability: An inclusive instrument pair for participatory age-friendly research and practice. *Gerontologist, 62*(1), E39–E47. https://doi.org/10.1093/geront/gnab079

Guthold, R., Stevens, G. A., Riley, L. M., & Bull, F. C. (2020). Global trends in insufficient physical activity among adolescents: A pooled analysis of 298 population-based surveys with 1·6 million participants. *The Lancet Child and Adolescent Health, 4*(1), 23–35. https://doi.org/10.1016/S2352-4642(19)30323-2

Hajek, A., Brettschneider, C., Mallon, T., Ernst, A., Mamone, S., Wiese, B., Weyerer, S., Werle, J., Pentzek, M., Fuchs, A., Stein, J., Luck, T., Bickel, H., Weeg, D., Wagner, M., Heser, K., Maier, W., Scherer, M., Riedel-Heller, S. G., et al. (2017). The impact of social engagement on health-related quality of life and depressive symptoms in old age – Evidence from a multicenter prospective cohort study in Germany. *Health and Quality of Life Outcomes, 15*(1), 1–8. https://doi.org/10.1186/s12955-017-0715-8

Hao, R., Zhang, Y., Cao, Z., Li, J., Xu, Q., Ye, L., Guo, X., Zheng, T., & Song, H. (2021). Control strategies and their effects on the COVID-19 pandemic in 2020 in representative countries. *Journal of Biosafety and Biosecurity, 3*(2), 76–81. https://doi.org/10.1016/j.jobb.2021.06.003

Henriques, G. R. (2004). Psychology defined. *Journal of Clinical Psychology, 60*(12), 1207–1221. https://doi.org/10.1002/jclp.20061

Jacobson, T. A. (2006). Overcoming "ageism" bias in the treatment of hypercholesterolaemia: A review of safety issues with statins in the elderly. *Drug Safety, 29*(5), 421–448. https://doi.org/10.2165/00002018-200629050-00005

Jagtap, S., Trollman, H., Trollman, F., Garcia-Garcia, G., Parra-López, C., Duong, L., Martindale, W., Munekata, P. E. S., Lorenzo, J. M., Hdaifeh, A., Hassoun, A., Salonitis, K., & Afy-Shararah, M. (2022). The Russia-Ukraine conflict: Its implications for the global food supply chains. *Food, 11*(14), 1–23. https://doi.org/10.3390/foods11142098

Keating, N. (2022). A research framework for the United Nations Decade of Healthy Ageing (2021–2030). *European Journal of Ageing, 19*(3), 775–787. https://doi.org/10.1007/s10433-021-00679-7

Khan, H. T. A. (2019). Population ageing in a globalized world: Risks and dilemmas? *Journal of Evaluation in Clinical Practice, 25*(5), 754–760. https://doi.org/10.1111/jep.13071

Khojasteh, D., Davani, E., Shamsipour, A., Haghani, M., & Glamore, W. (2022). Climate change and COVID-19: Interdisciplinary perspectives from two global crises. *Science of the Total Environment, 844*, 157142. https://doi.org/10.1016/j.scitotenv.2022.157142

Kivlahan, C., AlSharif, M., Elliott, I., Pereira, A. G., Hallak, Z., Yonso, R., Odaimi, A., AlHafez, N., & Aswad, M. (2024). Long-term physical and psychological symptoms in Syrian men subjected to detention, conflict-related sexual violence and torture: Cohort study of self-reported symptom evolution. *EClinicalMedicine, 67*, 102373. https://doi.org/10.1016/j.eclinm.2023.102373

Klin, A., & Clin, A. (2024). Assault on healthcare in conflict: A critical examination of attacks on medical facilities and personnel in occupied Palestinian territories and Gaza post-October 7 under the lens of international law Çatışma halinde sağlık hizmetlerine saldırı : İşgal a. 0–3. https://doi.org/10.21673/anadoluklin.1412404

Kohrt, B. A., Hruschka, D. J., Worthman, C. M., Kunz, R. D., Baldwin, J. L., Upadhaya, N., Acharya, N. R., Koirala, S., Thapa, S. B., Tol, W. A., Jordans, M. J. D., Robkin, N., Dev Sharma, V., & Nepal, M. K. (2012). Political violence and mental health in Nepal: Prospective study. *British Journal of Psychiatry, 201*(4), 268–275. https://doi.org/10.1192/bjp.bp.111.096222

Li, M., Li, C., & Zhang, M. (2018). Exploring the spatial spillover effects of industrialization and urbanization factors on pollutants emissions in China's Huang-Huai-Hai region. *Journal of Cleaner Production, 195*, 154–162. https://doi.org/10.1016/j.jclepro.2018.05.186

Lim, W. M., Chin, M. W. C., Ee, Y. S., Fung, C. Y., Giang, C. S., Heng, K. S., Kong, M. L. F., Lim, A. S. S., Lim, B. C. Y., Lim, R. T. H., Lim, T. Y., Ling, C. C., Mandrinos, S., Nwobodo, S., Phang, C. S. C., She, L., Sim, C. H., Su, S. I., Wee, G. W. E., & Weissmann, M. A. (2022). What is at stake in a war? A prospective evaluation of the Ukraine and Russia conflict for business and society. *Global Business and Organizational Excellence*, 1–14. https://doi.org/10.1002/joe.22162

Lowen, T., Davern, M. T., Mavoa, S., & Brasher, K. (2015). Age-friendly cities and communities: Access to services for older people. *Australian Planner, 52*(4), 255–265. https://doi.org/10.1080/07293682.2015.1047874

Mäkinen, T. E., Sippola, R., Borodulin, K., Rahkonen, O., Kunst, A., Klumbiene, J., Regidor, E., Ekholm, O., MacKenbach, J., & Prättälä, R. (2012). Explaining educational differences in leisure-time physical activity in Europe: The contribution of work-related factors. *Scandinavian Journal of Medicine and Science in Sports, 22*(3), 439–447. https://doi.org/10.1111/j.1600-0838.2010.01234.x

Oleksiyenko, A., Terepyshchyi, S., Gomilko, O., & Svyrydenko, D. (2021). 'What do you mean, you are a refugee in your own country?': Displaced scholars and identities in embattled Ukraine. *European Journal of Higher Education, 11*(2), 101–118. https://doi.org/10.1080/21568235.2020.1777446

Orakani, S. N., Officer, T. N., & Good, G. (2024). Systems are overstretched from the COVID-19 pandemic: An interpretive description of disabled people's access to healthcare and disability support in New Zealand. *Healthcare (Basel), 12*(3), 387.

Panter-Brick, C., Dajani, R., Eggerman, M., Hermosilla, S., Sancilio, A., & Ager, A. (2018). Insecurity, distress and mental health: Experimental and randomized controlled trials of a psychosocial intervention for youth affected by the Syrian crisis. *Journal of Child Psychology and Psychiatry and Allied Disciplines, 59*(5), 523–541. https://doi.org/10.1111/jcpp.12832

Pitas, N. A. D., Mowen, A. J., & Powers, S. L. (2021). Person-place relationships, social capital, and health outcomes at a nonprofit community wellness center. *Journal of Leisure Research, 52*(2), 247–264. https://doi.org/10.1080/00222216.2020.1776652

Quinn, V. J. M., Dhabalia, T. J., Roslycky, L. L., Wilson, V. J. M., Hansen, J. C., Hulchiy, O., Golubovskaya, O., Buriachyk, M., Vadim, K., Zauralskyy, R., Vyrva, O., Stepanskyi, D., Ivanovitch, P. S., Mironenko, A., Shportko, V., & McElligott, J. E. (2022). COVID-19 at war: The joint forces operation in Ukraine. *Disaster Medicine and Public Health Preparedness, 16*(5), 1753–1760. https://doi.org/10.1017/dmp.2021.88

Rudnicka, E., Napierała, P., Podfigurna, A., Męczekalski, B., Smolarczyk, R., & Grymowicz, M. (2020). The World Health Organization (WHO) approach to healthy ageing. *Maturitas, 139*, 6–11. https://doi.org/10.1016/j.maturitas.2020.05.018

Rutherford, A., Zwi, A. B., Grove, N. J., & Butchart, A. (2007). Violence: A priority for public health? (Part 2). *Journal of Epidemiology and Community Health, 61*(9), 764–770. https://doi.org/10.1136/jech.2006.049072

Sallis, J. F., Kerr, J., Carlson, J. A., Norman, G. J., Saelens, B. E., Durant, N., & Ainsworth, B. E. (2010). Evaluating a brief self-report measure of neighborhood environments for physical activity research and surveillance: Physical Activity Neighborhood Environment Scale (PANES). *Journal of Physical Activity and Health, 7*(4), 533–540. https://doi.org/10.1123/jpah.7.4.533

Saulnier, D. D., Brolin Ribacke, K., & Von Schreeb, J. (2017). No calm after the storm: A systematic review of human health following flood and storm disasters. *Prehospital and Disaster Medicine, 32*(5), 568–579. https://doi.org/10.1017/S1049023X17006574

Schulz, M., Romppel, M., & Grande, G. (2018). Built environment and health: A systematic review of studies in Germany. *Journal of Public Health (United Kingdom), 40*(1), 8–15. https://doi.org/10.1093/pubmed/fdw141

Shreim, N. (2014). War in Gaza: A multimodal analysis of the attacks on the UNRWA school. *Journal of War and Culture Studies, 7*(1), 54–81. https://doi.org/10.1179/1752628013Y.0000000010

Strong, J., Varady, C., Chahda, N., Doocy, S., & Burnham, G. (2015). Health status and health needs of older refugees from Syria in Lebanon. *Conflict and Health, 9*(1), 1–10. https://doi.org/10.1186/s13031-014-0029-y

Vale, M. T., Stanley, J. T., Houston, M. L., Villalba, A. A., & Turner, J. R. (2020). Ageism and behavior change during a health pandemic: A preregistered study. *Frontiers in Psychology, 11*, 1–12. https://doi.org/10.3389/fpsyg.2020.587911

Wahl, H. W., & Gerstorf, D. (2018). A conceptual framework for studying COntext Dynamics in Aging (CODA). *Developmental Review, 50*, 155–176. https://doi.org/10.1016/j.dr.2018.09.003

Wahl, H. W., & Gerstorf, D. (2020). Person-environment resources for aging well: Environmental docility and life space as conceptual pillars for future contextual gerontology. *Gerontologist, 60*(3), 368–375. https://doi.org/10.1093/geront/gnaa006

Wunsch, K., Kasten, N., & Fuchs, R. (2017). The effect of physical activity on sleep quality, well-being, and affect in academic stress periods. *Nature and Science of Sleep, 9*, 117–126. https://doi.org/10.2147/NSS.S132078

Yen, I. H., Michael, Y. L., & Perdue, L. (2009). Neighborhood environment in studies of health of older adults. A systematic review. *American Journal of Preventive Medicine, 37*(5), 455–463. https://doi.org/10.1016/j.amepre.2009.06.022

Yeung, J. W. K., Zhang, Z., & Kim, T. Y. (2017). Volunteering and health benefits in general adults: Cumulative effects and forms. *BMC Public Health, 18*(1), 1–8. https://doi.org/10.1186/s12889-017-4561-8

Chapter 3
Making the "Smart Cities" Agenda a Reality: The Role of a Proposed Integrated Model

Mariana Flores-García

Acronyms and Abbreviations

CODA	Context dynamics in ageing
COVID-19	Coronavirus disease 2019
P–E	Person–environment
SAN	Socially active neighbourhoods
WHO	World Health Organization

3.1 Introduction

Global crises such as the Coronavirus disease 2019 (COVID-19) and climate change have highlighted the vulnerability of current health systems, as well as housing and neighbourhoods, transportation, and services, where vulnerable groups such as older adults are those who lack greater opportunities to achieve adequate living conditions when finding themselves in higher risk situations. Projections towards 2050 indicate that the number of people aged 65 and over worldwide will be twice the number of children under 5 years of age and almost equivalent to the number of children under 12 years of age (United Nations, 2022b). The purpose of this chapter is to glimpse a new paradigm around healthy ageing and its potential in the planning and design processes of smart cities, where there is an important correlation between the premises of healthy ageing and the future of cities. To this end, an integrated is proposed as an instrument that facilitates the design and planning processes of smart cities from the perspective of healthy ageing. The proposed model, based on three models,

M. Flores-García (✉)
Universidad La Salle Bajío, Leon, Guanajuato, Mexico
e-mail: maryfg83@gmail.com; mfloresg@lasallebajio.edu.mx

N. Asiamah et al. (eds.), *Sustainable Ageing*,
https://doi.org/10.1007/978-3-031-69475-2_3

is utilised to identify implications for the Decade of Healthy Ageing 2021–2030. This framework can guide the development of new knowledge, instruments, methodologies, and new ways of building smart and sustainable age-friendly cities.

The World Health Organization (WHO) defines healthy ageing as the process of maintaining the functional capacity and well-being of ageing people (Rudnicka et al., 2020). Based on this, WHO establishes the Decade of Healthy Ageing 2021–2030 initiative with an international agenda. The action plans of the initiative include promoting public policy on healthy ageing in all countries, creating friendly environments, harmonising health systems with the needs of older people, developing sustainable and equitable long-term care delivery systems, and seeking to improve measurement, monitoring and research on ageing (OMSP-OMS, 2019). The Decade of Healthy Ageing initiative has emphasised the importance of promoting research actions and projects that inform the development of age-friendly cities and a resilient health system. One of the key priorities of the initiative that is of interest in this chapter is enhancing access to age-friendly communities and cities by extending the global network of age-friendly cities (Rudnicka et al., 2020; Buffel & Phillipson, 2018). This priority is analogous to the "smart cities" agenda that emphasises the provision of age-friendly ecosystems for ageing people.

The Decade of Healthy Ageing 2021–2030 was declared at the United Nations General Assembly in 2020 (Keating, 2022; Rudnicka et al., 2020; United Nations, 2022a). The four action plans of the initiative are to (1) change the way we think, feel or act regarding age and ageing; (2) ensure that communities foster the capabilities of older people; (3) offer integrated person-centred care and primary health services; and (4) provide access to long-term care for seniors who need it. These action plans imply seeking convergence between the adaptability of existing physically built infrastructures and the ability of people to cope with crises to foster healthy ageing for themselves (OPS, 2021). From this perspective, the development of a framework for understanding the structure of the ideal places to age in times of crises (e.g. COVID-19, war, and floods) and in the context of the Decade of Healthy Ageing campaign is imperative. This chapter is the first to develop such a framework by combining existing models and highlighting implications for policy and action in the context of the foregoing initiative.

The first section of this chapter identifies the aim and rationale of the discourse, setting a basis for the second section, where a theoretical framework is developed to explain the role of "smart cities" in healthy ageing. The third section explores three frameworks of healthy ageing, allowing for the formulation of the new integrated model. The fourth section discusses some implications of the model for policy and practice. Limitations and concluding remarks are presented in the fifth and sixth sections, respectively.

3.2 Theoretical Framework

Age-friendly Cities and Communities initiative arises from the WHO Global Network of Age-friendly Cities and Communities (Rudnicka et al., 2020). This network was established in 2010 to improve access to age-friendly communities

(Rudnicka et al., 2020; OPS, 2024). The network has 922 cities, and the Decade of Healthy Ageing 2020–2030 seeks to widen this network to enhance access to age-friendly neighbourhoods.

The age-friendly cities and communities initiative has been informed largely by person–environment (P–E) fit models. Noteworthy among them is Cantor's (1975) framework, which is based on a survey conducted in New York City. Cantor found that people are more likely to perform health-seeking behaviours (e.g. walking to a supermarket or hospital) if essential services are located close to their homes. The survey also highlights key social and physical environmental attributes that are inherent in a pro-health community. Even so, Cantor's work undermines many social environment attributes, which were later incorporated into the Context Dynamics in Ageing (CODA) framework.

The CODA model is an integrated model of built and social environment attributes (Wahl & Gerstorf, 2018). This model suggests that age-friendly neighbourhoods comprise a wide variety of social and physical environmental factors. Parks, traffic lights, and interconnected streets are some of the key built environment elements whereas services and psychosocial conditions (e.g. peace and safety) that encourage social inclusion are some of the social environmental factors inherent in these neighbourhoods. Thus, the model assumes that age-friendly neighbourhoods comprise physical and social factors that allow residents to remain engaged with life in their communities. On the other hand, there are other proposals like Masbe Model or Meavel Model, focused on analysing the interaction processes between person and environment, with a holistic approach based on promoting ageing in place in homes and neighbourhoods (Flores-García, 2021; Mercader-Moyano et al., 2020).

More recently, the socially active neighbourhood (SAN) framework (Asiamah et al., 2023) was developed to advance the CODA framework. This framework argues that healthy ageing occurs in a complex relationship between physical and social environmental factors as well as personal variables such as age and income. Whether streets and parks (physical environmental factors) would be used by residents depends on community peace and cohesion (social environmental factors) and the physical functional capacity (a personal factor) of individuals. Thus, age-friendliness cannot undermine personal circumstances.

A smart city, therefore, should provide access to all the physical and social environmental conditions necessary for performing health-seeking behaviours and maintaining well-being. In this chapter, the three models integrated into the proposed model comprise these social and physical environmental factors and, therefore, promise to serve as a reliable framework for designing or redesigning neighbourhoods to foster healthy ageing.

3.3 The Integrated Reference Model for Healthy Ageing

As mentioned earlier, the proposed model is a combination of three main frameworks encapsulating age-friendly community attributes. The proposed model is superior to the individual models from which it is made for some reasons. First, the

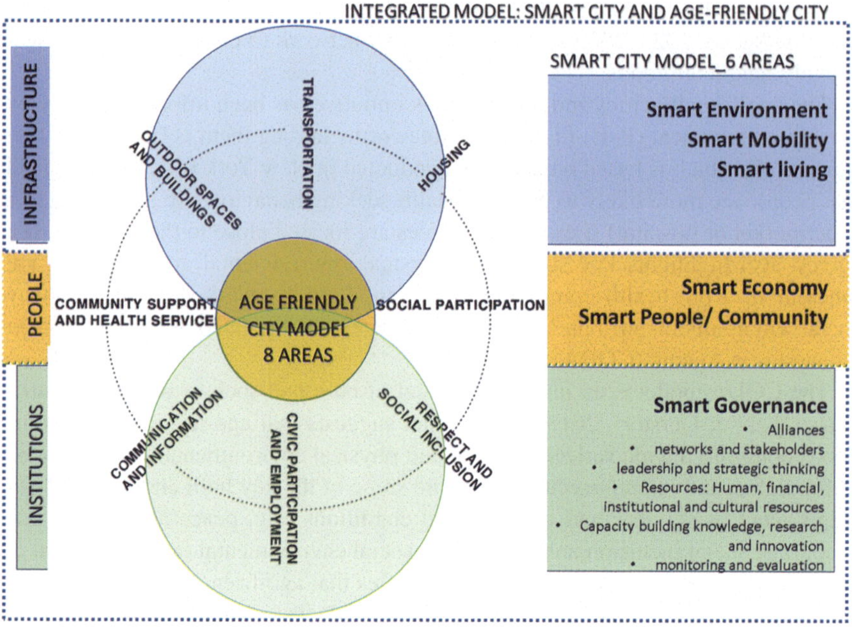

Fig. 3.1 Author's conceptualisation of a smart age-friendly context according to Pinheiro (2021) and the Age-Friendly Conceptual Model (PAHO, 2023)

proposed (integrated) model is consistent with more holistic and contemporary P–E fit models, such as the CODA and SAN frameworks, which means that it meets the theoretical requirements for healthy longevity. Second, the model is more exhaustive of social and environmental attributes that facilitate healthy ageing. These attributes encompass both social and physical environmental attributes that stakeholders of healthy ageing campaigns (e.g. the Decade of Healthy Ageing 2021–2030) should consider.

One of the three models underlying the proposed framework is the smart city framework developed by Pinheiro (2021) (see Fig. 3.1). This framework embodies a group of actors, their actions, and outcomes that influence healthy ageing. Actors include institutions (e.g. governments) and people who contribute to the infrastructure needed to encourage health-seeking behaviours. Outdoor spaces, transportation systems, and public spaces (e.g. parks and streets) are part of the infrastructure, which is expected to encourage social participation, physical activity, and healthcare utilisation. Institutions foster social inclusion and psychological conditions (e.g. safety and social cohesion) that facilitate health-seeking behaviours. Outcomes include smart people or individuals who utilise available social and physical resources in their communities to maintain health. Figure 3.1 shows the author's depiction of the interplay between elements of an age-friendly context, which is similar to the second model adapted.

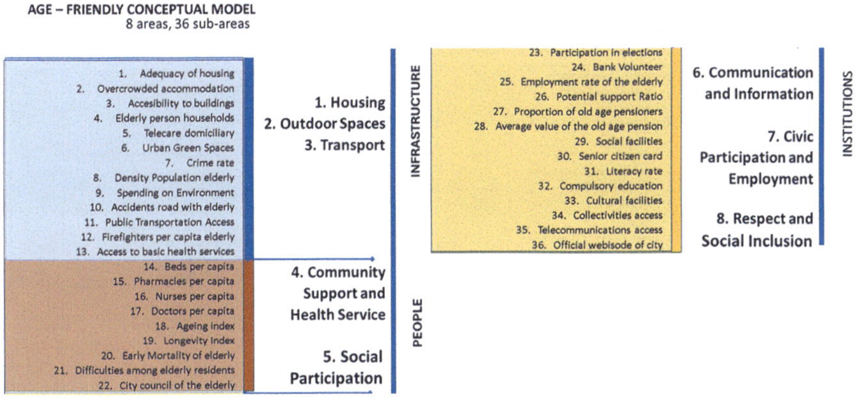

Fig. 3.2 Author's conceptualisation of the Age-Friendly Model (second model adapted)

The second model adapted (i.e. see Fig. 3.2) is the Age-friendly Model characterised by eight spatial determinants (hereby called areas) of healthy ageing (PAHO, 2023; Pinheiro, 2021). Like the model developed by Pinheiro (2021), this framework has three major areas, namely, people, infrastructure, and institutions. People as a dimension of the model characterises resources from individuals (e.g. social support) that translate into social participation and other pro-health behaviours. Infrastructure includes transport, housing, and outdoor spaces, whereas civic participation and employment are elements or outcomes of institutions. The worth of the model (see Fig. 3.2) is in the 36 sub-areas that represent specific features of an age-friendly community.

Complementing the above two models is the Smart City Model (ONTSI, 2015) (i.e. Figure 3.3), which shares features with the model developed by Pinheiro (2021). The common features between these two models are the six areas (i.e. smart environment, smart mobility, active living, smart economy, smart community, and smart government) that span three major dimensions (i.e. people, institutions, and infrastructure). As Fig. 3.3 depicts, the 29 sub-areas are the actions, statuses, or outcomes of the six areas. For instance, health is an outcome of smart living (e.g. participation in social and physical activities), whereas citizen collaboration is an action necessary for inclusion and health. Deductively, the areas and sub-areas in all the models are related in the sense that one action (e.g. strategic planning) may influence access to transportation and other services. Putting the above models together results in Fig. 3.4, the proposed model. Because this adapted model is unique and more exhaustive of the socio-environmental factors necessary for healthy longevity, it can be used as a lens for driving forward the smart cities agenda through the Decade of Healthy Ageing 2021–2030.

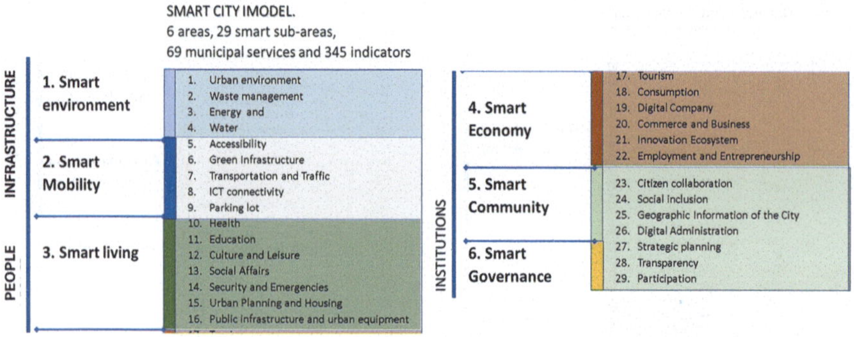

Fig. 3.3 Author's conceptualisation of the Smart City Model (third model adapted)

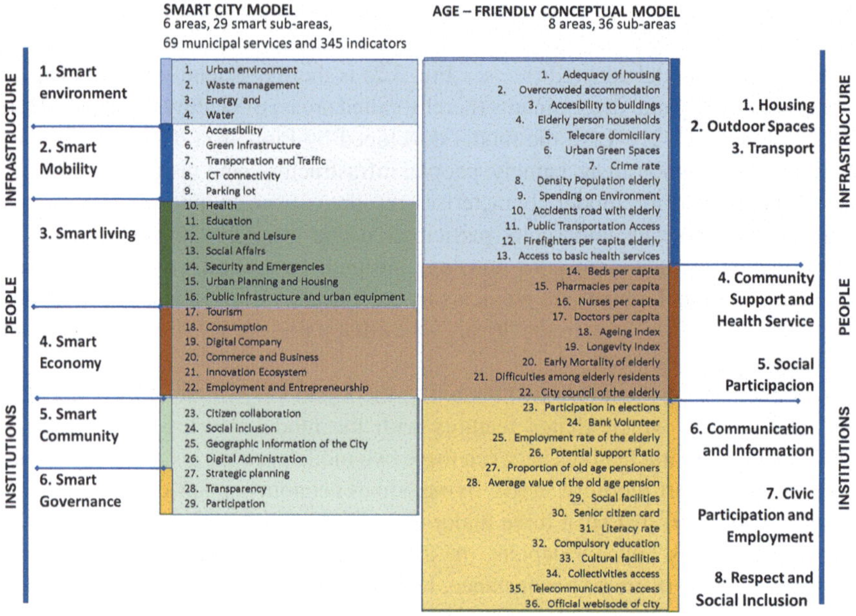

Fig. 3.4 The proposed Integrated Model of Smart and Age-Friendly Cities

3.4 Implications for Healthy Ageing and Policy

As the integrated framework suggests, the smart cities agenda is better approached in a way that engages or relishes multiple actors such as older adults, institutions, governments, and civil society organisations. The involvement of multiple actors maximises the chance of successfully taking all actions necessary for outcomes shown in the model (see Fig. 3.4). This view emphasises the role of older adults in designing communities to meet the requirements depicted in the integrated model.

Allowing older adults to influence the design of cities complies with the codesign principle, which advocates the inclusion of beneficiaries in the design of systems targeting them. This principle is central to the Decade of Healthy Ageing 2021–2030 initiative (Rudnicka et al., 2020; WHO, 2020), which emphasises taking everyone along as healthy ageing is fostered.

The inclusion of all stakeholders in fostering healthy ageing, nevertheless, is more complex than the foregoing thoughts imply. Institutions, people, and infrastructure are the dominant areas of the model that have various dimensions. Institutions include health organisations, community engagement groups, businesses, and other institutions that influence public health. People include older adults (beneficiaries), authorities in government, and individuals within institutions. Infrastructure comprises social and physical environmental factors implicit in the SAN and CODA frameworks. The complexity of engaging all actors means that all these components of the three dominant areas must work together to realise healthy ageing goals. This level of collaboration is ideal for "leaving no one behind" to support older adults and foster healthy longevity.

Admittedly, outcomes and actions in the proposed model are numerous and may be farfetched. For this reason, coordination of stakeholders and actions as well as routine monitoring of outcomes is necessary. This means that the Decade of Healthy Ageing 2021–2030, in terms of its age-friendly environment agenda, must aim at not only widening the network of age-friendly cities but also at monitoring how the subareas in the proposed model are maintained over time. Monitoring from this perspective would require sustained research and data analysis that provide insights into areas of age-friendly cities being sustained or lost over time. These insights would inform interventions for replenishing social and built environment resources, ensuring that the potential of communities and cities to positively influence healthy longevity is safeguarded.

The design of cities in harmony with the proposed model and monitoring the outcomes of this action should be policy driven. Policies provide a point of reference by which all stakeholders can act in harmony, ensuring that there are national or international best practices protected by legislation and established norms. From this viewpoint, the WHO should pursue its healthy ageing agenda through a policy-led approach where governments and other stakeholders play a role to develop policies that sustain and protect collective action. This thought is shared by Asiamah et al. (2023) who recognise policy as an essential requirement for institutionalising and realising age-friendly neighbourhood initiatives.

It is necessary for policies to recognise crises such as climate change and war as threats to age-friendly neighbourhoods. This recognition should accompany measures that maximise the resilience of the social and physical elements of cities and communities against crises. The measures can include robust design and construction of city infrastructure and the creation of opportunities for older adults and other vulnerable groups to remain engaged with service providers during crises. If neighbourhoods meeting the conditions in the proposed model cannot withstand the crises, investment in them would not have a lasting impact.

3.5 Limitations and Future Research

This chapter has some limitations, which future researchers must consider. First, the thoughts and ideas shared in this chapter are not based on a systematic review, so it is possible that complementary or divergent opinions in the literature are not considered to provide a more critical analysis of the proposed model. Moreover, this chapter aimed to produce an integrated model by drawing on existing models assumed to best encapsulate age-friendly attributes. This approach implies that this chapter may have overlooked other models and failed to draw on them to provide a more complete picture of age-friendly contexts. Future researchers are encouraged to build upon this work by positioning the proposed model within complementary and opposing debates, ideally through a systematic review of the literature. Finally, a discussion of many of the attributes (e.g. 69 municipal services and 345 indicators) of the proposed model was beyond the scope of this book. These components should be viewed as constituent elements of an age-friendly city or neighbourhood. To understand their role in a community, researchers and decision-makers are encouraged to evaluate their sources, which are Pinheiro (2021) and PAHO (2023).

3.6 Conclusion

The Integrated Model proposed provides opportunities for research, planning, and (re)design of cities and neighbourhoods. It is worth mentioning that the framework developed would inform dialogues that throw light on what the ideal place to age during crises is. The different components of the model might provide insights into pathways to realising the smart cities agenda, which is being pursued through the Decade of Healthy Ageing 2021–2030. Thus, the proposed model presents attributes of an age-friendly city or community and, therefore, mirrors a model of smart cities that meet the expectations of stakeholders of the Decade of Healthy Ageing campaign. Even so, the model does not necessarily encapsulate all essential features of a smart city in every context; hence, it needs to be expanded, if possible, and empirically tested.

Review Questions

1. Identify the key components of the integrated model of age-friendly cities and discuss their role in healthy ageing.
2. How does the proposed integrated model align with P–E fit models such as the Socially Active Neighbourhoods and Context Dynamics in Ageing frameworks?
3. What may be the limitations of the integrated model of age-friendly cities?
4. In which ways can the integrated model of age-friendly cities guide policymakers, including stakeholders of the Decade of Healthy Ageing initiative?

References

Asiamah, N., Bateman, A., Hjorth, P., Khan, H. T. A., & Danquah, E. (2023). Socially active neighborhoods: Construct operationalization for ageing in place, health promotion and psychometric testing. *Health Promotion International, 38*(1), 1–10.

Buffel, T., & Phillipson, C. (2018). A manifesto for the age-friendly movement: Developing a new urban agenda. *Journal of Ageing & Social Policy*. https://doi.org/10.1080/08959420.2018.1430414

Cantor, M. H. (1975). Life space and the social support system of the inner-city elderly of New York. *Gerontologist, 15*(1), 23–27. https://doi.org/10.1093/geront/15.1_Part_1.23

Flores-Garcia, M. (2021). La atractividad de la vivienda para propiciar el envejecimiento en el Lugar: modelo Meavel. Obtenido de https://idus.us.es/handle/11441/105375

Keating, N. (2022). A research framework for the United Nations Decade of Healthy Ageing (2021–2030). *European Journal of Ageing*. https://doi.org/10.1007/s10433-021-00679-7

Mercader-Moyano, P., Flores-García, M., & Serrano-Jiménez, A. (2020). Housing and neighbourhood diagnosis for ageing in place: Multidimensional Assessment System of the Built Environment (MASBE). *Sustain Cities and Society, 62*. https://doi.org/10.1016/j.scs.2020.102422

OMSP-OMS. (2019). Envejecimiento saludable. Obtenido de https://www.paho.org/es/envejecimiento-saludable

ONTSI. (2015). *Estudio y Guía Metodológica sobre Ciudades Inteligentes*. Gobierno de España. Obtenido de https://www.ontsi.es/sites/ontsi/files/destacados_ciudades_inteligentes.pdf

OPS. (2021). Década del Envejecimiento Saludable en las Américas (2021–2030). Obtenido de https://www.paho.org/es/decada-envejecimiento-saludable-americas-2021-2030

OPS. (2024). Organización Panamericana de la Salud. Ciudades y comunidades amigables con las personas mayores. Obtenido de https://www.paho.org/es/temas/ciudades-comunidades-amigables-con-personas-mayores

PAHO. (2023). *National programmes for age-friendly cities and communities: A guide*. Pan-American Health Organization. https://doi.org/10.37774/9789275327975

Pinheiro, F. A. (2021). Age-friendly cities performance index: Proposal of model. *Revista Kairós-Gerontologia*. https://doi.org/10.23925/2176-901X.2021v24i2p39-64

Rudnicka, E., Napierał, P., Podfigurna, A., Męczekalski, B., Smolarczyk, R., & Grymowicza, M. (2020). The World Health Organization (WHO) approach to healthy ageing. *Maturitas, 139*, 6–11. https://doi.org/10.1016/j.maturitas.2020.05.018

United Nations. (2022a). *The UN decade of healthy ageing 2021–2030 in a climate-changing world*. United Nations. Obtenido de https://www.who.int/initiatives/decade-of-healthy-ageing

United Nations. (2022b). *World population prospects 2022*. United Nations, Department of Economic and Social Affairs Population Division. Obtenido de https://www.un.org/development/desa/pd/sites/www.un.org.development.desa.pd/files/wpp2022_summary_of_results.pdf

Wahl, H. W., & Gerstorf, D. (2018). A conceptual framework for studying COntext Dynamics in Ageing (CODA). *Developmental Review, 50*, 155–176. https://doi.org/10.1016/j.dr.2018.09.003

WHO. (2020). UN decade of healthy ageing: World Health Organization. Obtenido de https://www.who.int/initiatives/decade-of-healt

Chapter 4
A Systematic-Narrative Review of the Determinants of Green Purchasing Capabilities in Developing Countries: Healthy Aging Perspective

James Peprah Adu and John Amoah

Acronyms and Abbreviations

GP	Green purchasing
EPP	Environmentally preferable purchasing
CSR	Corporate social responsibility
CPOs	Chief purchasing officers
GSCM	Green supply chain management
SDGs	Sustainable development goals
SERP	Socially and environmentally responsible procurement
KWT	Women farmers group (Kelompok Wanita Tani)
MSMEs	Micro, small, and medium enterprises
WHO	World Health Organization
UNDP	United Nations Development Programme

4.1 Introduction

Green purchasing (GP), also known as environmentally preferable purchasing (EPP), has become increasingly important due to growing environmental worries (Suleiman, economic instability). It encompasses making environmentally aware choices throughout the procurement cycle, from product and process design to

J. P. Adu (✉)
Department of Procurement and Supply Chain, Takoradi Technical University, Takoradi, Ghana
e-mail: jamespeprah2000@gmail.com

J. Amoah
Department of Marketing and Strategy, Takoradi Technical University, Takoradi, Ghana

N. Asiamah et al. (eds.), *Sustainable Ageing*,
https://doi.org/10.1007/978-3-031-69475-2_4

product disposal, according to the Institute for Supply Management (ISM) (Yusoff et al., 2023). These strategies blend environmental concerns with traditional factors such as product cost and supplier location in supply management decisions (Lasuin & Ng, 2014). With materials expenses constituting approximately 59% of revenue in emerging countries, purchasing holds a pivotal role in the upstream supply chain activities of most organizations (Kaufmann et al., 2012). Consequently, embracing GP aligns with firms' broader corporate social responsibility (CSR) goals. Hence, it has emerged as a focal point for purchasing managers striving to exhibit CSR within their supply chains (Ji et al., 2015). According to Galeazzo et al. (2021), sustainability has emerged as a significant focus for purchasing managers, joining price, quality, and time as a key dimension of their initiatives. Furthermore, the Principles of Sustainability and Social Responsibility outlined by the ISM provide a framework for supply professionals, emphasizing social responsibility and sustainability practices. Consequently, an increasing number of companies are acknowledging their role in sustainability efforts with suppliers (Joshi & Rahman, 2015). For instance, major corporations like Puma, Coca-Cola, and McDonald's have introduced Sustainability Scorecards, incorporating environmental responsibility into their supply chain management (Yook et al., 2018). Walmart's implementation of the "CO_2 scorecard" led to savings exceeding $3.4 billion through reduced packaging materials. Anheuser-Busch collaborated with lid suppliers to decrease can–lid diameter, resulting in savings of 20 million pounds of aluminum and energy annually. Accor Hotels' adoption of energy-efficient lighting across 2300 hotels led to electricity savings of 72 million kWh in 1 year (Yook et al., 2018).

Green purchasing promotes healthier products, age-friendly environments, and environmental sustainability, enhancing overall health and well-being, particularly for older adults (Suleiman, 2023). It encourages the purchase of organic foods and minimal chemical additives, supporting healthier dietary choices (Yusoff et al., 2023). Additionally, green purchasing supports sustainability in housing and transportation, promoting age-appropriate housing and transportation options that reduce exposure to pollutants and environmental hazards (Lasuin & Ng, 2014). Moreover, it fosters community engagement, and social responsibility and provides educational opportunities, empowering older adults to make informed choices about their health and well-being (Ji et al., 2015). Apart from providing immediate assistance to senior citizens, promoting sustainable procurement initiatives in developing nations enhances the sustainability and general well-being of societies (Rudnicka et al., 2020; Chou et al., 2019; Malanowski et al., 2008). This includes ensuring the availability of wholesome and secure food options, easily accessible transportation, and age-appropriate housing, all crucial elements for healthy aging. Therefore, comprehending the dynamics of green purchasing capabilities development in emerging countries is imperative for advancing sustainable procurement agendas globally, addressing urgent environmental concerns, and directly supporting older individuals' healthy aging.

Presently, a significant portion of firms delegate their operations to suppliers, leading to the company's overall environmental footprint being increasingly influenced by the environmental practices of its supply chain partners (Khan & Qianli,

2017). With the broadening scope of procurement, chief purchasing officers (CPOs) and purchasing managers have embraced additional dimensions beyond traditional criteria like price, quality, reliability, and timeliness (Lintukangas et al., 2015). Sustainable purchasing and supply management have emerged as one such new dimension. Essentially, the environmental impact of a firm is shaped by its purchasing capability (Paulraj, 2011). There is a growing interest in sustainable purchasing and supply management within academia as well. Green purchasing has become a prominent research area, mirroring the concerns of industry practitioners (Liu et al., 2017a). Numerous studies have explored various aspects of green purchasing, yet the focus has primarily been on identifying green purchasing practices, engaging existing suppliers in environmental initiatives, selecting, managing, and assessing environmentally conscious suppliers, and redefining the role of the purchasing department in environmental matters (Ahmad & Zhang, 2020; Amoako et al., 2020; Hazaea et al., 2022; Mazar & Zhong, 2010). There has been limited research exploring how the ability to make green purchases affects both environmental and economic outcomes. Recent studies in organizational research have shown significant interest in understanding the connection between environmental and economic performance and green supply chain management (GSCM) practices (Singh & El-Kassar, 2019). However, there is inconsistency in the constructs or variables used to measure environmental and economic performance, making it challenging to define these aspects due to a lack of consensus and established norms regarding which constructs or variables should be used for analysis (Sarkis et al., 2011).

The development of green purchasing capabilities in emerging countries represents a significant yet understudied aspect of sustainable procurement practices (Gliedt & Parker, 2010). Despite the growing recognition of the importance of integrating environmental considerations into procurement decision-making, there is a significant disparity in comprehending the precise factors that impact the advancement of these abilities in the framework of developing nations (Foo et al., 2019). While extensive literature exists on green purchase intention and behavior in developed nations, research focusing on the process of cultivating green purchasing capabilities in emerging countries is limited (Yee et al., 2021). This disparity holds notable importance considering the distinctive socio-economic, cultural, and institutional environments found in developing nations, which can greatly impact the acceptance and execution of sustainable procurement methods. Understanding the dynamics of green purchasing capability development in these contexts is crucial for advancing sustainable procurement agendas globally and addressing pressing environmental challenges. Therefore, filling this gap in the literature is essential for guiding policymakers, businesses, and other stakeholders in fostering effective and contextually relevant strategies to promote green purchasing capabilities in emerging countries.

This systematic review aims to comprehensively analyze the factors influencing green purchasing capabilities within the context of emerging countries. With a focus on examining empirical studies published between 2000 and 2023, this review seeks to fill a notable gap in the existing literature by providing an intricate understanding of the development of green purchasing competencies in regions undergoing significant economic and social transformations. By systematically reviewing the available literature, this study aims to identify key external, organizational, and individual factors shaping green purchasing capabilities, highlighting their role in addressing pressing environmental challenges, particularly in regions where sustainable procurement practices are crucial for fostering cleaner and more sustainable urban environments. Through this attempt, the systematic review aims to provide valuable insights for practitioners and policymakers, enabling the formulation of evidence-based strategies and policies to promote environmentally conscious consumer behavior and sustainable development in emerging economies. This systematic review of green purchasing capabilities in emerging countries holds substantial global significance and aligns closely with multiple sustainable development goals (SDGs), particularly SDGs 3, 12, and 13. Green purchasing directly contributes to SDG 3 by ensuring healthy lives and supporting well-being for all ages through the promotion of healthier products and environments (Fernandez, 2020). It also supports healthy aging, a crucial aspect of SDG 3, by promoting age-friendly housing and transport options (Fong et al., 2022). Additionally, by reducing environmental impact and preserving resources, green purchasing promotes responsible patterns of consumption and production—a critical component of attaining SDG 12 (Schröder et al., 2019). Green purchasing also contributes to SDG 13's goals of climate action and resilience building (Freihat et al., 2023) by reducing emissions and increasing sustainability in procurement.

This chapter is structured into eight sections. The first section outlines the aim, rationale, and significance of the chapter, while the second section details the methods employed in the literature review. Section 4.3 presents the results of the literature review, laying the foundation for discussing the factors influencing green purchasing capabilities in the fourth section. Section 4.5 delves into the intersection of green purchasing capabilities, healthy aging, and climate change. Sections 4.6 and 4.7 address the implications for research and limitations, respectively. Finally, concluding remarks are provided in the eighth section.

4.2 Methods

4.2.1 Overview of a Systematic-Narrative Review

A systematic-narrative hybrid literature review combines elements of both systematic and narrative approaches to comprehensively synthesize existing literature on a particular topic (Turnbull et al., 2023). This method begins with a systematic search strategy, meticulously identifying and screening relevant studies based on predetermined criteria. Following this rigorous process, the review integrates the findings into a coherent narrative, allowing for a nuanced understanding of the subject matter by contextualizing empirical evidence within broader theoretical frameworks (Parviz, 2023). By maintaining the systematic rigor of traditional systematic reviews while incorporating the flexibility and interpretive depth of narrative reviews, this hybrid approach offers a balanced synthesis that enhances the depth and richness of the analysis.

4.2.2 Selection Criteria for Studies

Studies were screened using the following criteria: (1) Publication Year: Studies must have been published between 2000 and 2023 to ensure relevance to contemporary issues and recent developments in green purchasing capabilities; (2) Empirical Nature: Only empirical studies will be included, ensuring that the research is based on systematic observation or experimentation, providing evidence-based insights into green purchasing capabilities; (3) Focus on Factors: Included studies must specifically discuss factors influencing green purchasing capabilities, such as external influences (economic conditions, cultural factors, governmental policies), organizational variables (sustainable business practices, corporate environmental responsibility), and individual drivers (awareness, attitudes, values); and (4) Relevance to developing countries: Studies selected should focus on or have implications for developing countries, providing insights into the development of green purchasing capabilities within these contexts.

4.2.3 Data Sources and Search Strategy

This study adheres to a network analysis of scientific publications in Scopus, Web of Science, and Google Scholar to maintain objectivity and transparency to determine which important papers were about determinants of green purchasing capabilities. To explore the latest advancements in factors influencing green purchasing abilities research, the period under scrutiny ranged from 2006 to 2023, with a focus on primary articles as the preferred publication type. The search string for literature search on Scopus, Web of Scopus, and Google Scholar databases was: ALL ("green purchasing" OR "sustainable procurement" OR "environmentally conscious procurement") AND ALL ("capabilities" OR "competence" OR "factors" OR "determinants") AND ALL ("emerging countries" OR "developing nations") AND PUBYEAR >2005 AND PUBYEAR <2024 AND (LIMIT-TO (SRCTYPE, "j")) AND (LIMIT-TO (LANGUAGE, "English")) AND (LIMIT-TO (DOCTYPE, "ar")). All identified records were downloaded from the Scopus database on February 11, 2024, for further analysis.

To ensure the retrieval of sufficient and manageable data, specific criteria were established. The inclusion of only journal articles was determined for several reasons. First, journal articles represent the most comprehensive and current repository of knowledge within academic disciplines. Second, they serve to maintain adherence to research standards within the academic community. Additionally, journal articles are esteemed as reliable data sources due to the rigorous peer review process they undergo before publication. Given the systematic nature of this literature review, review articles were deliberately omitted to prevent result duplication. By excluding review articles, the literature review ensures that the analysis focuses solely on original empirical studies, thereby providing a more thorough examination of the factors influencing green purchasing capabilities in emerging countries without redundant information from review articles. Furthermore, the search was restricted to English-language journal articles. A total of 946 bibliographic records were identified and collected for analysis. The research methodology framework is depicted in Fig. 4.1.

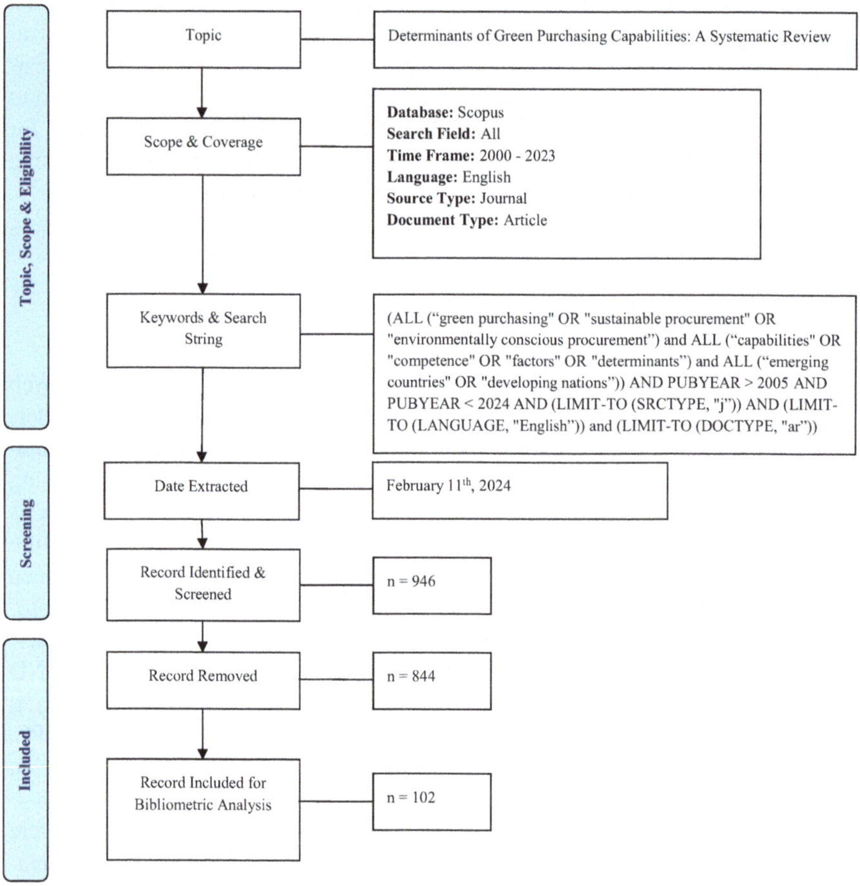

Fig. 4.1 Flow diagram of the search strategy

4.2.4 Inclusion/Exclusion Criteria

The screening process assessed article relevance against eligibility criteria across three tiers: title, abstract, and full text. Initially, articles were assessed based on their titles, aiming for inclusivity within the research scope. Articles deemed relevant after abstract evaluation underwent full-text screening for final eligibility. Specifically, studies conducted solely in English, focusing on determinants of green purchasing capabilities, were included. Exclusions comprised duplicate studies, non-original research (e.g. literature reviews, letters, opinions, conference abstracts, dissertations, theses), studies lacking relevance in title/abstract or inaccessible full text, or not assessing determinants of green purchasing capabilities. Only articles from developing countries were downloaded and used for this study. The exclusion of 844 articles was found not useful toward the objectives of the study while 102 articles used meet the objectives set for the study.

4.2.5 Data Extraction and Analysis

The data retrieved included information about results and research discoveries. Every piece of extracted data underwent quality checks. To ensure reproducibility, one author initially extracted entries, which were then reviewed by another author. Any discrepancies among team members were addressed through discussion, leading to adjustments and clarifications in the coding scheme. Any absent data were labeled as "not stated." The collected metadata was analyzed to extract valuable insights from the scientific literature. The outcomes were visualized using the Bibliometrics package in R version 4.1.3, along with its biblioshiny web interface. The R bibliometrics package improves the communication of scientific literature by offering a full suite of bibliometric analysis capabilities. It makes it possible to thoroughly analyze keyword co-occurrence, citation patterns, and co-authorship networks. Integrating using R improves customization, transparency, and repeatability, all of which strengthen the validity of study findings (Martín Martín et al., 2021)

4.2.6 Addressing Potential Biases

Publication bias occurs when statistically significant findings are disproportionately represented in published literature, potentially skewing the outcomes of a systematic review. Various approaches have been devised to address the potential impact of publication bias. In this study, to minimize or prevent publication bias, the search strategy was designed to be comprehensive, encompassing relevant keywords, subject headings, and filters tailored to the research question. The authors consulted with subject experts to ensure the inclusion of relevant terms and employed appropriate Boolean operators to refine searches.

4.3 Results

4.3.1 Attributes of Included Studies

The analysis encompassed a wide timespan from 2006 to 2023, drawing from 357 sources and 935 documents, reflecting a substantial annual growth rate of 39.06% (Table 4.1). Documents were relatively recent, with an average age of 2.86 years, and received an impressive average of 28.75 citations each. Notably, the dataset contained no references, indicating a focus on primary research. Across the documents, a total of 2089 Keywords Plus (ID) and 2584 Author's Keywords (DE) were identified, suggesting a diverse range of topics and themes. The dataset comprised 2503 unique authors, with a minority (49) contributing to single-authored documents, while collaboration was common, evidenced by an average of 3.47 co-authors per document and approximately 36.58% of documents involving international co-authorships. Predominantly, the dataset consisted of articles (926) with a few categorized as "articles" (9), underlining the emphasis on empirical research in understanding the determinants of green purchasing in emerging countries.

Table 4.1 Descriptive Statistics

Description	Results
Main information about data	
Time span	2006:2023
Sources (Journals, Books, etc.)	357
Documents	935
Annual growth rate %	39.06
Document average age	2.86
Average citations per doc	28.75
References	0
Document contents	
Keywords plus (ID)	2089
Author's keywords (DE)	2584
Authors	
Authors	2503
Authors of single-authored docs	49
Authors collaboration	
Single-authored docs	53
Co-authors per doc	3.47
International co-authorships %	36.58
Document types	
Article	935

Table 4.2 Details of journal sources

Sources	Articles
Sustainability (Switzerland)	100
Journal of Cleaner Production	76
Business Strategy and the Environment	30
Frontiers in Psychology	26
Journal of Retailing and Consumer Services	21
Environmental Science and Pollution Research	19
Resources, Conservation, and Recycling	13
Environment, Development and Sustainability	12
Management of Environmental Quality: An International Journal	12
Young Consumers	11

4.3.2 Sources of Publications on Determinants of Green Purchasing in Emerging Countries

The analysis of sources contributing to the literature on determinants of green purchasing in emerging countries revealed a variety of academic journals (Table 4.2). The most prominent source was the Journal of Cleaner Production, with 76 articles identified in the dataset. Following closely behind was Business Strategy and the Environment, contributing 30 articles, indicating a significant interest in the intersection of business strategies and environmental concerns in emerging economies. Additionally, Frontiers in Psychology emerged as a notable source, with 26 articles addressing psychological aspects that influence green purchasing behavior. The Journal of Retailing and Consumer Services also made a substantial contribution to the literature with 21 articles exploring consumer behavior and retail strategies in the context of green purchasing. Further examination of the dataset revealed other journals with noteworthy contributions. Environmental Science and Pollution Research published 19 articles, while Resources, Conservation, and Recycling focused on environmental conservation and recycling practices with 13 articles. Journals such as Environment, Development and Sustainability and Management of Environmental Quality: An International Journal each contributed 12 articles, providing insights into the sustainable development and environmental management aspects relevant to emerging economies. Furthermore, Young Consumers addressed the unique perspectives of younger demographics in green purchasing behavior with 11 articles. These findings underscore the multidisciplinary nature of research on determinants of green purchasing in emerging countries, with contributions spanning environmental science, psychology, business strategy, retail management, and consumer behavior.

Table 4.3 The most cited publications, including year, authors, sources, and total citations

Paper	Total citations (TC)	TC per year	Normalized TC
Yadav R, 2016, *J Clean Prod*	783	87.00	3.69
Yadav R, 2017, *Ecol Econ*	651	81.38	6.67
Jaiswal D, 2018, *J Retail Consum Serv*	400	57.14	3.91
Sreen N, 2018, *J Retail Consum Serv*	365	52.14	3.56
Maichum K, 2016, *Sustainability*	365	40.56	1.72
Mangla SK, 2018, *Prod Plann Control*	329	47.00	3.21
Hsu CC, 2013, *Int J Oper Prod Manage*	298	24.83	1.00
Chekima BC, 2016, *J Clean Prod*	298	33.11	1.40
Abdul-Rashid SH, 2017, *Int J Oper Prod Manage*	291	36.38	2.98
Liobikiene G, 2016, *Ecol Econ*	286	31.78	1.35

4.3.3 The Most Cited Publications, Including Year, Authors, Sources, and Total citations

Table 4.3 shows bibliometric information about the papers included in this review. The determinants of green purchasing in emerging countries were explored through an analysis of citation metrics for ten key papers. Among these, Yadav et al. (2017), published in Ecological Economics, garnered the highest total citations (651) and normalized total citations (6.67), suggesting significant impact and visibility within the field. This was followed by Yadav and Pathak (2016) in the Journal of Cleaner Production with 783 total citations. Papers such as Jaiswal and Kant (2018) and Mangla et al. (2018) also demonstrated notable influence, receiving 400 and 329 total citations, respectively. However, variations in citation counts and rates across the papers highlight the diverse contributions and impact levels within the research landscape of green purchasing determinants in emerging countries.

4.3.4 Thematic Map Clusters

The thematic analysis of determinants influencing green purchasing capabilities in emerging countries revealed four distinct clusters: sustainable development, consumption behavior, consumer behavior, and human influences. The sustainable development cluster emerged as the most central and densely interconnected theme, indicating a strong emphasis on environmentally sustainable practices and products in consumer decision-making. Consumption behavior and consumer behavior clusters highlighted the significance of consumer preferences and choices in driving green purchasing, albeit with differences in centrality and prevalence. The human cluster focused on human influences on green purchasing behavior, such as social norms and attitudes. These findings underscore the multifaceted nature of green purchasing behavior in emerging countries, emphasizing the importance of sustainability considerations alongside consumer attitudes and societal influences.

4.4 Factors Influencing Green Purchasing Capabilities

4.4.1 External Factors

4.4.1.1 Economic Conditions

Scholars have challenged the belief among some practitioners that engaging in environmentally friendly supply chain practices leads to increased production costs and reduced profits (Yee et al., 2021). Instead, numerous studies have explored the impact of GP initiatives on firm performance. For instance, El-Garaihy et al. (2022) conducted research using surveys and archival data, showing a positive relationship between environmental purchasing and firm performance. Similarly, Galeazzo et al. (2021) found that firms with formal environmental management systems tend to perform better across various operational aspects. Pinto (2023) discovered that adopting green purchasing practices improves both environmental and financial performance. Moreover, studies such as Kabra et al. (2023) have highlighted the interconnectedness between socially and environmentally responsible procurement (SERP) and firm performance, suggesting that certain drivers influence SERP, which, in turn, affects firm performance. Other researchers, like Singh and El-Kassar (2019) have confirmed the positive impact of GSCM activities, including green purchasing, on corporate performance. Additionally, studies conducted in different countries, such as Malaysia and Japan, have consistently shown that environmental purchasing positively correlates with operational and economic performances (Yu et al., 2018; Zorzini et al., 2015). However, despite these findings, there remains uncertainty about what exactly constitutes "performance" attributable to GP. While many studies have focused on specific aspects of green purchasing performance, such as financial or environmental outcomes, this present study aims to address this gap by considering five key performance variables: operational, financial, social, environmental, and market-related metrics.

4.4.1.2 Cultural Influences

Understanding and forecasting the impact of culture plays a pivotal role in shaping consumer purchasing behavior (Khan & Qianli, 2017). Given the diverse cultural landscapes across nations, scholars have proposed various dimensions to delineate cultural orientations (EL Baz et al., 2022). These dimensions encompass people's connections to nature and the world, their interpersonal relationships, predominant activities, and their temporal and spatial orientations (Liu et al., 2017a, b). The research underscores substantial disparities in environmental values and attitudes among collectivist versus individualistic cultures, materialistic versus post-materialist cultures, past-oriented versus future-oriented cultures, and externally versus internally controlled cultures (Grossmann & Santos, 2020).

4.4.1.3 Governmental Policies

In many emerging countries, the government plays a pivotal role in responding to market demands and fostering sustainable practices, especially in sectors like agriculture, which face challenges due to aging populations (Gupta et al., 2021). For instance, initiatives such as forming farmer groups and promoting organic agriculture are essential not only for meeting market demands but also for addressing the aging workforce in agriculture (Liu et al., 2017a, b). In Bantul Regency, the Women Farmers Group (KWT) Lestari stands as a testament to such initiatives, cultivating non-pesticide plants amidst challenges posed by limited land and an aging workforce. The government's support, particularly through policies aimed at promoting environmentally friendly practices, catalyzes organizations like KWT Lestari (ElTayeb et al., 2010). By aligning with governmental policies promoting organic agriculture, KWT Lestari navigates challenges posed by an aging workforce and dwindling resources (Gil & Jacob, 2018). This includes efforts to source quality seeds, organic fertilizers, and environmentally friendly packaging despite challenges such as increased costs and logistical constraints (Sharma & Foropon, 2019). Despite facing obstacles such as increased costs and logistical challenges, organizations like KWT Lestari understand the importance of adhering to environmentally friendly practices and governmental regulations (Schaper, 2002). Their commitment not only contributes to environmental sustainability but also addresses concerns related to the aging agricultural workforce. As such, enhancing green capabilities through sustainable practices and governmental support becomes paramount for improving the performance of organizations in emerging countries, particularly in sectors affected by aging demographics (Mahmood et al., 2023).

4.4.1.4 Regulatory Frameworks

Green purchasing practices are motivated by a range of factors, which can be divided into internal and external influences (Wu et al., 2015). Internally, factors such as strong endorsement from company owners or founders and active participation from top and middle management in initiatives aimed at environmental protection play a significant role (Moser, 2015). Moreover, employee awareness and concern regarding environmental impacts contribute to cost savings through waste reduction, enhanced quality, and increased efficiency. Externally, factors include adherence to regulatory standards, competition for market advantage, customer demand for environmentally friendly supply chains, collaboration with suppliers, and societal pressure from environmental advocacy groups (Nguyen et al., 2019). Prior research indicates that external drivers exert greater influence on environmental supply chain management practices compared to internal factors.

For example, ElTayeb et al. (2010) discovered in their examination of 132 Malaysian manufacturing companies that the adoption of GP is driven by factors such as regulations, social responsibility, customer demands, and anticipated business advantages. Hoejmose and Adrien-Kirby (2012) emphasized the significance of top management support and trust in driving GSCM in Taiwanese electronics manufacturing firms, alongside factors like collaboration with suppliers and customer pressure. Research on micro, small, and medium enterprises (MSMEs) in India revealed by Huma et al. (2023) indicated that both external and internal pressures motivate the adoption of GSCM initiatives. In a more recent investigation focusing on Malaysian manufacturing firms with 150 or fewer employees, Yildiz Çankaya and Sezen (2019) observed that government regulations, customer demands, and perceived benefits play a significant role in influencing GP adoption. While there may be variances among scholars regarding the factors influencing GP initiatives, there are also shared findings across multiple research studies.

4.4.2 *Organizational Factors*

4.4.2.1 Sustainable Business Practices

Effectively adopting green initiatives is often challenging for firms, especially when constrained by limited resources and capabilities (Borah et al., 2023). However, aligning resources and capabilities with supply chain partners can facilitate green initiatives. Capabilities play a crucial role in driving sustainable practices (Dagher & Itani, 2014). These include manufacturing capabilities, financial capabilities, innovation capabilities, intra-organizational capabilities, and integrative capabilities (Kwabena Anin et al., 2023). Manufacturing capabilities optimize manufacturing systems for improved performance and efficiency. Intra-organizational capabilities empower high-performance teams to achieve long-term sustainability objectives (Nkrumah et al., 2021). Integration capabilities facilitate close collaboration with suppliers and customers, reducing environmental impact and creating competitive advantages (Bowen et al., 2001). Financial capabilities enable investments in green technology and cost management, essential for effective supplier control. Innovative capabilities drive product design aimed at reducing environmental impact and long-term investments in sustainable practices (Min et al., 2014). These capabilities create value for customers and financial returns for firms, leading to lower costs and increased income. In conclusion, sustainable business practices depend on various organizational factors, including supplier selection and collaboration, organizational capabilities, financial management, and innovation. By aligning resources and capabilities with sustainability goals, firms can achieve long-term competitive advantages while minimizing environmental impact.

4.4.2.2 Corporate Environmental Responsibility

The triple bottom line, initially proposed by Richardson (2013), comprises three main aspects: the natural environment, society, and economic performance. Scholars advocate for companies to assess their performance beyond just economic metrics, taking into account ecological and social impacts (Gleim et al., 2013). Integrating sustainability principles into supply chain management is increasingly seen as essential for long-term success, aligning economic, environmental, and intangible goals (Yee et al., 2021). This holistic approach, termed sustainability performance, aims to enhance competitiveness in the market. Leppelt et al. (2013) emphasize the need for firms to manage suppliers' sustainability performance to ensure long-term sustainability. The incorporation of the triple bottom line concept into supply chain management, as highlighted by Archel et al. (2008), facilitates sustainability promotion within companies. By considering economic, environmental, and social factors, organizations can establish lasting competitive advantages and foster cross-functional collaboration (Chkanikova, 2016). Environmental performance involves reducing material usage and hazardous materials, while economic performance focuses on minimizing costs related to materials, energy consumption, and waste treatment while increasing profitability and productivity (Fauzi et al., 2010). Intangible performance encompasses aspects such as corporate image and customer satisfaction, which are essential but challenging to quantify. Isil and Hernke (2017) underscore the increasing reliance of firms on their supply base to gain competitive advantages and the necessity to address social and environmental concerns alongside financial performance. Collaborative efforts with suppliers can enhance environmental performance, as demonstrated by Hubbard (2009), who found that personnel knowledgeable in green purchasing facilitate improved collaboration and environmental outcomes.

4.4.2.3 Personal Attitudes

Personal attitude refers to an individual's unfavorable or favorable assessment of a specific behavior (Gimenez et al., 2012). When it comes to green products, attitude concerns whether an individual believes the product contributes positively to environmental protection (Gliedt & Parker, 2010). It reflects how much someone values the act of purchasing environmentally friendly items. Green purchase capability, on the other hand, refers to consumers' ability to buy such products (Yusoff et al., 2023). A positive attitude toward green products is expected to translate into actual purchases (Amoako et al., 2020). Research supports a positive correlation between attitude and capability regarding green product purchases (Yadav & Pathak, 2017). Psychologically, attitudes toward green purchases are shaped by ecological knowledge and affect, albeit to varying extents (Fatoki, 2023). The literature suggests that these two factors exert an asymmetric influence, indicating that an individual's emotional responses and cognitive understanding of environmental issues play distinct roles in shaping attitudes toward green purchases. Notably, attitudes toward green purchases are significantly more influenced by ecological effects than ecological knowledge (Nguyen et al., 2019).

4.4.3 *Individual Drivers*

4.4.3.1 Awareness

Fundamental to environmental research is individuals' concern for the environment, defined by Jamal et al. (2016) as a global attitude indirectly influencing behavior. Environmental concern, noted Lintukangas et al. (2015), strongly relates to preserving the environment and is an enduring positive or negative feeling about environmental issues. This concern has been a significant predictor of environmentally conscious behaviors, including recycling and green purchasing, as seen in studies by Suleiman (2023), Ahmad and Zhang (2020), and others. Environmental awareness, as described Chaudhary and Bisai (2018), encompasses an individual's understanding of human behavior's impact on the environment, while local awareness focuses on community-specific environmental issues. Studies have shown a positive correlation between environmental awareness and pro-environmental behavior, with Jamal et al. (2016) highlighting its role in differentiating green consumers. Moreover, Kaufmann et al. (2012) found that heightened awareness correlates with increased pro-social and pro-environmental behavior. The degree of environmental concern directly influences consumers' inclination to buy environmentally friendly products. AlNuaimi et al. (2021) argued that stronger environmental concern leads to increased purchasing of environmentally friendly products, corroborated by Hamner (2006). Additionally, environmental attitudes have been instrumental in predicting behaviors such as energy conservation, as evidenced by studies like those of Nguyen et al. (2017) and Naalchi Kashi (2020). While some studies have shown a strong association between environmental attitudes and behaviors, others have found only a moderate or weak relationship. Nonetheless, environmental attitude significantly impacts consumer environmental purchasing behavior, as highlighted by Moser (2015) and Kaufmann et al. (2012).

4.4.3.2 Attitudes

Attitudes, rooted in past experiences, significantly influence individuals' responses to various objects, persons, institutions, or events, as defined by Professor Icek Ajzen in "Attitude, Personality and Behavior" (Ajzen, 2005). These attitudes play a pivotal role in shaping consumer behavior, yet there has been a lack of emphasis on understanding attitudes toward green purchasing behavior (Ghosh, 2019). Research has indicated a strong interrelation between ecological consciousness and behavior, with emotions and personalities also influencing individuals' engagement with environmental issues (Alberg Mosgaard, 2015). Despite these influences, attitudes remain a key driver of involvement in ecological matters, shaping human activities and purchasing decisions aligned with ecological goals. In the emerging countries context, studies have demonstrated a positive association between attitudes toward green products and actual green purchasing behaviors (Song et al., 2015). For instance, AlNuaimi and Khan (2019) found a positive relationship between past green attitudes and green buying behavior among consumers in metropolitan cities. Similarly, Blome et al. (2014) observed that attitudes toward green practices in the lodging industry significantly influence consumers' choices to stay in environmentally friendly hotels. Conversely, Ji et al. (2015) did not find a significant association between attitudes toward environmental consequences and green purchasing capability. Understanding the underlying motives and values behind attitudes toward ecological matters could enhance efforts toward environmental conservation.

4.4.3.3 Values

The theoretical and empirical basis for incorporating perceived value defined perceived value as the overall assessment of a product's utility based on what is received compared to what is given (Foo et al., 2021). Typically, green products are priced higher than their conventional counterparts, and consumers often prioritize functionality over environmental considerations (Gliedt & Parker, 2010). When faced with a choice between product attributes and environmental friendliness, consumers tend to prioritize attributes, necessitating effective green marketing strategies to enhance perceived value concerning environmental concerns (Large & Gimenez Thomsen, 2011). By improving product values, companies can increase consumer purchase intention, as perceived value significantly predicts customer purchasing behavior. Perceived value plays a crucial role in the consumer decision-making process, with consumers favoring products with higher perceived value (Yook et al., 2018). Moreover, perceived green value positively influences purchase intention for environmentally friendly products. Zhuang et al. (2021) explored environmentally responsible behavior in ecotourism and found that perceived value positively influences such behavior. Moreover, personal values such as prioritizing health and safety, alongside indulging in pleasurable experiences such as enjoying food, have a beneficial influence on consumers' decisions to buy environmentally friendly products, with a specific emphasis on green food items (Chaudhary & Bisai, 2018). Yadav and Pathak (2017) discovered that both moral and individual norms play a substantial role in affecting purchase intentions and actual buying behavior. Consequently, it can be inferred that consumers' inclinations toward environmental, social, and ethical values, as well as their values, contribute positively to their ability to make green purchases.

4.5 Intersection of Green Purchasing Capabilities, Healthy Aging, and Climate Change

4.5.1 Implications for Healthy Aging in Developing Nations

The results highlight how important green buying methods are for healthy aging, especially in emerging economies. Green purchasing helps to create healthier work conditions by reducing the use of hazardous chemicals and encouraging cleaner environments through lower air emissions (AlNuaimi & Khan, 2019; Liu et al., 2020). The impact of these practices can be especially significant in emerging economies where environmental regulations are less strict, as older adults often have limited access to resources, including healthcare, and are, therefore, more susceptible to the negative effects of pollution and exposure to hazardous substances (WHO, 2018). Furthermore, the implementation of sustainable business practices and the creation of eco-friendly goods and services meet the needs of the aging population and enhance their quality of life (Muralidharan & Muralidharan, 2021). The availability of age-friendly goods and services is crucial for preserving the health and independence of senior citizens in areas with quickly aging populations and inadequate healthcare infrastructure (WHO, 2023). Hence, the quality of life for senior citizens in these environments can be greatly enhanced by environmentally friendly purchasing programs that give top priority to the creation of such goods and services. Additionally, green activities promote a sustainable and comfortable living environment for older individuals by reducing the environmental impact of climate change (Galeazzo et al., 2021). This indirectly supports healthy aging. Environmental degradation and disasters linked to climate change disproportionately affect older persons in many emerging economies. This can worsen preexisting health conditions and lead to social isolation and economic instability (Mezzina et al., 2022). Green procurement initiatives can lessen environmental hazards and build more resilient communities for senior citizens by encouraging sustainable activities. Moreover, green purchasing and sustainable procurement practices contribute to environmental sustainability by reducing resource consumption, minimizing waste generation, and mitigating climate change. Examining the determinants of green purchasing capabilities sheds light on how organizations can adopt more environmentally responsible practices, thereby addressing the environmental crises outlined in the Sustainable Aging framework and creating a more sustainable future for all generations (Fang et al., 2023).

4.5.2 Alignment with the Healthy Aging Initiatives

This review strongly aligns with the goals of current healthy aging initiatives, such as the Decade of Healthy Ageing 2020–2030, as well as with the SDGs mentioned earlier. The results are consistent with the objectives of these programs since they highlight the role that environmental sustainability plays in encouraging healthy aging. A fundamental component of healthy aging initiatives is the creation of age-friendly surroundings that emphasize sustainable practices, safe workplaces, and clean air (Bull et al., 2020). The integration of green purchasing capabilities becomes even more critical in emerging economies, where limited resources and infrastructure can exacerbate the issues of an aging population. Green procurement efforts help campaigns like the Decade of Healthy Ageing, Age-Friendly Cities and Communities, Nutrition and Healthy Eating Campaigns, etc. achieve their goals by creating age-friendly products and services, safer workplaces, and lower air pollution—all of which promote healthy aging. Furthermore, green purchasing initiatives in developing nations support the likes of Age-Friendly Cities and Communities, Nutrition and Healthy Eating Campaigns, Decade of Healthy Ageing's overarching objectives of fostering environments that allow older people to live longer, healthier, and more fulfilling lives by addressing the environmental determinants of health and encouraging sustainable practices (Bull et al., 2020). Thus, the incorporation of green purchasing capabilities in developing nations not only contributes to the overall goals of initiatives such as the Decade of Healthy Ageing but also marks a significant milestone in the construction of more age-friendly and sustainable societies for older adults in the present and the future. Green purchasing initiatives play a key role in promoting age-friendly environments, ensuring access to healthier products, sustainable housing options, and safe transportation. By identifying determinants that enable green purchasing capabilities in developing countries, the study provides insights into how organizations can integrate environmental considerations into their procurement processes, ultimately contributing to creating healthier and safer environments for older adults.

4.5.3 Actions for Stakeholders to Foster Healthy Aging

By implementing laws and policies that encourage environmentally friendly purchasing behaviors and the advancement of age-friendly goods and services, governments can significantly contribute to the promotion of healthy aging. This involves providing tax breaks, grants, or other financial aid to companies that put the needs of senior citizens and sustainability first (Dubey et al., 2013; Hoejmose & Adrien-Kirby, 2012). Governments can also fund infrastructure initiatives that create age-friendly surroundings, like affordable housing options that are suited to the requirements of older persons, pedestrian-friendly streets, and accessible public transportation. The creation of more inclusive and livable communities for older individuals can be facilitated by governments by giving infrastructure expenditures that promote healthy aging a top priority. Incorporating environmental factors into company plans and operations is another important way that organizations support healthy aging. According to Borah et al. (2023), this entails putting in place green purchasing procedures, cutting carbon emissions, and making investments in environmentally friendly technology and procedures. In addition, organizations could create and promote age-appropriate goods and services that address the requirements of senior citizens. Examples of these include easily navigable and accessible products, individualized medical treatment, and workplace and public area amenities that help seniors. Individuals can promote age-friendly policies and programs in their communities and places of employment, as well as support sustainable enterprises by making ecologically responsible purchase decisions (Gimenez et al., 2012). Stakeholders may foster a more inclusive and supportive environment for healthy aging, advancing the health, well-being, and dignity of older individuals in the present and the future by putting resources into age-friendly policies and environmental sustainability at the top of the priority list.

4.6 Implications for Future Research

The implications for future research stemming from this study are multifaceted. First, further investigation is warranted to delve deeper into the specific mechanisms through which external factors, organizational variables, and individual drivers interact to shape green purchasing capabilities in emerging countries. This could involve longitudinal studies or cross-sectional analyses to capture changes over time and across different contexts. Additionally, comparative research across multiple emerging economies could provide valuable insights into the relative importance of various factors and the effectiveness of different policy interventions. Furthermore, exploring the role of technology, innovation, and digital platforms in facilitating green purchasing capabilities represents a promising avenue for future inquiry. Future research on green consumerism presents numerous avenues for exploration and analysis. One key area of focus could particularly be to investigate customer attitudes across diverse locations and cultures within emerging countries. Cross-country analyses of green consumer capabilities offer another compelling aspect to explore, providing valuable insights for both practitioners and academics alike. Additionally, future research should aim to uncover the conditions and circumstances that prompt consumers to modify their environmentally conscious capabilities

4.7 Limitations

Although this study offers insightful information about how green purchasing practices impact healthy aging, it is crucial to recognize some of its limitations. The study may have missed significant articles from other databases because the researchers limited their review to only the Scopus, Web of Science, and Google Scholar databases, suggesting future research could conduct thorough literature searches. The hybrid methodology used, systematic-narrative reviews, may be subjective, less quantitative, and difficult to integrate. To ensure comprehensive coverage and reduce bias, future research should use a more rigorous approach, like traditional systematic reviews.

Notwithstanding these drawbacks, this study advances the knowledge of the possible effects of environmentally friendly purchasing methods on long-term healthy aging. The researchers have emphasized the important consequences of green purchasing for fostering healthier communities and surroundings for aging citizens by combining the results of the extant research. By addressing the aforementioned limits and instituting systematic review methods in future research endeavors, the robustness and reliability of understanding in this domain can be further improved.

4.8 Conclusion

This systematic narrative review fills a crucial gap in understanding green purchasing capabilities in emerging countries, highlighting external influences, organizational variables, and individual drivers as key factors. It emphasizes the potential of green purchasing to address climate change and cater to aging populations' needs. This study's conclusion emphasizes the diverse effects of green purchasing skills in emerging economies, especially when it comes to tackling environmental sustainability and the issues brought on by an aging population. The researchers have emphasized the critical role that sustainable business practices, corporate environmental responsibility, and individual attitudes play in influencing environmentally conscious consumer behavior through a thorough analysis of the factors that influence green purchasing, including economic, cultural, governmental, regulatory, organizational, and individual drivers. Moreover, the researchers have explained how green purchasing promotes social cohesion and economic progress in emerging countries in addition to helping to preserve the environment. Emerging nations can strike a healthy balance between environmental concerns, societal well-being, and economic progress by supporting sustainable procurement practices that meet the demands of aging populations while also aligning with environmental objectives. In addition, the incorporation of green purchasing capabilities has the potential to significantly reduce greenhouse gas emissions, increase resource efficiency, and cultivate a sustainable culture in developing nations. Developing nations can pave a sustainable route to an eco-friendly future by embracing eco-friendly goods and services and establishing laws and regulations that encourage them. This study emphasizes how critical it is to build green purchasing skills in emerging nations to accomplish all-encompassing and sustainable growth and open the door to a future that is more socially, environmentally, and economically affluent.

This review emphasizes the significance of incorporating environmental considerations into purchasing decisions in emerging countries, particularly for the aging population. Sustainable business practices and corporate environmental responsibility offer economic opportunities and support while addressing climate change is crucial. However, the journey toward green purchasing capabilities is ongoing and requires adaptation to evolving socio-economic, cultural, and environmental landscapes.

Review Questions

1. What are the main determinants influencing green purchasing behaviors in developing countries, and how do they differ from those in developed nations?
2. How does the socio-economic context of developing countries impact individuals' ability and willingness to engage in green purchasing practices?
3. In what ways can promoting green purchasing behaviors contribute to healthier aging populations in developing countries? Provide specific examples or case studies.
4. What role do cultural factors play in influencing attitudes and behaviors toward green purchasing in different regions of the world?
5. How can governments and businesses in developing countries encourage and support the adoption of green purchasing practices among both younger and older populations?
6. What are some potential challenges or barriers to implementing sustainable consumption initiatives in developing countries, particularly in the context of promoting healthy aging?

References

Ahmad, W., & Zhang, Q. (2020). Green purchase intention: Effects of electronic service quality and customer green psychology. *Journal of Cleaner Production, 267*, 122053. https://doi.org/10.1016/j.jclepro.2020.122053

Ajogwu, A., & Odeyemi, K. (2021). Active ageing: Process and determinants among middle-aged men in rural and urban communities in Lagos state, Nigeria. *Pan African Medical Journal, 39*, 39. https://doi.org/10.11604/pamj.2021.39.195.27546

Alberg Mosgaard, M. (2015). Improving the practices of green procurement of minor items. *Journal of Cleaner Production, 90*, 264–274. https://doi.org/10.1016/j.jclepro.2014.11.077

AlNuaimi, B. K., & Khan, M. (2019). Public-sector green procurement in The United Arab Emirates: Innovation capability and commitment to change. *Journal of Cleaner Production, 233*, 482–489. https://doi.org/10.1016/j.jclepro.2019.06.090

AlNuaimi, B. K., Singh, S. K., & Harney, B. (2021). Unpacking the role of innovation capability: Exploring the impact of leadership style on green procurement via a natural resource-based perspective. *Journal of Business Research, 134*, 78–88. https://doi.org/10.1016/j.jbusres.2021.05.026

Amoako, G. K., Dzogbenuku, R. K., & Abubakari, A. (2020). Do green knowledge and attitudes influence the youth's green purchasing? Theory of planned behavior. *International Journal of Productivity and Performance Management, 69*(8), 1609–1626.

Ajzen, I. (2005). *Attitudes, personality and behaviour*. McGraw-hill education (UK).

Archel, P., Fernández, M., & Larrinaga, C. (2008). The organizational and operational boundaries of triple bottom line reporting: A survey. *Environmental Management, 41*, 106–117.

Balin, A. I., & Sari, K. (2023). The effect of green purchasing practices on financial performance under the mediating role of environmental performance: Evidence from Türkiye. *Sustain, 15*. https://doi.org/10.3390/su15043617

Benameur, K. B., Mostafa, M. M., Hassanein, A., Shariff, M. Z., & Al-Shattarat, W. (2023). Sustainability reporting scholarly research: A bibliometric review and a future research agenda. *Management Review Quarterly, 74*, 823–866.

Blome, C., Hollos, D., & Paulraj, A. (2014). Green procurement and green supplier development: Antecedents and effects on supplier performance. *International Journal of Production Research, 52*, 32–49. https://doi.org/10.1080/00207543.2013.825748

Borah, P. S., Dogbe, C. S. K., Pomegbe, W. W. K., et al. (2023). Green market orientation, green innovation capability, green knowledge acquisition and green brand positioning as determinants of new product success. *European Journal of Innovation Management, 26*, 364–385. https://doi.org/10.1108/EJIM-09-2020-0345

Bowen, F. E., Cousins, P. D., Lamming, R. C., & Faruk, A. C. (2001). The role of supply management capabilities in green supply. *Production and Operations Management, 10*, 174–189. https://doi.org/10.1111/j.1937-5956.2001.tb00077.x

Bull, F. C., Al-Ansari, S. S., Biddle, S., Borodulin, K., Buman, M. P., Cardon, G., & Willumsen, J. F. (2020). World Health Organization 2020 guidelines on physical activity and sedentary behaviour. *British Journal of Sports Medicine, 54*(24), 1451–1462.

Chaudhary, R., & Bisai, S. (2018). Factors influencing green purchase behavior of millennials in India. *Management of Environmental Quality: An International Journal, 29*, 798–812. https://doi.org/10.1108/MEQ-02-2018-0023

Chkanikova, O. (2016). Sustainable purchasing in food retailing: Interorganizational relationship management to green product supply. *Business Strategy and the Environment, 25*, 478–494. https://doi.org/10.1002/bse.1877

Chou, J.-J., Shih, C.-S., Wang, W.-D., & Huang, K.-C. (2019). IoT sensing networks for gait velocity measurement. *International Journal of Applied Mathematics and Computer Science, 2019*(29), 245–259.

Dagher, G. K., & Itani, O. (2014). Factors influencing green purchasing behaviour: Empirical evidence from the Lebanese consumers. *Journal of Consumer Behaviour, 13*, 188–195. https://doi.org/10.1002/cb.1482

Dasanayake, D. M. S. M., & Amarasena, T. S. M. (2022). Impact of green procurement on purchasing performance (Special reference to the Apparel Manufacturing Industry in Sri Lanka). *International Journal of Innovative Research and Publications*. https://doi.org/10.51430/ijirp.2022.25.002

Dubey, R., Bag, S., Ali, S. S., & Venkatesh, V. G. (2013). Green purchasing is key to superior performance: An empirical study. *International Journal of Procurement Management, 6*, 187–210. https://doi.org/10.1504/IJPM.2013.052469

EL Baz, J., Jebli, F., Cherrafi, A., Akenroye, T., & Iddik, S. (2022). The cultural dimensions in supply chain management research: A state-of-the-art review and research agenda. *European Business Review, 34*(2), 171–190.

El-Garaihy, W. H., Badawi, U. A., Seddik, W. A., & Torky, M. S. (2022). Investigating performance outcomes under institutional pressures and environmental orientation motivated green supply chain management practices. *Sustainability, 14*(3), 1523.

ElTayeb, T. K., Zailani, S., & Jayaraman, K. (2010). The examination on the drivers for green purchasing adoption among EMS 14001 certified companies in Malaysia. *Journal of Manufacturing Technology Management, 21*, 206–225. https://doi.org/10.1108/17410381011014378

Fang, M. L., Sixsmith, J., Hamilton-Pryde, A., Rogowsky, R., Scrutton, P., Pengelly, R., & Creaney, R. (2023). Co-creating inclusive spaces and places: Towards an intergenerational and age-friendly living ecosystem. *Frontiers in Public Health, 10*, 996520.

Fatoki, O. (2023). Determinants Of Green Purchase Behaviour Of University Students In South Africa. *Environmental Economics, 86*, 556–582. https://doi.org/10.34659/eis.2023.86.3.607

Fauzi, H., Svensson, G., & Rahman, A. A. (2010). "Triple bottom line" as "sustainable corporate performance": A proposition for the future. *Sustainability, 2*, 1345–1360. https://doi.org/10.3390/su2051345

Fernandez, R. M. (2020). SDG3 good health and well-being: integration and connection with other SDGs. In *Good health and well-being* (pp. 629–636). Springer.

Fong, B. Y., Law, V. T., Leung, T. C., Lo, M. F., Ng, T. K., & Yee, H. H. (2022). *Sustainable development goal 3: Health and well-being of ageing in Hong Kong* (p. 104). Taylor & Francis.

Foo, M. Y., Kanapathy, K., Zailani, S., & Shaharudin, M. R. (2019). Green purchasing capabilities, practices and institutional pressure. *Management of Environmental Quality: An International Journal, 30*, 1171–1189. https://doi.org/10.1108/MEQ-07-2018-0133

Foo, M. Y. E. E., Kanapathy, K., Zailani, S., & Shaharudin, M. R. (2021). Green Purchasing: Capabilities, practices and effects on firms' triple bottom line performance. *Estudios de Economía, 39*, 1–22. https://doi.org/10.25115/eea.v39i3.4160Freihat

Freihat, L., Al-Qaaida, M. S., Abbod, M., & Huneiti, Z. A. (2023). Green Human Resource Management/Supply Chain Management/Regulation and Legislation and its Effects on Sustainable Development Goals in Jordan. *Sustainability, 16*(7), 2769.

Galeazzo, A., Ortiz-de-Mandojana, N., & Delgado-Ceballos, J. (2021). Green procurement and financial performance in the tourism industry: The moderating role of tourists' green purchasing behaviour. *Current Issues in Tourism, 24*, 700–716. https://doi.org/10.1080/13683500.2020.1734546

Ghosh, M. (2019). Determinants of green procurement implementation and its impact on firm performance. *Journal of Manufacturing Technology Management, 30*, 462–482. https://doi.org/10.1108/JMTM-06-2018-0168

Gil, M. T., & Jacob, J. (2018). The relationship between green perceived quality and green purchase intention: A three-path mediation approach using green satisfaction and green trust. *International Journal of Business Innovation and Research, 15*, 301–319. https://doi.org/10.1504/IJBIR.2018.089750

Gimenez, C., Sierra, V., & Rodon, J. (2012). Sustainable operations: Their impact on the triple bottom line. *International Journal of Production Economics, 140*, 149–159. https://doi.org/10.1016/j.ijpe.2012.01.035

Gleim, M. R., Smith, J. S., Andrews, D., & Cronin, J. J. (2013). Against the green: A multi-method examination of the barriers to green consumption. *Journal of Retailing, 89*, 44–61. https://doi.org/10.1016/j.jretai.2012.10.001

Gliedt, T., & Parker, P. (2010). Dynamic capabilities for strategic green advantage: Green electricity purchasing in North American firms, SMEs, NGOs, and agencies. *Global Business and Economic Review, 12*, 171–195. https://doi.org/10.1504/GBER.2010.034892

González-Benito, J., Lannelongue, G., Ferreira, L. M., & Gonzalez-Zapatero, C. (2016). The effect of green purchasing on purchasing performance: The moderating role played by long-term relationships and strategic integration. *The Journal of Business and Industrial Marketing, 31*, 312–324. https://doi.org/10.1108/JBIM-09-2014-0188

Grossmann, I., & Santos, H. C. (2020). Individualistic cultures. In *Encyclopedia of personality and individual differences* (pp. 2238–2241). Sprigner.

Gupta, N., Pradhan, S., Jain, A., & Patel, N. (2021). *Sustainable agriculture in India 2021*. Council on Energy, Environment and Water.

Hamner, B. (2006). Effects of green purchasing strategies on supplier behaviour. In *Greening the supply chain* (pp. 25–37). London: Springer London.

Hazaea, S. A., Al-Matari, E. M., Zedan, K., Khatib, S. F., Zhu, J., & Al Amosh, H. (2022). Green purchasing: Past, present, and future. *Sustainability, 14*(9), 5008. https://doi.org/10.3390/su14095008

Hoejmose, S. U., & Adrien-Kirby, A. J. (2012). Socially and environmentally responsible procurement: A literature review and future research agenda of a managerial issue in the 21st century. *Journal of Purchasing and Supply Management, 18*, 232–242. https://doi.org/10.1016/j.pursup.2012.06.002

Hubbard, G. (2009). Measuring organizational performance: Beyond the triple bottom line. *Business Strategy and the Environment, 18*, 177–191. https://doi.org/10.1002/bse.564

Huma, S., Ahmed Siddiqui, D., & Ahmed, W. (2023). Understanding the impact of Green supply chain management practices on operational competitive capabilities. *The TQM Journal, 35*, 796–815. https://doi.org/10.1108/TQM-08-2021-0246

Isil, O., & Hernke, M. T. (2017). The triple bottom line: A critical review from a transdisciplinary perspective. *Business Strategy and the Environment, 26*, 1235–1251. https://doi.org/10.1002/bse.1982

Jaiswal, D., & Kant, R. (2018). Green purchasing behaviour: A conceptual framework and empirical investigation of Indian consumers. *Journal of Retailing and Consumer Services, 41*, 60–69.

Jamal, Z. B., Islam, S., & Barua, P. (2016). Analyzing factors that affect green purchase behavior: From the context of Bangladeshi consumers. *Journal of Economics, Business and Management, 4*, 611–617. https://doi.org/10.18178/joebm.2016.4.10.461

Ji, P., Ma, X., & Li, G. (2015). Developing green purchasing relationships for the manufacturing industry: An evolutionary game theory perspective. *International Journal of Production Economics, 166*, 155–162. https://doi.org/10.1016/j.ijpe.2014.10.009

Joshi, Y., & Rahman, Z. (2015). Factors affecting green purchase behaviour and future research directions. *International Strategic Management Review, 3*, 128–143. https://doi.org/10.1016/j.ism.2015.04.001

Kabra, G., Srivastava, S. K., & Ghosh, V. (2023). Mapping the field of sustainable procurement: A bibliometric analysis. *Benchmarking: An International Journal, 30*(10), 4370–4396.

Kaufmann, H. R., Panni, M. F. A. K., & Orphanidou, Y. (2012). Factors affecting consumers' green purchasing behavior: An integrated conceptual framework. *Amfiteatru Economic, 14*, 50–69.

Khan, S. A. R., & Qianli, D. (2017). Impact of green supply chain management practices on firms' performance: An empirical study from the perspective of Pakistan. *Environmental Science and Pollution Research, 24*, 16829–16844. https://doi.org/10.1007/s11356-017-9172-5

Kwabena Anin, E., Ataburo, H., Effah Ampong, G., & Osei Bempah, N. D. (2023). A resource orchestration perspective of the link between environmental orientation and green purchasing: Empirical evidence from an emerging economy. *Cogent Business & Management, 10*, 2215576. https://doi.org/10.1080/23311975.2023.221557

Kyomuhendo, C., & Adeola, R. (2021). Green and grey: Nutritional lifestyle and healthful ageing in rural and urban areas of three sub-Saharan African countries. *Business Strategy and Development, 4*, 22–33. https://doi.org/10.1002/bsd2.153

Large, R. O., & Gimenez Thomsen, C. (2011). Drivers of green supply management performance: Evidence from Germany. *Journal of Purchasing and Supply Management, 17*, 176–184. https://doi.org/10.1016/j.pursup.2011.04.00

Lasuin, C. A., & Ng, Y. C. (2014). Factors influencing green purchase intention among university students. *Malaysian Journal of Business and Economics (MJBE), 1*(2), 1–14.

Leppelt, T., Foerstl, K., & Hartmann, E. (2013). Corporate social responsibility in buyer-supplier relationships: is it beneficial for top-tier suppliers to market their capability to ensure a responsible supply chain?. *Business Research, 6*, 126–152.

Lintukangas, K., Hallikas, J., & Kähkönen, A. K. (2015). The role of green supply management in the development of a sustainable supply chain. *Corporate Social Responsibility and Environmental Management, 22*(6), 321–333.

Liu, Y., Srai, J. S., & Evans, S. (2016). Environmental management: The role of supply chain capabilities in the auto sector. *Supply Chain Management, 21*, 1–19. https://doi.org/10.1108/SCM-01-2015-0026

Liu, Y., Zhu, Q., & Seuring, S. (2017a). Linking capabilities to green operations strategies: The moderating role of corporate environmental proactivity. *International Journal of Production Economics, 187*, 182–195. https://doi.org/10.1016/j.ijpe.2017.03.007

Liu, Y., Segev, S., & Villar, M. E. (2017b). Comparing two mechanisms for green consumption: cognitive-affect behavior vs theory of reasoned action. *Journal of Consumer Marketing, 34*(5), 442–454.

Liu, J., Liu, Y., & Yang, L. (2020). Uncovering the influence mechanism between top management support and green procurement: The effect of green training. *Journal of Cleaner Production, 251*, 119674. https://doi.org/10.1016/j.jclepro.2019.119674

Mahmood, F., Al-Shattarat, W., Hamed, R., Al-Shattarat, B., Benameur, K., Hassanein, A., & Tahat, Y. (2023). The influence of urbanization and environmental factors on the financial performance of retail and automotive industries in China. *Sustainability, 15*(23), 16138.

Malanowski, N., Ozcivelek, R., & Cabrera, M. (2008). Active ageing and independent living services: The role of information and communication technology. *European Community, 39*, 1–42.

Mangla, S. K., Luthra, S., Mishra, N., Singh, A., Rana, N. P., Dora, M., & Dwivedi, Y. (2018). Barriers to effective circular supply chain management in a developing country context. *Production Planning & Control, 29*(6), 551–569.

Martín-Martín, A., Thelwall, M., Orduna-Malea, E., & Delgado López-Cózar, E. (2021). Google Scholar, Microsoft Academic, Scopus, Dimensions, Web of Science, and OpenCitations' COCI: A multidisciplinary comparison of coverage via citations. *Scientometrics, 126*(1), 871–906.

Mazar, N., & Zhong, C. B. (2010). Do green products make us better people? *Psychological Science, 21*(4), 494–498.

Mezzina, R., Gopikumar, V., Jenkins, J., Saraceno, B., & Sashidharan, S. P. (2022). Social vulnerability and mental health inequalities in the "Syndemic": Call for action. *Frontiers in Psychiatry, 13*, 894370.

Michelsen, O., & de Boer, L. (2009). Green procurement in Norway; a survey of practices at the municipal and county level. *Journal of Environmental Management, 91*, 160–167. https://doi.org/10.1016/j.jenvman.2009.08.001

Min, S. H., Im, S. B., & Kogan, T. T. (2014). Mediating effects of green purchasing capability on the organizational characteristics-firm performance relationship. *Asia Marketing Journal, 16*. https://doi.org/10.53728/2765-6500.1525

Moser, A. K. (2015). Thinking green, buying green? Drivers of pro-environmental purchasing behavior. *Journal of Consumer Marketing, 32*, 167–175. https://doi.org/10.1108/JCM-10-2014-1179

Muralidharan, K., & Muralidharan. (2021). *Sustainable development and quality of life*. Springer Singapore.

Naalchi Kashi, A. (2020). Green purchase intention: A conceptual model of factors influencing green purchase of Iranian consumers. *Journal of Islamic Marketing, 11*, 1389–1403. https://doi.org/10.1108/JIMA-06-2019-0120

Nguyen, T. N., Lobo, A., & Greenland, S. (2017). The influence of cultural values on green purchase behaviour. *Marketing Intelligence & Planning, 35*, 377–396. https://doi.org/10.1108/MIP-08-2016-0131

Nguyen, T. T. H., Yang, Z., Nguyen, N., et al. (2019). Greenwash and green purchase intention: The mediating role of green skepticism. *Sustainability, 11*, 1–16. https://doi.org/10.3390/su11092653

Nkrumah, S. K., Asamoah, D., Annan, J., & Agyei-Owusu, B. (2021). Examining green capabilities as drivers of green supply chain management adoption. *Management Research Review, 44*, 94–111. https://doi.org/10.1108/MRR 01 2020 0015

Parviz, M. (2023). Reflecting on the consequences of the Iranian university entrance examination: A systematic-narrative hybrid literature review. *Discover Education, 2*, 1–11. https://doi.org/10.1007/s44217-023-00046-x

Paulraj, A. (2011). Understanding the relationships between internal resources and capabilities, sustainable supply management and organizational sustainability. *Journal of Supply Chain Management, 47*, 19–37. https://doi.org/10.1111/j.1745-493X.2010.03212.x

Pinto, L. (2023). Investigating the relationship between green supply chain purchasing practices and firms' performance. *J Ind Eng Manag, 16*, 78–101. https://doi.org/10.3926/jiem.3686

Richardson, J. (2013). *The triple bottom line: Does it all add up?: Assessing the sustainability of business and CSR*. Taylor and Francis.

Rudnicka, E., Napierała, P., Podfigurna, A., Męczekalski, B., Smolarczyk, R., & Grymowicz, M. (2020). The World Health Organization (WHO) approach to healthy ageing. *Maturitas, 139*, 6–11.

Santos, C. J., Paciência, I., & Ribeiro, A. I. (2022). Neighbourhood socioeconomic processes and dynamics and healthy ageing: A scoping review. *International Journal of Environmental Research and Public Health, 19*. https://doi.org/10.3390/ijerph19116745

Sarkis, J., Zhu, Q., & Lai, K. H. (2011). An organizational theoretic review of green supply chain management literature. *International Journal of Production Economics, 130*(1), 1–15.

Schaper, M. (2002). Introduction: The essence of ecopreneurship. *Greener Management International, 38*, 26–30.

Schröder, P., Antonarakis, A. S., Brauer, J., Conteh, A., Kohsaka, R., Uchiyama, Y., & Pacheco, P. (2019). SDG 12: Responsible consumption and production–Potential Benefits and impacts on forests and livelihoods. Sustainable development goals: Their impacts on forests and people, 386–418. Cambridge University Press

Sharma, A., & Foropon, C. (2019). Green product attributes and green purchase behavior: A theory of planned behavior perspective with implications for circular economy. *Management Decision, 57*(4), 1018–1042.

Singh, S. K., & El-Kassar, A. N. (2019). Role of big data analytics in developing sustainable capabilities. *Journal of Cleaner Production, 213*, 1264–1273.

Slastanova, N., Palus, H., Sulek, R., et al. (2021). The benefits of applying green purchasing. *SHS Web of Conferences, 92*, 06037. https://doi.org/10.1051/shsconf/20219206037

Song, H., Yu, K., & Zhang, S. (2015). Green procurement, stakeholder satisfaction and operational performance. *The International Journal of Logistics Management, 28*(4), 1054–1077. https://doi.org/10.1108/IJLM-12-2015-0234

Suleiman, M. A. (2023). The impact of the tourism supply chain on sustainable performance in sub-Saharan Africa: evidence from Tanzania. *Management of Environmental Quality: An International Journal, 34*(2), 492–510.

Tondolo, V., de Otero, L. O., Garcia, D. R., et al. (2023). Effect of supplier environmental damage on environmental concern and green purchase dynamic capabilities. *Life Style, 10*, e01553. https://doi.org/10.19141/2237-3756.lifestyle.v10.n00.pe01553

Turnbull, D., Chugh, R., & Luck, J. (2023). Systematic-narrative hybrid literature review: A strategy for integrating a concise methodology into a manuscript. *Social Sciences & Humanities Open, 7*(1), 100381.

World Health Organization. (2018). WHO report on surveillance of antibiotic consumption: 2016-2018 early implementation.

World Health Organization. (2023). National programmes for age-friendly cities and communities: A guide. World Health Organization.

Wu, J. H., Wu, C. W., Lee, C. T., & Lee, H. J. (2015). Green purchase intentions: An exploratory study of the Taiwanese electric motorcycle market. *Journal of Business Research, 68*, 829–833. https://doi.org/10.1016/j.jbusres.2014.11.036

Yadav, R., & Pathak, G. S. (2016). Young consumers' intention towards buying green products in a developing nation: Extending the theory of planned behavior. *Journal of Cleaner Production, 135*, 732–739.

Yadav, R., & Pathak, G. S. (2017). Determinants of consumers' green purchase behavior in a developing nation: Applying and extending the theory of planned behavior. *Ecological Economics, 134*, 114–122.

Yee Foo, M., Kanapathy, K., Zailani, S., & Shaharudin, M. R. (2019). The impact of green purchasing capabilities and practices on firm sustainability. *Science Proceedings Series, 1*, 16–21. https://doi.org/10.31580/sps.v1i1.513

Yee, F. M., Shaharudin, M. R., Ma, G., et al. (2021). Green purchasing capabilities and practices towards Firm's triple bottom line in Malaysia. *Journal of Cleaner Production, 307*, 127268. https://doi.org/10.1016/j.jclepro.2021.127268

Yildiz Çankaya, S., & Sezen, B. (2019). Effects of green supply chain management practices on sustainability performance. *Journal of Manufacturing Technology Management, 30*, 98–121. https://doi.org/10.1108/JMTM-03-2018-0099

Yook, K. H., Choi, J. H., & Suresh, N. C. (2018). Linking green purchasing capabilities to environmental and economic performance: The moderating role of firm size. *Journal of Purchasing and Supply Management, 24*(4), 326–337. https://doi.org/10.1016/j.pursup.2017.09.001

Yu, Z., Golpira, H., & Khan, S. A. R. (2018). The relationship between green supply chain performance, energy demand, economic growth, and environmental sustainability: An empirical evidence from developed countries. *LogForum, 14*(4), 479–494.

Yusoff, N., Alias, M., & Ismail, N. (2023). Drivers of green purchasing behaviour: A systematic review and a research agenda. *F1000Research, 12*. https://doi.org/10.12688/f1000research.140765.1

Zhuang, W., Luo, X., & Riaz, M. U. (2021). On the factors influencing green purchase intention: A meta-analysis approach. *Frontiers in Psychology, 12*, 644020. https://doi.org/10.3389/fpsyg.2021.644020

Zorzini, M., Hendry, L. C., Huq, F. A., & Stevenson, M. (2015). Socially responsible sourcing: Reviewing the literature and its use of theory. *International Journal of Operations & Production Management, 35*(1), 60–109.

Part II
Innovation, Planning, and Change

Chapter 5
The Future of Healthy Ageing Amidst Threats: The Role of Innovation for Nigerian Older Adults

Jacinta C. Ene, Henry T. Ajibo, and Uzoma O. Okoye

Acronyms and Abbreviations

ADL	Activities of daily living
COVID-19	Coronavirus Disease 2019
CSSA	Child survival sustainability assessment
LGA	Local government area
NHIS	National Health Insurance Scheme
NSCCA	National Senior Citizen Center Act
SDGs	Sustainable development goals
SMS	Short message services
STRACEP	Strategic contacts ethics publications
UN	United Nations
UNDESA	United Nations Department of Economics and Social Affairs
WHO	World Health Organization

J. C. Ene (✉) · H. T. Ajibo
Department of Social Work, Faculty of the Social Sciences, University of Nigeria, Nsukka, Enugu State, Nigeria
e-mail: jacinta.ene@unn.edu.ng; henry.ajibo@unn.edu.ng

U. O. Okoye
Department of Social Work, Faculty of the Social Sciences, University of Nigeria, Nsukka, Enugu State, Nigeria

School of Humanities, Social Sciences and Law, University of Dundee, Dundee, UK

Department of Social Work and Social Administration, College of Social Sciences, Makerere University, Kampala, Uganda
e-mail: uzoma.okoye@unn.edu.ng

N. Asiamah et al. (eds.), *Sustainable Ageing*,
https://doi.org/10.1007/978-3-031-69475-2_5

5.1 Introduction

The United Nations (UN) decade of healthy ageing for older adults entails achieving the Sustainable Development Goals (SDGs): 1–3. This signifies that older adults have the right to a dignified life, which includes providing support to end poverty and hunger and ensure healthy lives by adding health to years (United Nations Department of Economics and Social Affairs [UNDESA], 2016). Healthy ageing requires keeping up with the functional capacity that ensures well-being in older adults (World Health Organization [WHO], 2017). This is a major policy priority for the UN and its Part States because population ageing is a trend of significant policy concern in the contemporary time and for the coming decade (UNDESA, 2020). This stems from the fact that since healthy ageing is connected to a scope of safety development, health and environmental agendas, there is a developing interest in investigating diverse and creative ways to deal with strategies that will proactively support sustainable ageing.

In every society, there are older adults. These are persons aged 60 years and older, with the worldwide projection to reach 9.8 billion in 2050 and 11.2 billion in 2100 (UNDESA, 2017). In sub-Saharan Africa, population ageing is projected to reach 67 million by 2025 and 163 million by 2050 (WHO, 2023), while in Nigeria, it is expected to hit 16 million by 2050 and 74 million by 2100 (UNDESA, 2019). With the increasing population ageing despite their ages, older adults contribute to the development of society. This could be within their family, local community, or society more broadly. However, the extent of these human and social resources and the opportunities available to them as they age depend on their health status. Hence, if people are experiencing extra years in good health, their ability to do the things they value will have few limits (WHO, 2017). On the contrary, if these added years are dominated by declines in physical and mental capacities, the implications for older adults and society may be negative. Hence, with increasing population ageing and health conditions, challenges constraining the efficiency of the well-being of older adults may pose a threat to healthy ageing.

Ageing is a global phenomenon which may involve frailty and disengagement from various formal and informal activities. In a changing world, we need sustainable ageing, with societies responding to the imminent ageing challenges by instituting ageing programmes to prepare and protect people as they grow older and live longer. As people age, they often experience a gradual decline in health and may become susceptible to illnesses. Mcgregor et al. (2018) reported that most health conditions associated with ageing are often chronic illnesses, including cancer, diabetes, and osteoarthritis, among others. They may require assistance with the management of their health needs and personal care, such as bathing, dressing, toileting, cooking, feeding, and other activities of daily living (ADL). Providing care assistance for older adults is perceived to be a filial responsibility in African countries, including Nigeria (Ene et al., 2022a). Thus, caregiving assistance for older adults should be friendly, helpful, available, and sensitive to the needs of recipients, irrespective of the negative and positive aspects (Ene & Nnama-Okechukwu, 2022). Some positive and negative aspects of caregiving include a feeling of affection, the extent of closeness, a sense of personal satisfaction, and often overwhelming, constantly demanding, and always challenging (Faronbi & Olagun, 2017). To this end, strategising measures for healthy ageing requires concentration on technology and innovative health management services.

Ageing innovations are new opportunities and resources targeted to reinvent or preserve a sense of self (LaFave et al., 2021). This becomes significant in that the world today is powered by technological advancement and innovative ideas. Employing technological innovations will ensure available comprehensive data, artificial intelligence to improve healthy life expectancy and meet the demands of an ageing population. This will benefit healthy ageing and longevity by enabling people to live healthier, more fulfilling lives at all ages. For example, technological innovations have been deployed to keep people physically active, enable independent living, ensure paid careers programme availability, early detection of diseases and management of disease conditions, maintenance of social connections by reducing social isolation and continued engagement in the workforce, to name a few (Nolte, 2018). During the COVID-19 pandemic, technological innovations were adopted to trace people's contacts with disease carriers, log their location, provide health information, and keep track of vaccination records and infection histories.

Therefore, it has become essential that Nigerians can deploy technological innovation in their social service sector to erode the existing threat in caregiving and improve healthy living for older adults. Evidently, innovative interventions can be adopted to accomplish healthy ageing by further developing proficiency, expanding efficiency, and optimising patient outcomes (Pal et al., 2021). For instance, there is an increasing concentration on innovative health technology such as computerised heart monitor machines, remote wheelchairs, hip protectors, and many more. Other interventions include a community-centred paid careers programme, mainstreaming ageing management into the educational curriculum, utilisation of social workers, and use of religion and social media to develop an interactive platform (adopting online interviews and videos) that offers opportunities to find, share, and provide the knowledge needed on healthy ageing. More so, access to internet services has been increased by the use of mobile devices. For example, cell phone applications can offer types of assistance like heart and internal health level screens and electrocardiograms, among others (Ene & Ajibo, 2023). Cell phones can be used to make mindfulness and updates through the Short Message Service (SMS) Administration, YouTube, Instagram, Google, Twitter, Facebook, and WhatsApp (Nolte, 2018). Others are web-internet services that offer internet-based pharmacopoeia assistance, data to comprehend and oversee infection conditions, and different conventional options in contrast to exorbitant medications. These services eventually improve healthy living, which is the space this chapter desires to fill.

In this chapter, we endeavoured to investigate worries about reimagining healthy ageing through the lens of flagship campaigns. This is of the essence because contemporary society is characterised by various global crises such as climate change, extreme industrialisation, infectious diseases, and cases of insecurity and war. Specifically, innovative interventions on reimagining healthy ageing become realistic through the flagship campaigns on adopting an age-friendly environment, strength-based approach, delivering person-centred integrated care, long−/short-term care, adopting religion, and ageing policies. While Shipalana (2020) suggested the diffusion of innovation initiatives in the public health sector for the enhancement of healthcare services, Pal et al. (2021) expressed that innovative interventions in medical care can drive monitoring development by further developing proficiency, expanding efficiency, and upgrading patient results. More so, it will address shortages in older adults' medical service cost, security, and quality, while offering better and improved approaches to deal with finding, treatment, and taking care of oneself during health crisis diagnosis (Nolte, 2018). Further, ageing innovation can be directed by a framework designated at accomplishing healthy living through the coordinated effort of social work experts and all partners in the wide world mission to battle ageism.

Indeed, numerous studies abound that have discussed innovation in health service delivery, particularly in sub-Saharan Africa (Ene & Ajibo, 2023; Nolte, 2018; Pal et al., 2021; Shipalana, 2020). Of all these studies, one issue that became significant in this chapter was incorporating innovative solutions tailored to the Nigerian context that can help improve healthy living for older adults. To fill this gap in the literature, this chapter becomes vital as it contributes to the scarce but vital literature on ageing innovations, advocates for sustainable ageing, and ensures the inclusion of social workers for the future of healthy ageing amidst threats. It is against this background that this chapter poses the following research questions: (1) what are the existing trends and threats in healthy ageing, (2) what is the role of innovation in promoting healthy ageing, and (3) what are the innovative interventions that can help improve the lives of older adults in Nigeria.

This chapter comprises seven sections. First is an introductory section that provides a background of the subject matter. The second section demonstrates a theoretical framework that advocates for sustainable ageing through innovation. Following the theoretical framework is the third section that dwells on the methodology. This section provides a basis for the methods of data collection and analyses. In the fourth section, we displayed our findings first, with the summary of the socio-demographic characteristics of the participants represented in Table 5.1, and the existing trends and threats in healthy ageing. More so, issues including the role of innovation in promoting healthy ageing and innovative interventions to improve the lives of older adults were presented in this fourth section. Discussion on how these findings influence healthy ageing appeared in the fifth section. The limitations and policy implications of the chapter can be seen in section six, with concluding remarks presented in section seven.

Table 5.1 Summary of the socio-demographic characteristics of the participants of the study

Respondent	Gender	Age	Level of education	Last occupation
Older adult 1	Male	76	Secondary school completed	Civil servant
Older adult 2	Female	79	Secondary school completed	Civil servant
Older adult 3	Male	81	Primary school completed	Businessman
Older adult 4	Male	78	Primary school not completed	Artisan
Older adult 5	Female	80	Secondary school not completed	Businesswoman
Older adult 6	Male	76	Higher institution completed	Civil servant
Older adult 7	Female	75	Primary school completed	Trader
Older adult 8	Female	77	Higher institution completed	Civil servant
Older adult 9	Male	83	Primary school not completed	Businessman
Older adult 10	Female	82	Secondary school completed	Civil servant
Older adult 11	Male	74	Primary school not completed	Businessman
Older adult 12	Female	84	Secondary school not completed	Businesswoman

5.2 Theoretical Framework

Regarding a theoretical framework for this study, we adopted the diffusion of innovation theory propounded by Rogers, E. M in 1962. This theory has been utilised in the Child Survival Sustainability Assessment (CSSA) to examine the implementation of health programmes (Fox et al., 2014). The tenant of this theory is that it seeks to make sense of how, why and at what rate flagship campaigns and healthcare inventive technology spread; with the outcome that individuals as a feature of the social framework embrace groundbreaking thoughts and innovation for healthy ageing. The objective of the adoption of this theory is that older adults should see the thought, conduct or procedure as innovative for dispersion to be conceivable (Mohammed et al., 2018).

A reception of innovation does not occur at the same time; however, there is a steady interaction. For instance, older adults may experience difficulties in adopting ageing innovations owing to threats, including the attitude of the older adult, financial constraints, and cultural health beliefs. Against these backdrops, we recommend intercessions through which healthy ageing innovation can diffuse and be utilised to achieve sustainable ageing. They include the establishment of a coordinating (formal) caregiving agency, older adults' interactive platforms, advocating for a community-based care system, providing an age-friendly environment, and long-/short-term nursing homes. These interventions, with the involvement of social workers, will ensure sustainable ageing.

5.3 Methodology

5.3.1 Study Design

The qualitative approach was adopted for this study to systematically explain a phenomenon, situation, or population (Crossman, 2020). To guarantee an explicit description in the chapter, the authors also employed a phenomenological study design. This study design was able to describe in detail the existing trends and threats to healthy ageing. In furtherance, the researchers employed the study design to describe in detail the role of innovation in promoting healthy ageing and innovative interventions that can help improve the lives of older adults from their perspectives in Nigeria.

5.3.2 Study Participants and Sampling Procedure

Data were collected from twelve (12) older adults, comprising six males and six females. The justification is that these participants served as key informants and people who were able to share their experiences. These participants were selected from three health facilities in Nsukka, Enugu State. Two males and females aged 74–88 years were selected from each health facility for gender balancing. The justification for selecting the age range was that most health outcomes associated with ageing often manifest with an increase in age (Mcgregor et al., 2018). Again, these participants have witnessed the situation and are willing to share their experiences in relation to the future of healthy ageing amidst threats. Among the various sampling procedures, availability sampling was deployed for selecting the study participants. The researchers adopted this sampling procedure because a unique target population was needed for the study. More so, the availability sampling procedure was employed to ensure that participants who were available and willing to participate in the study were recruited based on convenience.

5.3.3 Study Area

Our study participants were drawn from three health facilities in Nsukka, Enugu State. The justification is associated with the fact that as people age, they may become more susceptible to health challenges and may have an increased demand for healthcare utilisation (Mcgregor et al., 2018). Nsukka Local Government Area (LGA) was used for this study because it is a semi-urban area made up of 17 rural communities with a major urban area, which is Nsukka town (Ugwuishiwu et al., 2016). The choice for selecting the study area could be attributed to the fact that most rural indigenes migrate to the town for healthcare services. There are ten major health facilities in the study area (Uzochukwu et al., 2014). The health facilities in the study locality function at the primary, secondary, and tertiary levels and are unevenly distributed politically (Ndibuagu et al., 2015). The researchers purposively selected one government-owned health facility from each of the three levels of health institutions in the locality. The reason is that the government-owned health facility service charge is subsidised. Their names are withheld for confidentiality.

5.3.4 Data Collection and Analyses

The instrument for data collection from the participants was a structured, in-depth interview guide. The rationale for the instrument was to enable the researchers to elicit answers from the respondents from a pre-designed structured research question. The data collection period lasted for two weeks, from 15 to 28 January 2024. We selected two research assistants from undergraduate students of the Department of Social Work, in the University of Nigeria, Nsukka. One of the research assistants served as the note-taker while the other monitored the recording device. The researchers served as the interviewer and timekeeper during the interview. The interview sessions lasted between 40 and 60 minutes to circumvent burnout and fatigue associated with longer durations.

The data analysis technique began with note-taking and care audio-recording of all the interviews. Data were manually analysed after transcribing the interviews in English. Although the interviews were conducted using the local language, there was no need for an interpreter as the researcher was familiar with the language. Data immersion commenced by repeatedly hearing the audio and reading the transcribed discussion and field notes for familiarisation. The data analysis process followed the qualitative procedure of data reduction, data display and conclusion (Neubauer et al., 2019). We compared the contents of the transcript with the field notes and recorded information to ensure coherence. An inductive coding approach was utilised to provide meaning to the coded qualitative data. Codes with similar characteristics were grouped thematically. Thematic analysis was employed to categorise the data into themes for easy comprehension (Creswell & Creswell, 2018). To add more rigour to our data analysis, the transcripts generated were read for content validity by two academic peers who were not part of the research for further examination. Their insights contributed to the final checks on the analysis. These exercises are in line with Crossman (2020) overview of the qualitative research method.

5.3.5 Ethics Approval and Consent to Participate

Ethical approval for the study was obtained from the institutional review board of the Strategic Contacts Ethics Publications (STRACEP) of the University of Nigeria, Nsukka campus, Enugu State. All methods of data collected were carried out by relevant institutional guidelines and regulations. The need for written informed consent was waived by the institutional review board of the Strategic Contacts Ethics Publications (STRACEP) of the University of Nigeria, Nsukka campus, Enugu State. The justification for the waived informed consent was that it was deemed unnecessary as the older adults volunteered to participate in the study. The participants were informed of their freedom to withdraw at any time during the study. In all, they were assured of anonymity and confidentiality (Carey, 2017).

5.4 Findings

The findings are presented in themes and sub-themes. First, the researchers started by presenting the socio-demographic features of the study participants.

5.4.1 Socio-demographic Characteristics of Respondents

5.4.2 Existing Trends and Threats in Healthy Ageing

In this section, the participants narrated existing trends and threats to healthy ageing. Concerning ageing trends, they explained that caring for older adults has been an enduring social norm. It is considered to be an obligation of grown offspring and spouses with some assistance from the extended family networks. Hence, offspring or spouse who abandons their older adults is reproached by society and viewed as savage. The participants explained that care for parents in old age is a reciprocal obligation that compensates old parents for caring for their children. It is seen as a mark of respect and ensures abundant blessings for the offspring and family members. The participants further narrated that the traditional society is governed on a gerontology premise. This demonstrates that they are the overseer of traditional values, and consequently, respect and care should be accorded to them. However, nearly all the participants agreed that this existing trend is gradually fading with possible threats.

Reported threats associated with care for older adults in healthy ageing include modernisation, economic situation, the attitude, and cultural health behaviour of older adults. Except for a few, most participants agreed that society has changed owing to the quest for (female) education, job opportunities and a family life system. For instance, a 74-year-old businessperson said, "*The contemporary society adopts the nuclear family system. Most family members are not easily eager to accommodate their older parents where they reside in the cities, neither are they willing to reside in the village with their older parents*".

Regarding the economic situation and healthy living for older adults, a participant lamented the high inflation level in the country. She was of the view that the economic condition of family caregivers raises above their financial capacity to provide adequate health needs of older adults. According to her, a neighbour once said to her, "*Why not consider the choice of utilizing non-institutional health facilities so that your children will not venture into debt in paying your medical bills*".

Yet another participant blamed the situation on supposed attitude of older adults which is usually not their fault. She explained that because ageing is often accompanied by various changes including memory loss (dementia), fatigue, and fragility among others, older adults experiencing these body changes may indirectly exhibit certain attitudinal changes which may be negative such as excessive demand or complaint. These attitudinal changes may often lead to loss of dignity, isolation, stereotyping and labelling of the older adult. In her words, she said, "*...there are times when I may request assistance. My daughter will often tell me that I am self-centered and demanding. I do not know how this occurs*". Yet another participant said, "*Today I am strong, but tomorrow I may be sick, then my daughter will say that I behave like a witch*".

In our study, a participant narrated the cultural health behaviour of older adults as ageing sets in. She stressed that older adults rarely visit health institutions for regular medical examinations. They allow for prolonged illness before healthcare visitation. According to her, "*We have the culture of allowing illness to get worse before we go for treatment. This is discouraging for persons at this stage in life*". A related response was narrated by another participant who reported on poor hygiene and unsafe medication prevalent among older adults. Hear her:

> Indeed, we fall short of basic social services in our country. For instance, water is scarce and so there is poor usage owing to supply. Hence, poor sanitation and hygiene become prevalent among older adults who may not have access to these essential needs **[Male/74 years/ Businessman]**.

5.4.3 Role of Innovation in Promoting Healthy Ageing

From the discussions, innovation advancement was ensnared as a significant worry in promoting healthy ageing. A considerable number of male participants felt that innovation would promote effective coordination of care assistance, particularly with activities of daily living. One of the men in the urban location had this to say:

> The world today is powered by innovation in technology. This can help improve care assistance especially when experiencing difficulty in mobility. Technical systems can be adapted to deliver services such as transportation facilities (Uber), home delivery services, and Meals on Wheels, among other services to provide help with everyday living **[Male/76 years/ Civil servant]**.

In the course of our interview, a male participant talked about innovation in the health sector, including internet services that offer online prescribed medication. The participant further explained that this service can provide data to comprehend and oversee sickness conditions and different options in contrast to expensive medications. He stressed the role of advancement in the health sector during the COVID-19 pandemic. Below are his exact words:

> The use of online services enabled me to cope with the COVID-19 pandemic. Essential information such as awareness of the existence and prevention of the diseases was communicated. This helped me to protect myself adequately against infection **[Male/81 years/Businessman]**.

The participants further narrated the importance of smartphone applications. While some explained that it can aid health services like heart and body temperature monitors, others stated that smartphone devices can be used to serve as reminders through short message services, WhatsApp, and Google applications. Yet, a male participant reported that it will improve adherence to safe hygiene practices, particularly in times of infectious diseases and climate change. Below are some illustrative quotes:

> You see, one can search online to obtain essential health knowledge required to manage health conditions. Oftentimes, when I may be unable to go for my routine health visit, I will use my phone to make calls to my physician **[Male/78 years/Artisan]**.
>
> This era calls for the adoption of innovation in healthy ageing. From our experience during the coronavirus pandemic, it has become important to adopt innovations like health monitor devices to monitor and regulate the body system **[Male/74 years/Businessman]**.
>
> From our experience during the coronavirus pandemic, it has become important to adopt innovative technology. A major one is the cell phones that serve numerous purposes like increasing health awareness, serving as reminders and improving knowledge on other health/environmental related issues **[Male/76 years/Civil servant]**.

5.4.4 Innovative Interventions to Improve the Lives of Older Adults

The participants mentioned various innovative interventions that can improve their lives. A significant point from the respondents unveils evidence of a formal coordinating agency with a clear budget line for the care of older adults. According to a participant, this agency should comprise professionals who specialise in the field of health management for older adults. They should be able to recommend trained staff who can provide paid care assistance to older adults. The quote below contains the exact view of the participant:

> There is a need for a formal caregiving agency that can recommend trained paid caregivers to older adults who have the need. The reason is that it is difficult to live alone, so one must have a companion. The employed caregiver can come and deliver services and maybe go at the close of work. At the end of the week/month, remunerations can be given to the employed staff **[Male/83 years/Businessman]**.

Few participants gave suggestions on the adoption of adult nursing homes. Though a female participant mentioned long-term nursing homes, most of the participants particularly the males were against this view. According to a male participant residing in the rural locality, he suggested that a place where older adults could stay temporarily for two to three hours and interact with other cohorts would be perfect. This could be a village square or a common centre where they can go periodically to meet one another. See his exact words below:

> Oftentimes we (the male folks) go to the bar where we can drink and discuss certain life issues. Again, (for those who wish) there is the central square (called 'Otobo' in the local dialect) which has a big Iroko tree that serves as a shade. This place is specifically for men who are aged and have participated in the village masquerade. We also go there and interact with one another **[Male/78 years/Artisan]**.

Religious solace was also mentioned by the participants. They explained how religious faith can serve as an intervention to ensure sustainable ageing. Narratives illustrate that older adults belong to various religious associations, including Order of Knights, Christian Men, and Women associations among other pious groups. These organisations periodically organise programmes on family life, healthy living and medical examination for awareness creation and early dictation of chronic illnesses. The quotes below show how religion can impact healthy ageing:

> I am 75 years now and I am really happy that I have lived a fulfilled life. Attending the Church service regularly is very important for me to feel good about myself. It also enables me to be able to face death whenever it comes **[Female/75 years/Trader]**.
>
> I am a member of St. Anthony in my church. Our members, on the second Sunday of every month pay a visit to all the association's older adults. They not only keep us company but they also give us money and foodstuff. I always look forward to this visit **[Female/80 years/Business woman]**.
>
> It is expected that every Christian woman should be a member of this association. Oftentimes, health programmes are organized for members. Also, this group collaborates with health professionals and organizes health examinations for members at a subsidized cost. More so, lessons are learned and experiences shared by the members so that the young ones can learn and take preventive measures **[Male/83 years/Businessman]**.

Furthermore, participants explained how a community-based care system and a community-centred paid career programme can serve as innovative interventions for sustainable ageing. Concerning community-based care systems, a participant was of the view that various age groups, including men, women, and youth, can periodically provide collective assistance to older adults. This, she said, has been practiced in the past, but it is no longer obtained recently. Regarding the community-centred paid careers programme, another female participant explained that formal caregiving programmes can be organised by women and youths in communities. They could establish a legal institution where older adults could apply for paid caregivers who have some degree of training and good conduct. These caregivers when employed, would be monitored periodically by the institution's supervisors.

5.5 Discussion

Regardless of the headway in science and innovation, the future of healthy ageing remains a threat. With a rising ageing populace in Nigeria (UNDESA, 2017, 2020) and with older adults' susceptibility to illness; the role of ageing innovation becomes paramount to achieving sustainable ageing. Given this fact, the UN decade of healthy ageing 2021–2030 entails keeping up with the useful capacity that ensures prosperity in older adults (WHO, 2017). In Nigeria, like other African countries, care for older adults has been a traditional norm (Ene et al., 2022b). In this study, however, it was found that this existing trend is gradually fading. This finding corroborates with the study by Ene et al. (2022a), which poses that filial care for older adults in Nigeria is threatened. This raises the future of healthy ageing amidst threats in Nigeria and beyond.

A novel finding in this book chapter is that possible threats in providing care for older adults were associated with modernisation, economic situation, and the attitude and cultural health behaviour of older adults. These worries influence the protection, welfare, and well-being of older adults in Nigeria. Subsequently, a pivotal move toward settling this issue is to highlight the worries that compromise care for older adults. Concerns about modernisation were anchored on the responsibility of the family in providing caregiving for older adults. While findings indicate that the high economic inflation in the country results to increasing obligations for family caregivers in providing healthy ageing for older adults; it was found that the attitude of older adults often leads to loss of dignity, isolation, stereotyping, and labelling. In furtherance, the cultural health behaviour of older adults considers delayed diseases before healthcare administration service commences. These threats to healthy ageing are compounded by poor available social services which often result in unfortunate cleanliness and hazardous drug rehearses in times of infectious diseases and climate change.

From this study, another novel finding is the role of innovations in promoting healthy ageing. This finding upholds the way that times are changing as is our current circumstance. This finding depended on their encounter during the worldwide coronavirus pandemic. Our data indicated that ageing innovation would promote effective coordination of care assistance, particularly with activities of daily living. This becomes essential in web-internet services, which provide data to comprehend and oversee illness conditions, provide online medical consultations, and different options in contrast to expensive medications. We see in this study that participants advocate for a mechanically creative environment, especially in the use of smartphone devices to serve as a reminder through short message services, WhatsApp and Google applications. Others include the utilisation of health monitors to examine health status. Advocating for the adoption of a technologically innovative environment will not only improve awareness and information on cleanliness and safe drug rehearses especially in times of infectious diseases, war, industrialisation, and climate change but will fill the gap in increasing health demands. In literature, the unprecedented contribution of innovation advancement in the health sector has been adulated by scholars including Pal et al. (2021) and Shipalana (2020). The reason according to the diffusion of innovation theory is that it will ensure how, why, and what rate innovative ideas spread. This will lead to people embracing these concepts for healthy ageing. This finding is an obvious sign that ageing innovation has become essential to tackle the future of healthy ageing amidst threats in Nigeria.

Notwithstanding the strong contextual emphasis on the institutionalisation of older adults in our society (Adisa, 2019), participants did not rule out the option of a coordinating agency with a clear budget line for the care of older adults. This agency, as was suggested, should comprise of experts who work in the field of health management for older adults or be able to recommend trained staff who can provide paid care assistance to older adults. An additional innovative intervention was a short-term residential care system option, which could serve as a meeting centre for older adults to interact with one another. More so, since most older adults rely on religious consolation, religious doctrine can serve as an innovative intervention to ensure sustainable ageing. This can be done through religious interactive programmes organised by members of these pious groups with a concentration on family healthy living and health awareness. Above all, a community-based care system and a community-centred paid career programme can serve as innovative interventions for sustainable ageing. This could serve as a legal institution where older adults could apply for paid caregivers who have some degree of training and good conduct. These innovative approaches are in line with the Nigerian context of healthy ageing.

It is vital to note that, in the soul of our research objective in qualitative research, we did not explore the perceptions of the study participants concerning government mediation in providing healthy ageing for older adults. However, we discovered that intervention from the Nigerian government was never mentioned by any of the participants. This indicates that there is a rising indifference towards the government's assistance since this has not been approaching. The Nigerian government can key into healthy ageing for older adults by mainstreaming the rights of older adults in the constitution and implementing health/social policies that cover their welfare. For instance, the National Health Insurance Scheme (NHIS) will grant free healthcare management services for all older Nigerians, and the implementation of the National Senior Citizen Centre Act (NSCCA) in all 36 states of the federation will safely guard their welfare. These policies have been suggested by Adebajo (2019) and Mbam et al. (2022).

In this chapter, a unique recommendation on the future of healthy ageing amidst threats is on social work professional involvement as an intervention measure for sustainable ageing. Observation of our data indicates that the participants require urgent assistance from learned professionals. It is evident that the social work profession promotes social change, cohesion, empowerment and liberation of susceptible groups; one of which is older adults. Unlike countries in the Global North, the profession of social work with older adults in Nigeria is very much in its early stage of development (Okoye et al., 2017). Since older adults comprise a positive power in every society, it is essential to incorporate a society where they reside in pride, receive respect, and have access to a dignified life. Hence, social work proficient contribution fills in as a mediation measure for sustainable ageing. One of the ways to guarantee sufficient survival technique is through the idea of 'self-improvement' development in old age. Through this idea, older adults can be urged to take on a 'strength-based approach' that demonstrates a conviction that they can adapt to the real factors and requests of life related with ageing process (Portraj, 2016). This should be possible through support of a difference in disposition that dodges correlation with different ages, demoralisation of negative explanations about self and usage of self-strength, the need to foster great relational abilities and all that can empower one to remain socially associated (Olason, 2012).

In the families, social workers work with older adults and their caregivers. They provide person-centred, integrated care to deal with possible health challenges that may compound problems in caregiving. The professionals adopt a multi-dimensional approach to evaluate the competencies of caregivers, their willingness to provide care, and their acceptability of older adults, particularly those who are distraught as a result of an unwelcome health diagnosis (Wolff et al., 2020). Social workers can diffuse the sense of crisis for caregivers by assisting in planning with other health professionals, rendering effective therapeutic services, and providing follow-up programmes. Although Nigerian society does not support institutionalised homes for older adults (Adisa, 2019), short-term care homes can utilise the services of social workers. They supervise services provided by various care agencies and can aid in the provision of health services. It is envisaged that care agencies' collaboration with social workers will serve as a platform for recommending competent careers and help them in providing appropriate health care management services for older adults.

Overall, it is not exaggerating to state that social workers'intervention in reimagining healthy ageing becomes realistic through the flagship campaigns on adopting an age-friendly environment. This entails a society free from ageing stereotyping. Ensuring an age-friendly environment entails mainstreaming health management of the aged into the educational curriculum and the use of various social media to develop an interactive platform that provides the knowledge needed for sustainable ageing. This knowledge will provide a positive perception of ageing, increase awareness of ageing innovations, and erode existing threats in the future of healthy ageing.

5.6 Limitations and Policy Implications

Employing a qualitative research method, the information gathered is used to describe the opinions of older adults who as key informants, undergo experiences in caregiving. A quantitative study may be used for a wider range of older adults conceivably as a feature of an assessment of the effect of innovative interventions being executed by stakeholders. This includes the advancement of pertinent inquiries or items that will be computer-analysed and statistically tested. Again, the translation of interview responses to the English language posed a challenge as some exact words may be omitted. This chapter failed to recognise the views of caregivers who assist older adults. Their views become essential to assess the level of awareness, utilisation, and types of technological innovation they adopt for older adults' healthcare management services. Also, notwithstanding that the study area concentrated on a particular locality, the information gathered therein remains valid.

Considering the threats associated with caregiving, older adults may be vulnerable in times of global crisis, including war, infectious diseases, and climate change. This allows for prolonged illnesses that may pose a danger to their healthy lives. For this reason, the Nigerian government, with the collaboration of social workers and different partners, should prioritise the safety of older adults in future interventions. Innovative intervention in this regard includes health and social policies that will ensure resilience against global crises. The aim of partners might be to roll out strategies that would cause older adults to have a solid sense of reassurance in their homes during emergencies.

Our framework only portrays a few innovative interventions and flagship campaigns for achieving sustainable ageing. These types mentioned are predominant in our society and describe a gradient of social statuses determined by traditional values. We were unable to make references to explicit models obtained in Western countries, yet future examination is urged to do this and to confirm their reasonableness in our conventional society.

5.7 Conclusion

Change is a common element of life that occurs with the right help and support services. Hence, promoting technology innovation support for older adults can contribute to healthy ageing if sensitively developed and applied.

This study produced several insights into the sample. First, concerns about possible threats to healthy ageing could jeopardise the protection, welfare, and well-being of older adults in Nigeria. It is then crucial to resolve these concerns that threaten care for older adults. This effort will ensure adequate care management and treatment to prevent the rapid spread of infectious diseases and ensure future healthy ageing for all older adults. Second, times are changing as is our current circumstance. There is a need for a high contribution of innovation and development particularly in the healthcare sector, that will promote healthy ageing amidst ageing threats in Nigeria. Promoting technological innovation will not only improve living conditions for older adults, especially in times of infectious diseases, war, industrialisation, and climate change but will also fill the gap in health demands. Third, despite our traditional norms, it has become essential to adopt the option of a coordinating agency with a clear budget line for the care of older adults. This can be done by good-spirited individuals, religious groups, and cooperate bodies. Such agencies can operate long–/short-term care homes and serve as legal institutions where paid formal caregivers can be recommended by professionals for older adults in need of their services.

Fourth, since most older adults experience fragility as they age, they are often economically vulnerable. Consequently, the Nigerian government must key into healthy ageing for older adults by mainstreaming the rights of older adults and implementing health/social policies that cover their welfare. These policies, when implemented, should be monitored for the effective welfare of all older adults in the country. Lastly, healthcare assistance could emanate from social workers' involvement as an intervention measure for healthy ageing. Their professional role in reimagining healthy ageing becomes realistic through the flagship campaigns on adopting an age-friendly environment, increasing awareness of ageing innovations through various interactive platforms, and eroding threats that will jeopardise the efficacy of sustainable ageing.

Review Questions

1. Discuss at least two factors that pose threats to healthy ageing?
2. List two innovative technology devices adopted in the healthcare sector.
3. How do you think these devices can create a technologically innovative environment for older adults?
4. Describe the concept of "coordinating agency for the care of older adults" and how it can influence healthy ageing.
5. What do you think the Nigerian government can do to ensure healthy ageing for its older adults?
6. Describe one measure social workers can adopt to ensure an adequate campaign on achieving sustainable ageing?

References

Adebajo, K. (2019, October 1). Older person's day: Eight months after the law's passage, Nigerian senior citizens are still out of sight. *Premium Times Newspaper*, p. 5. https://www.premiumtimesng.com/features-andinterviews/287659-older-persons-day-8-months-after-law-nigerias-senior-citizens

Adisa, O. (2019). Why are some older persons economically vulnerable and others not? The role of socio-demographic factors and economic resources in the Nigerian context. *Ageing International, 44*(2), 202–222. https://doi.org/10.1007/s12126-019-09348-8

Carey, M. (2017). *Qualitative research skills for social work (theory and practice)* (1st ed.). Routledge, Publishers, Taylor and Francis.

Creswell, J., & Creswell, J. (2018). *Research design: Qualitative, quantitative and mixed methods approach* (5th ed.). SAGE Publications.

Crossman, A. (2020). *An overview of qualitative research method*. https://www.thoughtsco.com/qualitative-research-methods-302655537

Ene, J., & Ajibo, H. (2023). Covid-19 recovery and growth: Promoting technology innovation in healthcare sector on hygiene and safe medication practices in low-resourced Nigerian societies. *Journal of Scientific African, 19*, e01542. https://doi.org/10.1016/j.sciaf.2023.e01542

Ene, J., & Nnama-Okechukwu, C. (2022). COVID-19 pandemic in Nigeria: Caregivers lived experiences in healthcare management of older adults. *Social Work in Health Care, 61*(5), 1–17. https://doi.org/10.1080/00981389.2022.2140743

Ene, J., Agwu, P., Ekoh, P., & Okoye, U. (2022a). Is filial care for older adults in Nigeria threatened? Examining concerns from adult offspring providing care. *Journal of Aging Studies, 63*, 1–7. https://doi.org/10.1016/j.jaging.2022.101078

Ene, J., Chukwu, N., & Ajibo, H. (2022b). Exploring care management for older adults with illnesses as family members' responsibility. *European Journal of Mental Health, 17*(3), 38–51. https://doi.org/10.5708/EJMH.17.2022.3.3

Faronbi, J., & Olagun, A. (2017). The influence of caregivers' burden on the quality of life of caregivers of older adults in Nigeria. *International Psychogeriatric Journal, 29*(7), 1085–1093. https://doi.org/10.1017/S1041610216002295

Fox, A., Gardner, G., & Osborne, S. (2014). A theoretical framework to support the research of health service innovation. *Australian Health Review, PubMed, 39*(1), 1–8. https://doi.org/10.1071/AH14031

LaFave, S. E., Szanton, S. L., & Gitlin, L. N. (2021). *Handbook on aging and the social sciences* (9th ed., pp. 337–354). https://doi.org/10.1016/B978-0-12-815970-5.00021-8. Chapter 21.

Mbam, K. C., Halvorsen, C. J., & Okoye, U. O. (2022). Aging in Nigeria: A growing population of older adults requires the implementation of national ageing policies. *The Gerontologist, 62*(9), 1243–1250. https://doi.org/10.1093/geront/gnac121

Mcgregor, J., Mercer, S. W., & Harris, F. M. (2018). Healthcare benefits of primary care social work for adults with complex health and social needs: A systematic review. *Health and Social Care in Community, 26*(1), 1–13. https://doi.org/10.1111/hsc.12337

Mohammed, S., Kang, B., & Conejar, R. (2018). A conceptual framework for innovative E-Healthcare system. *International Journal of Software Engineering and its Application, 12*(1), 47–56. https://doi.org/10.21742/ijseia.2018.12.1.04

Ndibuagu, E., Nwobi, E., Onok, C., & Arinze-Onyia, S. (2015). Knowledge, attitude and practices of Enugu State district health system by public primary health care workers. *International Research Journal of Medical Science, 3*(4), 1–10.

Neubauer, B. E., Witkop, C. T., & Varpo, L. (2019). How phenomenology can help us learn from the experience of others perspective. *Medical Education, 8*(2), 90–97. https://doi.org/10.1007/s40037-019-0509-2

Nolte, E. (2018). How do we ensure that innovation in health service delivery and organization is implemented, sustained and spread? In H. Kluge & J. Figueras (Eds.), *Health system for prosperity and solidarity*. WHO Regional Office for Europe UN City, Copenhagen Ø, Denmark, 2018 Marmorvej 51 DK-2100. http://www.euro.who.int/pubrecuest

Okoye, U. O., Ebimgbo, S., & Ene, J. (2017). Social work with older adults. In U. Okoye, N. Chukwu, & P. Agwu (Eds.), *Social work in Nigeria: Book of readings* (pp. 160–171). University of Nigeria Press.

Olason, K. (2012). *Social workers' idea on health promotion among older adults* (Master's thesis). St. Catherine's University, SOPHIA. https://sophia.stkate.edu/msw_papers/68

Pal, P., Sambhakar, S., Dave, V., Paliwal, S. K., Paliwal, S., Sharma, M., Kumar, A., & Dhama, N. (2021). A review of emerging smart technological innovations in the healthcare sector for increasing patient medication adherence. *Global Health Journal, 5*, 183–189. https://doi.org/10.1016/j.glohj.2021.11.006

Portraj, J. A. (2016). *Importance of medical social workers*. Retrieved from https://www.ajmc.com.julie.potyraj-2016/03

Shipalana, M. L. (2020). Diffusion of innovation initiative in the public health sector: Towards enhancement of healthcare services. *International Journal of Innovative Sciences and Research Technology, 5*(5), 1574–1581. https://www.ijisrt.com

Ugwuishiwu, B. O., Nwodo, J. C., & Echiegu, E. (2016). Municipal solid waste characterization in Nsukka urban in South-East Nigeria. *Special issue, Transylvanian Review, 24*(7), 808–815.

United Nations Department of Economics and Social Affairs (UNDESA). (2016). *Sustainable Development Goals (SDGs): 2030 Agenda*. https://www.un.org/development/desa/disabilities/envision2030-goals3.html

United Nations Department of Economics and Social Affairs (UNDESA). (2019). *World population prospects 2019*. https://population.un.org/wpp/

United Nations Department of Economics and Social Affairs (UNDESA). (2020). *World population ageing 2020 highlights*. https://www.un.org/development/desa/pd/sites/www.un.org.development.desa.pd/files/files/documents/2020/Sep/un_pop_2020_pf_ageing_10_key_messages.pdf

United Nations Department of Economics and Social Affairs, Population Division (UNDESA). (2017). *World Population projection to reach 9.8 billion in 2050 and 11.2 billion in 2100*. https://www.un.org/development/desa/en/news/population/world-population-prospects-2017.html

Uzochukwu, B. S. C., Onwujekwe, O. E., & Ezumah, N. (2014). The district health system in Enugu State, Nigeria: An analysis of policy development and implementation. *African Journal of Health Economics, 3*(2), 1–14. https://doi.org/10.35202/AJHE.2014.3203

Wolff, J. L., Freedman, V. A., Mulcahy, J. F., & Kasper, J. D. (2020). Family caregivers' experiences with health care workers in the care of older adults with activity limitations. *JAMA Network Open, 3*(1), e1919866. https://doi.org/10.1001/jamanetworkopen.2019.19866

World Health Organization. (2017). *World Health Report Executive Summary: Achieving health* for all. http://www.who.int/whr/1998/media.center/executive summary 6/en/

World Health Organization (2023). *Ageing*. WHO Regional Office for Africa. https://www.afro.who.int/health-topics/ageing

Chapter 6
Global Social Policy Reform of Healthy Ageing: A Comparison of China and India

Jamie P. Halsall, Liping Mei, James Stockton, Kalim Siddiqui, Chloe Holland, Michael Sarfo, and Michael Snowden

Acronyms and Abbreviations

COVID-19	Coronavirus disease 2019
GPS	Global social policy
OECD	Organisation for Economic Co-operation and Development
SDGs	Sustainable development goals
UN	United Nations
WHO	World Health Organization

J. P. Halsall (✉) · J. Stockton · M. Sarfo · M. Snowden
School of Human and Health Sciences, University of Huddersfield, Queensgate, Huddersfield, UK
e-mail: j.p.halsall@hud.ac.uk; James.Stockton@hud.ac.uk; Michael.Sarfo@hud.ac.uk; m.a.snowden@hud.ac.uk

L. Mei
Beijing Youth Politics College, Beijing, China
e-mail: meiliping@bjypc.edu.cn

K. Siddiqui
Huddersfield Business School, University of Huddersfield, Queensgate, Huddersfield, UK
e-mail: K.U.Siddiqui@hud.ac.uk

C. Holland
Kirklees College, Huddersfield, UK
e-mail: cholland@kirkleescollege.ac.uk

N. Asiamah et al. (eds.), *Sustainable Ageing*,
https://doi.org/10.1007/978-3-031-69475-2_6

6.1 Introduction

The demographic landscape of the world is rapidly evolving, with profound implications for social policy and economic development. According to the World Health Organization (WHO, 2022), the global population aged 60 years and over is projected to increase significantly in the coming decades, reaching 1.4 billion by 2030 and a staggering 2.1 billion by 2050. This demographic shift is driven by a combination of factors, including declining fertility rates and increased life expectancy, which are reshaping the age structure of societies worldwide (Partridge et al., 2018).

Traditionally, the phenomenon of population ageing has been associated with developed nations, where advances in healthcare and living standards have led to longer lifespans. However, this narrative is rapidly changing, with low- and middle-income countries now experiencing a rapid increase in their elderly populations. By 2050, it is estimated that two-thirds of the world's population aged 60 years and over will reside in these countries, highlighting the global nature of the ageing phenomenon (WHO, 2022).

While improvements in healthcare have undoubtedly contributed to the increased longevity of individuals worldwide, the ageing population also presents significant challenges that must be addressed. One of the most pressing issues is the economic burden associated with an ageing population, stemming from changes in the labour market and increased healthcare expenditure (International Monetary Fund, 2023). As the labour force ages and shrinks, there is growing concern about the sustainability of social welfare systems and the ability of economies to support an increasing number of retirees (Sciubba, 2020).

In response to these potential challenges, there is growing recognition of the need for innovative solutions to support ageing populations and ensure their well-being and economic participation (Lee & Mason, 2011; Lutz et al., 2008). Initiatives aimed at promoting entrepreneurship and innovation among older adults have gained traction as a means of addressing the unique needs and opportunities associated with an ageing society. By empowering older individuals to engage in entrepreneurial activities and fostering innovation in products and services targeted towards older consumers, societies can unlock the potential of their ageing populations and promote active and healthy ageing.

The intersection of global social policy (GSP) reform, ageing populations, entrepreneurship, and innovation is a rich and complex area of study that requires interdisciplinary approaches and collaboration across sectors. This desk-based study seeks to explore the evolving landscape of social policy reform in ageing societies, with a specific focus on initiatives that aim to initiate entrepreneurship and innovation among older individuals. Existing research and empirical evidence will be synthesised to provide insights into the opportunities and challenges of promoting entrepreneurship and innovation in the context of global ageing.

The significance of this chapter lies in its demonstration of how social policy debates shift within the context of ageing and the greater impact these have on the United Nations' SDGs—specifically, the Decade of Healthy Ageing campaign. To date, there has been little academic and policy discussion on the key relationships between healthy ageing and social enterprise. The most notable pieces of work in this area are by Law (2022), who examines the landscape of social enterprises in Hong Kong and their responsibilities in community social care for older citizens, and Henderson et al. (2020) in the United Kingdom, who explore social enterprise actions for the health and well-being of citizens aged over 50. This approach can also provide critical insights into how emergent and ongoing climate change issues are adversely affecting the ability to age in place, and the associated ramifications for the ageing population.

Hence, the aim of this chapter is to provide an up-to-date viewpoint of GSP reform on ageing within a healthy ageing innovation perspective. This chapter is divided into five parts. Part one of the chapter provides a discussion of the changing dynamics of GSP in the contemporary world. Here, there is a strong emphasis on how climate change has affected and altered the GSP context. The second part explores the academic debates on climate change and provides a justification for why this is a crucial consideration in an ageing society. Moving on from this, part three examines how climate change has had a real influence on driving GSP. Then, the authors discuss very briefly the methodological framework that was applied for this narrative literature review before Sect. 6.5 presents the two case study examples: China and India. In these sections, there is a strong emphasis on social policy frameworks that pertain to ageing within the context of innovative policy ideas in today's contemporary world. Finally, the chapter provides a summary of the key points made and suggests areas for future research.

6.2 Global Social Policy

Global Social Policy (GSP) challenges the notion that social welfare is solely tied to national power structures (Yeates, 2014). GSP sees that intergovernmental and transnational organisations are able to influence social policy on a national level while working to improve socioeconomic outcomes on a global level (Deacon, 2006). GSP thus embodies the global redistribution of social resources, global social regulation, and global social rights (Holden, 2018).

GSP differs from national welfare states. Holden (2018) suggests that GSP stems from the integration of post-WW2 institutions and the global economy. Globalisation has led to national governments needing to be more responsive to the interconnectedness of labour markets. There is a 'competition state' model of social policy in play on a national level, which sees national welfare policy aligning with the needs of a competitive economy rather than with the needs of the population; GSP, on the other hand, emphasises the needs for mechanisms of regulation and governance that operate on a global level (Holden, 2018).

The World Bank (2024) notes that the Coronavirus disease 2019 (COVID-19) pandemic led to invaluable lessons regarding the implementation of social protection. There is a need for countries to build strategic, universal social protections, which safeguard populations in terms of their health, education, and ability to cope with crises and develop resilience (World Bank, 2024). This links to sustainable development goal one, which aims to end poverty and implement nationally appropriate social protection measures (United Nations Development Programme, 2012). In 2016, the World Bank and the International Labour Organisation joined forces to create the Global Partnership for Universal Social Protection to Achieve the SDGS (USP2030, 2022). USP2030 is a global alliance that brings together social partners, governments, organisations, and civil society organisations with the aim of implementing nationally appropriate social protection measures for all (USP2030, 2022). The rationale behind USP is to reduce poverty, promote social inclusion, expand economic growth, and build political stability and peace (USP2030, 2022). Theoretically, this initiative may be the answer to solving the disparities in intentions between national-level social welfare and GSP.

USP2030 acknowledges that since the COVID-19 outbreak, there have been some beneficial social protection responses; however, this is simply not enough to decrease vulnerabilities that are faced by individuals worldwide (USP2030, 2022). Universal social protection is beneficial to the ageing population because there is emphasis placed on establishing social protection systems that are present through legislation throughout the life cycle (USP2030, 2022). USP2030 aims to guarantee access to healthcare and social assistance, as it is acknowledged that all people may need such support regardless of their background (USP2030, 2022). Likewise, USP2030 also intends to improve human productivity by enhancing productive assets and human capital (USP2030, 2022).

GSP is vital in global contemporary society. Put simply, people are living longer. There is a need for adaptations to be made at both national and global levels to meet the needs of the ageing population; this includes governments having an awareness of the physical, social, and environmental barriers faced by the ageing population (Buffel et al., 2018). The elderly face a multitude of pressures across the globe, including an increase in social inequalities, the implication of social expectations, and stigmas placed upon age (Walsh et al., 2021). Walsh et al. (2021) suggest that the way a nation prioritises and implements social policy for the elderly demographic says a lot about how much society prioritises and values age and ageing. Age-friendly policy adopts a design that identifies environmental barriers, physical needs, and solution-based approaches (Buffel et al., 2018). That said, there are global disparities in what countries are able to achieve in their responses to the needs of the ageing population.

To contextualise this, the World Bank supported the rollout of vaccinations and emergency assistance to 100 developing countries during the height of the COVID-19 pandemic (World Bank, n.d.). This suggests that while in theory, GSP would be beneficial, there is not always the practical means for all countries to utilise these strategies due to an underdeveloped public health infrastructure. Pham and Vo (2019) argue that the ageing population (those aged 65 and above) causes issues for both developed and developing countries, in terms of population increase and how this impacts health and social care policy. In developed, richer countries, these issues can be solved through policy implementation, whereas developing countries simply do not have the resources for a boom in population (Pham & Vo, 2019). That said, USP2030 acknowledges the differences in the resources of developing countries and aims to provide equitable access to all people to reduce global poverty (USP2030, 2022).

In order to meet these aims, there is a collaboration between myriad organisations; this includes the United Nations (UN) and the World Health Organization (WHO). The UN has an initiative called 'A Decade of Healthy Ageing', which is a global initiative that is aimed at combatting ageism, establishing age-friendly environments, and supporting long-term and integrated care (WHO, 2024).

Overall, there is currently a global push towards healthy ageing. GSP is prevalent with the implementation of initiatives through organisations such as the UN, and the WHO. The real question is the extent to which these initiatives are successful. A Decade of Healthy Ageing is continuing until 2030, as is the push for universal social protection. This means that it is difficult to measure the impact of these initiatives until that point. The SDGs also push towards favourable policy outcomes for the ageing population, especially in relation to poverty, equality, innovation, and health outcomes (UNDP, 2012). What does remain prevalent is the issue of globalisation and social welfare being designed to meet capitalist means (Holden, 2018). This begs the question, in a 'competition state', is there room to provide for the social injustices faced by the elderly and whose responsibility is it to meet their needs? How does this differ from country to country?

6.3 The Climate Change Agenda

Climate change has always been an important geopolitical issue; however, debates surrounding climate change are becoming increasingly prevalent within political discourse. Accompanying this discourse is the ever-expanding scope of sustainable practices, designed to address the rapid change in both environment and domestic demographics (Soergel et al., 2021). Across both the developed and developing world, environmental catastrophes are becoming increasingly common, with the resulting damages causing substantial economic and domestic impacts. These impacts often include the mass disruption of populations due to unsustainable living environments and the widespread destruction of homes and properties (Woodward, 2019). Despite humanity's apparent success in domesticating the natural world, the 'goldilocks effect' (i.e. not too hot and not too cold), or our need for the living environment to be balanced (Woodward, 2019) remains a chief limitation in our ability to successfully age in place. Worryingly, projections generated from historical data show that year-on-year increases in global temperatures and climate disruption are expected to continue, with developed countries expected to endure more social consequences relating to the disruption of goldilocks zones (Tschumi & Zscheischler, 2020).

In response to these issues, both local and global political agencies have ramped up climate change legislation and are actively working on the achievement of SDGs.

The most visible of these agencies is the UN, who hold an annual conference of the parties (COP) meeting wherein member states meet to discuss, debate, and agree upon common global targets. At the time of writing, the most recent COP conference was held in 2023, where 200 parties agreed to make efforts to cut greenhouse gas emissions by 43% by 2030 to limit global warming to a 1.5c increase (United Nations Climate Change Conference, , 2023). Whilst strict guidelines may be necessary to curtail climate change, such stringent guidelines require both short- and long-term commitments, as well as potentially radical changes to the way that countries utilise technological solutions, as without robust adaptations progress towards the 1.5c cap is likely to stall. To match the requirements, many strategies have been proposed, including reduction of greenhouse gas emissions, expansion of renewable energy technology, expansion of restrictive climate change policies, and improved utilisation of unavoidable pollutants (Omoregbe et al., 2020). Despite an exciting range of opportunities available, it seems that much of the current literature has focused on the reduction of post-combustion carbon emissions to the exclusion of other options (Omoregbe et al., 2020).

Whilst many countries are focusing on combating climate change via the capping of emissions and limiting global temperature increases, space has also been carved out for sustainable development and ageing. Developmental insights all suggest that ageing within certain developed countries is set to become a crisis as the aged population becomes increasingly dependent on a decreasing younger population. Despite advances, healthy ageing remains an often-overlooked area of development; however, increasing focus on the correlation between environmental catastrophes and population trends has forced healthy ageing into the sphere of discussion.

When considering climate change, development, and healthy ageing as connected issues, population displacement shows overlap across all three areas. Interestingly, population displacement can both negatively and positively affect both those displaced and those who reside in areas that the displaced move to. There is then an exciting and prescient opportunity to broaden and deepen our understanding of how climate change affects population development. This can cross multiple avenues, including natural and man-made environmental disasters, decreased habitability, desertification, and depletion of natural resources, as well as means and methods of safeguarding an ageing population in the face of these challenges. When considering the latter, there are many different pathways available; however, as the climate continues to deteriorate and the elderly population grows, preventative action may need to be rapidly taken whilst opportunities are available. Based on these opportunities and barriers, the remaining sections of this chapter explore several case studies from global locations in order to highlight important occurrences and pathways for development.

6.4 Methodology

The chapter applies a narrative literature review approach with two geographical case studies: China and India. The two countries have been chosen because the authors have conducted extensive social research in these countries (Halsall et al., 2023a, b, c; Cook et al., 2015; Cook & Halsall, 2012), and these countries also demonstrate the interlocking characteristics of ageing and novel social policy approaches when it comes to entrepreneurship, innovation, and sustainability. When undertaking the literature searches for peer-reviewed publications (i.e. books and journal articles), the authors used the following databases: Google Scholar, JSTOR, Scopus, and Summon. The content of the articles that have been found in this search forms the basis of this chapter.

6.5 Case Studies

6.5.1 China's Healthy Ageing Policy Reforms

China has undergone a rapid transition into a moderately aged society since the year 2000, escalating to a significantly aged society within just over two decades (Cook & Halsall, 2012). In recent years, China has progressively developed its own concepts and policies in response to population ageing, drawing from the ideas of active ageing, healthy ageing, and sustainable development proposed by international organisations such as the UN and the WHO, as well as the policy and practical experiences of developed countries. Combining these with China's national conditions and traditions, China has gradually established its own policy system for active responses to population ageing, making significant progress in various aspects such as improving the regulatory framework for ageing policies, constructing eldercare service systems, enhancing elderly health services, promoting elderly social participation, fostering an elderly friendly society, optimising the silver economy development environment, and effectively implementing prevention and treatment measures for the elderly during the COVID-19 pandemic.

China's current eldercare service system, referred to as community and home-based elderly care, is the result of extensive consultation of international experiences and adaptation to national eldercare customs. This system emphasises that the vast majority of elderly people will receive basic eldercare services at home or within their communities. Due to China's millennia-old tradition of family eldercare, rooted in Confucian values promoting 'filial piety', this cultural tradition continues to deeply influence the eldercare preferences and choices of elderly people and their families. The majority of elderly people prefer to age at home, with data indicating that currently, only about 1.4% of elderly people reside in various types of eldercare institutions out of a total elderly population of approximately 280 million (China News Service, 2023). However, due to significant societal changes in

China over the past 40 years, including urbanisation, the implementation of family planning policies, and changes in family structure, elderly people in China are increasingly unable to rely on family and children for eldercare. Therefore, since 2006, China has been exploring the community and home-based care model and continuously adjusting and improving its implementation. The latest iteration of this model clarifies the relationship among home-based, community-based, and institutional eldercare services with home-based care being the foundation, and where over 90% of elderly people are expected to reside in their own homes for eldercare (Du & Wu, 2023). Nevertheless, the model also emphasises the socialised provision of eldercare services, whereby even if the vast majority of elderly people reside at home, they do not rely solely on family members or self-care but instead have access to a range of eldercare services provided by various stakeholders including the government, society, and families (Ji, 2022).

In the implementation of this model, various regions have actively explored and innovated around key questions such as: who provides the services? what services are provided? and how to sustainably provide services? resulting in the development of diverse community-based home care service models. Some typical examples include Beijing's 'Elderly Care Stations' model and Shanghai's 'Embedded Elderly Care' model.

Beijing's Elderly Care Stations model considers these stations as the foundation of constructing a four-tier elderly care service system at the municipal, district, street (township), and community (village) levels. The layout of these stations follows the principle of a 15-minute service circle, with each station typically serving a population of 20,000. From 2016 to 2023, more than 1000 elderly care stations have been established in Beijing (People's Daily, 2022). The construction of these stations is supported by government incentives, including land, facilities, policies, and funding. Essentially, the government provides housing, facilities, and equipment without charge, and these are operated and managed by social organisations, mainly non-profit private entities. Social organisations simply need to provide services and cover daily operational expenses, with the government offering subsidies for their operation. Simultaneously, the government sets specific and clear requirements for the services provided by these organisations, defining six primary functions of elderly care stations: daytime care, emergency services, meal assistance, health guidance, cultural and recreational activities, and psychological support. These stations are mandated to undertake the task of basic elderly care, providing the six aforementioned services to the basic elderly care service recipients for whom the government assumes the responsibility. The primary recipients include three categories of individuals with Beijing household registration: urban and rural elderly in extreme poverty; disabled or cognitively impaired elderly in low-income families; and elderly individuals in special families with disabilities, cognitive impairments, and under family planning restrictions. Only after fulfilling these basic service requirements can the stations expand to offer market-oriented activities to general elderly people. In essence, the stations must accomplish the prescribed actions set by the government before engaging in optional actions.

According to the government's policy vision, as long as the stations provide satisfactory basic services to the designated recipients, they can sustain themselves. However, the reality is more complex, and the majority of elderly care stations do not survive beyond 3 years, with some even closing within 3 months. The main challenges stem from three factors: the limited market capabilities of the social organisations operating the stations due to their non-profit nature, the restrictive regulations and limitations imposed by the government on the services provided by the stations, and the public's and regulatory authorities' limited understanding of elderly care services and stations. Public perception often assumes that elderly care stations, being government-run facilities, should provide services to the public for free. Regulatory authorities similarly believe that since these stations are government-provided facilities, they must be strictly regulated and should not engage in market-oriented activities. These perceptions place the stations in a dilemma, facing challenges from both sides. In recent years, the government has adjusted its policies. In 2021, Beijing Municipality explicitly lifted excessive regulations on elderly care stations, freeing up more space for development and encouraging the market-oriented operations of these stations. However, the policy still requires the stations to fulfil basic duties, including providing services to the designated basic elderly care service recipients. In summary, despite the new policies lifting restrictions on market-oriented operations, the fundamental issue of social organisations operating the stations lacking market capabilities remains.

Shanghai's community-embedded eldercare service refers to the integration of functional facilities, adaptive services, and emotional support around the basic needs of elderly individuals, such as daily care, rehabilitation, and spiritual comfort, within the community. This model enables communities experiencing profound ageing to sustainably provide care, allowing elderly individuals to age in place within familiar environments, supported by familial companionship. Widely adopted by provinces and municipalities including Beijing, Chongqing, Zhejiang, Jiangsu, Anhui, Hebei, and Hubei, this model was further elucidated and explained in 2019 by Shanghai through policy documents detailing its connotations, service functions, facilities, institutions, and innovations.

Community-embedded eldercare primarily operates in central urban areas and urbanised regions of the municipality, with layouts organised at the street offices and township levels following the principle of 15-minute service circles. In each service circle, the model relies on one community elderly care complex and several neighbourhood service stations to form a two-tiered service supply, ensuring that elderly care facilities are accessible and services are available. Within the service circle, elderly individuals at home can receive services such as daily care, meal assistance, bathing assistance, cleaning assistance, medical assistance, urgent assistance, and mobility assistance. At neighbourhood service stations, basic life care and mutual-assistance elderly care services are available, while community elderly care complexes offer more professional, comprehensive elderly care services. The operational models of eldercare complexes and neighbourhood service stations are diverse, encompassing public-operated, and privately operated models, with a predominant emphasis on public–private partnerships (Song, 2020). Private entities involved in these partnerships include both non-profit organisations and enterprises.

The Community-Embedded Elderly Care model exhibits distinct characteristics and advantages, yet it also faces numerous difficulties and challenges. The primary challenges arise from the market operational capability, profitability, and inconsistent government policies towards the operators of elderly care. For instance, non-profit organisations providing elderly care services can get government subsidies, while enterprises are not eligible; this leads to reduced enthusiasm among enterprises to participate in eldercare or incentivising them to register as non-profit organisations, thereby exacerbating the dilemma of insufficient market capability for non-profit organisations.

In summary, in recent years, China has elevated the active response to population ageing to a national strategy, continuously adjusting the policies and practices of community and home-based elderly care, aiming to make it a distinctive model and experience of care for the elderly in China. Throughout this process, from the policy's top-level design to its implementation, the government has demonstrated characteristics of strong national capability, yielding noticeable effects and enhancing the public's sense of gain. However, it cannot be denied that the overall market capacity of eldercare remains relatively inadequate. Given that eldercare possesses characteristics of both public welfare and marketisation, and considering the inherent market limitations of non-profit organisations, the prevailing model of community and home-based care, primarily reliant on non-profit organisations, faces widespread challenges in achieving sustainable development. Based on the experiences of the United Kingdom and other developed countries, the social enterprise, combining features of both public and market elements, may serve as a model for Chinese elderly care service operators to learn effective market operations. In the future, China may need to enact additional policies to promote the development of social enterprises and encourage their entry into the eldercare service sector. This could potentially be one of the pathways towards the sustainable development of community and home-based eldercare.

6.5.2 India's Healthy Ageing Policy Reforms

India's social order is rapidly changing due to the process of urbanisation, migration, and increasing participation of women in the workforce. Large numbers of people are leaving villages and migrating to either big cities or abroad to Gulf countries to find employment. All these factors have promoted the disintegration of the joint family system and the development of nuclear families. A joint family system is an extended family arrangement prevalent in India, where several generations of relatives live together in the same house, such as grandparents, parents, uncles, and aunties. The breakdown of the joint family system means that elders are left alone to look after themselves (Malik et al., 2022).

India has become the largest populated country in the world with a population of 1.4 billion people in 2023, with nearly 10% of its population made up of elderly people or people aged 60 years and above (Sahoo et al., 2023). Ageing presents a major challenge in the coming decades, given the global demographic shift. Consequently, the overall costs of healthcare will rise and involve huge, distinct socio-economic challenges through changes in labour supply, medicines, medical personnel, and increased health and social welfare expenditure.

It appears that India's elderly population is more vulnerable due to several socio-economic challenges in their lives, such as low literacy, high unemployment and poverty, and low labour force participation. The rise in the proportion of the elderly population will also hamper economic growth due to the associated rise in life expectancy and prolonged post-retirement period, coupled with a decreasing saving capability in a developing economy like India (Malik et al., 2022).

It is estimated that India will most likely be the country with the world's largest elderly population by 2050 (Sahoo et al., 2023), and this would create many possible challenges in terms of policymaking, needs, and the delivery of healthcare services. Currently, the elderly population (aged 60 and above) equals 133 million people in India [Organisation for Economic Co-operation and Development (OECD), 2020]. According to WHO projections, India's elderly population will double and reach 20% of its total by 2050, reaching more than 200 million by 2040, then 301 million by 2050 (OECD, 2020).

Demographic changes are reflected by factors such as life expectancy, mortality, and fertility. In recent years, low fertility and low mortality have led to a sharp rise in the elderly population in India. However, a greater proportion of the ageing population will create significant challenges for economic outcomes. It will create huge implications for a country like India. As Malik et al. note "[the elderly population] challenges through healthcare, economic burden and social well-being" (Malik et al., 2022, p. 3).

More than 70% of India's population lives in rural areas, and about 60% of its workforce relies on the agriculture sector for their livelihoods (Sahoo et al., 2023). Therefore, it is crucial to discuss environmental and agrarian issues briefly. The ideas are discussed broadly between two opposite views: the neoclassical economists' belief in the magic of the market to achieve human welfare, in contrast with the Malthusian view that human population growth would move towards suicide through overbreeding. While the former recognises no natural limits to economic development, the latter is obsessed with such limits (Siddiqui, 2021). According to Siddiqui (2018), some environmentalists take a more perceptive understanding of human hopes and argue that the excessive use of the earth could lead to ecological degradation and could threaten the future of humankind. The environmentalists are in favour of the sustainable use of natural resources and claim that industrial society is presently taken over by industrial needs and has wholly succumbed to the pursuit of wealth. They claim that protecting the ecology would benefit peasants. The environmentalists consider that humans should have an active but not dominant relationship with nature. The critics of the neoclassical approach of 'market knows best' oppose the increasing onslaught of commercialism and industrialisation. Rather, they propose to slow down the rapid growth of industrialisation and urbanisation and recommend a policy shift towards increased reliance on nature and lands (Siddiqui, 2018).

One of the most significant dimensions of global demographic change is population ageing. Specific attention should be paid to the unemployed and those who suffer financial insecurity and poor health. Across India, there has been a recent decline in poverty, which is believed to be a by-product of the acceleration in economic growth. That said, chronic poverty and increasing inequality are still a huge problem in India. Systems of social protection are in place, which suggests a significant step towards sustainability (Siddiqui, 2021). However, this social protection offers inadequate cover for those who are accessing it; despite numerous policy and healthcare initiatives, there is simply not enough being offered to provide for elderly people. Nevertheless, this does not account for the recent labour law reform in India, which represents a significant move forward in the way of sustainability.

In India, the provision of healthcare has come from both public and private sources since 1991. Neoliberal reforms have since led to greater reliance on market forces, which have made it more difficult for the poor to access healthcare. With the demographic changes taking place, a vast rise in demands for healthcare and expenditure is being experienced by India. Despite government-implemented subsidies for low-income groups and health schemes, due to low income and poverty, there is a significant amount of the Indian population who are unable to access healthcare. The schemes that have been implemented are ineffective at best, with the poorest 20% of the population only receiving 10% of the allotted subsidised healthcare. In contrast, the richest 20% of the population received 33% (Sahoo et al., 2023). Social security is not a well-developed system in India, and there is no health programme specifically aimed at the ageing population. As an example of this, COVID-19 saw India with an inadequate medical supply and limited availability of generalised medical care. The pandemic also saw the elderly population experiencing huge medical and food insecurities during the March 2020 lockdown (Sahoo et al., 2023).

A vast proportion of elderly people, equating to approximately 90% of the population, are generally from the unorganised sector, and they normally continue to work until health issues compel them to stop (Sahoo et al., 2023). The high costs of medical treatment and non-availability of public health services result in the poor health of most of the elderly in India. Those who can afford to and have reasonable savings can accommodate private medical expenses, but those with low savings, especially those from nonformal sectors, face financial constraints that prevent elders from seeking medical care once they are no longer in jobs.

In short, India needs to address the changing demands facing the healthcare sector due to the rising ageing population and advancing demographic shift. To accommodate these changes, India must reform their healthcare system to include strong government intervention as national policies, setting targets towards universal access to critical care, including geriatric and palliative care. The government can strengthen the support for the elderly through various state and community initiatives. The government can expand social security spending and establish a uniform, basic old-age insurance system in rural and urban areas. The government can also expand education, skills, and training for elderly people and encourage positive perceptions of elderly workers both in their communities and with employers.

6.6 Conclusion and Recommendations

Though the issue of healthy ageing has drawn attention in recent years, it remains a significant worldwide problem. It is evident that social welfare and approaches to ageing are tied to national power structures (Yeates, 2014). China's approach to community and home-based elderly care takes a distinctive approach and in some ways, does enhance the elderly communities' autonomy and preferences for ageing. That said, on a practical level, the insufficient market capability means that this approach cannot adequately meet needs due to an overreliance on non-profit organisations. Likewise, India faces similar needs in that there has been a distinct failure to address population growth and demographic shifts. The rise in population sees an inevitable increase in both communicable and non-communicable diseases and related healthcare demands. This has critical implications for India's medical financing.

There is a call for a more generalised GSP, one that sets a framework that truly supports the needs of the ageing population. There are so many global disparities to contend with; however, if there is one thing that this chapter has explored it is that there has been an increase in—and will continue to be an increase in—the elderly population worldwide. There is a need for a universal plan that recognises the physical, environmental, and social needs of the ageing population without an overreliance on non-profits. The aforementioned evidence suggests that healthcare financing based on a progressive taxation system is beneficial for sustaining an effective large-scale solution (Sahoo et al., 2023). This proposition would be impactful and could adopt a design that identifies solution-based approaches. Based on the evidence presented in this chapter, healthcare financing based on progressive taxation seems the most reasonable way to achieve sustainable development Goal 1 and provide nationally appropriate social protection.

Review Questions

1. How can global social policy develop a mode of governance to regulate mechanisms that operate on a global level?
2. Explain how climate change can influence healthy ageing.
3. Can China's community and home-based elderly care models be translated to other countries and regions?
4. In the cases of China and India, how successful have the health schemes implemented been in mitigating the access gap between groups and communities?

Acknowledgements This publication has been produced with the financial support of the China Scholarship Council, which has provided research assistance to Liping Mei. The contents of this publication are the sole responsibility of the authors and in no way reflect the views of the funder, China Scholarship Council. Special thanks go to Safa Ali (University of Huddersfield) who helped to undertake the academic literature searches, blind peer reviewers for their constructive observations, and to our proofreader Dr Stefanie El Madawi.

References

Buffel, T., Handler, S., & Phillipson, C. (2018). In T. Buffel, S. Handler, & C. Phillipson (Eds.), *Age-friendly cities and communities: A global perspective* (1st ed.). Policy Press.

China News Services. (2023). *White paper on the development of China's home care industry: The development of home care industry needs to focus on fundamentals*. http://www.wrsa.net/content_42383184.htm

Cook, I. G., & Halsall, J. P. (2012). *Aging in comparative perspective: Processes and policies*. Springer.

Cook, I. G., Halsall, J. P., & Wankhade, P. (2015). *Sociability, social capital, and community development: An international health perspective*. Springer.

Deacon, B. (2006). Global social policy reform. In P. Utting (Ed.), *Reclaiming development agendas: Knowledge, power and international policy making* (pp. 144–175). Palgrave.

Du, P., & Wu, Y. (2023). The transformation path, driving mechanism, and future transition of China's elderly care service policy. *Zhongzhou Journal, 03*, 82–90.

Halsall, J. P., Mei, L., Siddiqui, K., Snowden, M., & Stockton, J. (2023a). Demographic changes and ageing in China and India: A public policy perspective. In N. Asiamah, H. T. A. Khan, E. R. Vieira, R. Lowry, M. J. Koohsari, E. Mogaji, H. K. Mensah, & P. V. Dintrans (Eds.), *Sustainable neighbourhoods for ageing in place: An interdisciplinary voice against global crises* (pp. 197–216). Springer.

Halsall, J. P., Cook, I., Siddiqui, K., Kayama, D., Snowden, M., Stockton, J., & Holland, C. (2023b). Global public policy shifts: Comparative thoughts on aging and social care. In I. Rajan (Ed.), *Handbook of aging, health, and public policy* (pp. 1–22). Springer.

Halsall, J. P., Siddiqui, K., Oberoi, R., Snowden, M., & Holland, C. (2023c). The pandemic's economic consequences: A developing country case study of India. *Asian Profile, 51*(3), 231–248.

Henderson, F., Steiner, A., Mazzei, M., & Docherty, C. (2020). Social enterprises' impact on older people's health and wellbeing: Exploring Scottish experiences. *Health Promotion International, 35*(5), 1074–1084.

Holden, C. (2018). Global social policy: An application of welfare state theory. *Journal of International and Comparative Social Policy, 34*(1), 40–57. https://doi.org/10.1080/21699763.2017.1413993

International Monetary Fund. (2023). Population aging is the top global demographic trend; the pandemic can teach us how to prepare for it. *Finance & Development*. https://www.imf.org/en/Publications/fandd/issues/Series/Analytical-Series/aging-is-the-real-population-bomb-bloom-zucker

Ji, J. Y. (2022). Effect of home-based elderly care services on the quality of life for the elderly and policy implications in China. *Population and Development, 28*(03), 90–98.

Law, V. T. S. (2022). Social enterprises in elderly care. In V. T. S. Law & B. Y. F. Fong (Eds.), *Ageing with dignity in Hong Kong and Asia: Holistic and humanistic care* (Vol. 16). Springer Nature. https://doi.org/10.1007/978-981-19-3061-4_25

Lee, R., & Mason, A. (2011). The price of maturity: Aging populations mean countries have to find new ways to support their elderly. *Finance & Development, 48*(2), 6–11.

Lutz, W., Sanderson, W., & Scherbov, S. (2008). The coming acceleration of global population ageing. *Nature, 451*(7179), 716–719. https://doi.org/10.1038/nature06516

Malik, M. A., Singh, S. P., & Pattanaik, F. (2022). Economics of healthy aging in India: A multidimensional perspective. *Journal of Labour Policy, 12*(4), 1–23.

OECD/WHO. (2020). Ageing. In *Health at a glance: Asia/Pacific 2020: Measuring progress towards universal health coverage*. OECD Publishing. https://doi.org/10.1787/1ad1c42a-en

Omoregbe, O., Mustapha, A. N., Steinberger-Wilckens, R., El-Kharouf, A., & Onyeaka, H. (2020). Carbon capture technologies for climate change mitigation: A bibliometric analysis of the scientific discourse during 1998-2018. *Energy Reports, 6*, 1200–1212. https://doi.org/10.1016/j.egyr.2020.05.003

Partridge, L., Deelen, J., & Slagboom, P. E. (2018). Facing up to the global challenges of ageing. *Nature, 561*, 45–56. https://doi.org/10.1038/s41586-018-0457-8

People's Daily. (2022). The elderly care station provides heart-warming services. *Renmin Ribao*. http://paper.people.com.cn/rmrb/html/2022-03/18/nw.D110000renmrb_20220318_1-19.htm

Pham, T. N., & Vo, D. H. (2019). Aging population and economic growth in developing countries: A quantile regression approach. *Emerging Markets Finance & Trade, 57*(1), 108–122. https://doi.org/10.1080/1540496x.2019.1698418

Sahoo, P., Rout, H., & Jakovljevic, M. (2023). Consequences of India's population ageing to its healthcare financing and provision. *Journal of Medical Economics, 26*(1), 308–315.

Sciubba, J. D. (2020). *Population aging as a global issue*. Oxford Research Encyclopedia of International Studies. https://doi.org/10.1093/acrefore/9780190846626.013.559

Siddiqui, K. (2018). The political economy of India's post-planning economic reform: A critical review. *World Review of Political Economy, 9*(2), 235–264.

Siddiqui, K. (2021, January–February). *Agriculture, sustainable development, and government policy in developing countries* (pp. 44–59). World Financial Review.

Soergel, B., Kriegler, E., Weindl, I., Rauner, S., Dirnaichner, A., Ruhe, C., Hofmann, M., Bauer, N., Bertram, C., Bodirsky, B. L., Leimbach, M., Leininger, J., Levesque, A., Luderer, G., Pehl, M., Wingens, C., Baumstark, L., Beier, F., Dietrich, J. P., et al. (2021). A sustainable development pathway for climate action within the UN 2030 Agenda. *Nature Climate Change, 11*(8), 656–664. https://doi.org/10.1038/s41558-021-01098-3

Song, X. Y. (2020). Current situation and suggestion of embedded pension development in Shanghai community. *Scientific Development, 142*(09), 107–113.

The World Bank. (2024). *The World Bank on social protection*. https://www.worldbank.org/en/topic/socialprotection/overview

The World Bank. (n.d.). *World Bank Group's operational response to COVID-19 (coronavirus)—Projects List*. https://www.worldbank.org/en/about/what-we-do/brief/world-bank-group-operational-response-covid-19-coronavirus-projects-list

Tschumi, E., & Zscheischler, J. (2020). Countrywide climate features during recorded climate-related disasters. *Climatic Change, 158*(3–4), 593–609. https://doi.org/10.1007/s10584-019-02556-w

United Nations Climate Change Conference. (2023). *COP 28: What was achieved and qhat happens next*. https://unfccc.int/cop28/5-key-takeaways#end-of-fossil-fuels

United Nations Development Programme. (2012). *The SDGs in action*. https://www.undp.org/sustainable-development-goals

USP2030. (2022). *USP2030*.

Walsh, K., Scharf, T., Van Regenmortel, S., & Wanka, A. (Eds.). (2021). *Social exclusion in later life* (Vol. 28). Springer International Publishing. https://doi.org/10.1007/978-3-030-51406-8

Woodward, A. (2019). Climate change: Disruption, risk and opportunity. *Global Transitions, 1*, 44–49. https://doi.org/10.1016/j.glt.2019.02.001

World Health Organization. (2022). *Ageing and health*. https://www.who.int/news-room/fact-sheets/detail/ageing-and-health

World Health Organization. (2024). *WHO's work on the UN decade of healthy ageing*. https://www.who.int/initiatives/decade-of-healthyageing#:~:text=The%20United%20Nations%20Decade%20of,communities%20in%20which%20they%20live

Yeates, N. (2014). The idea of global social policy. In N. Yeates (Ed.), *Understanding global social policy* (pp. 1–18). Policy Press.

Chapter 7
A Health Promotion Perspective on the "Decade of Healthy Ageing" Initiative

Nestor Asiamah, Amar Kanekar, Peter Hjorth, Kyriakos Kouveliotis, and Thomas Rieger

Acronyms and Abbreviations

AFCCs	Age-friendly cities and communities
ATA	Activity theory of ageing
CTA	Continuity theory of ageing
DTA	Disengagement theory of ageing
SST	Socioemotional selectivity theory
UN	United Nations
WHO	World Health Organization

N. Asiamah (✉)
School of Health and Social Care, Colchester, Essex, UK

International Public Health Management Programme, University of Europe for Applied Sciences, Iserlohn, Germany

Department of Health Management, Berlin School of Business and Innovation, Berlin, Germany

Department of Gerontology and Geriatrics, Africa Centre for Epidemiology, Accra North, Accra, Ghana
e-mail: n.asiamah@essex.ac.uk; nestor.asiamah@ue-germany.de

A. Kanekar
School of Counselling, Human Performance and Rehabilitation, University of Arkansas at Little Rock, Little Rock, AR, USA
e-mail: axkanekar@ualr.edu

P. Hjorth
Institute of Regional Health Research, University of Southern Denmark, Odense, Denmark

N. Asiamah et al. (eds.), *Sustainable Ageing*,
https://doi.org/10.1007/978-3-031-69475-2_7

7.1 Introduction

The Decade of Healthy Ageing 2021–2030 is an initiative championed by the United Nations (UN) through the World Health Organization (WHO) to support older people, their familial social networks and neighbourhoods (Keating, 2022). It is a timely response to population ageing, which is expected to more than double the population of older adults by 2050 (Chang et al., 2019; Muszyńska & Rau, 2012). The rapidly increasing size of older adult populations around the world requires concerted efforts to support older adults in maintaining quality of life as well as autonomy, and the foregoing campaign is a strategic pathway along which these efforts are made. The burden of disease and its associated healthcare expenditure increase with population ageing (Chang et al., 2019), but the Decade of Healthy Ageing initiative is a framework of action plans with which the onset and progression of chronic conditions (e.g. diabetes, hypertension and dementia) requiring hospitalisation or healthcare can be delayed.

By aiming to support older adults, their families and the communities where they live, the Decade of Healthy Ageing campaign provides a basis for rolling out a salutogenic health promotion model that prioritises disease prevention over the life course in all segments of the population. This argument is based on the idea that life course approaches to preserving population health usually target the general population or communities (Baird et al., 2017; Kuruvilla et al., 2018). Unlike campaigns focused on older adults who may already be living with chronic conditions and disability, this life course approach can enable individuals to maintain prophylactic behaviours (e.g. preventive healthcare utilisation, physical activity and healthy diet) over the life course, thereby enhancing healthy life expectancy. A life course approach allows everyone to maintain health and eases the disease burden of every community.

Healthy ageing is about the maintenance of health in the general population over the life course (Menassa et al., 2023; Peel et al., 2004); hence, the Decade of Healthy Ageing campaign should ideally sustain health in the general population. We reason that action plans of the Decade of Healthy Ageing initiative can be utilised to realise healthy ageing through the foregoing health promotion approach. Yet, no study or scholarly work has provided a health promotion approach to the implementation of the Decade of Healthy Ageing campaign. This shortcoming is a major literature gap because the initiative's focus on older adults alone undermines most of the population.

K. Kouveliotis
Office of the Provost and Chief Academic Officer, Berlin School of Business and Innovation, Berlin, Germany
e-mail: kyriakos.kouveliotis@berlinsbi.com

T. Rieger
Faculty of Business, University of Europe for Applied Sciences, Iserlohn, Germany
e-mail: thomas.rieger@ue-germany.com

This chapter, therefore, aims to propose a health promotion approach to implementing the Decade of Healthy Ageing initiative. Our proposed framework is unique for attempting to provide insights into how to achieve healthy longevity for everyone, being operational through the Decade of Healthy Ageing campaign, and enabling individuals to maintain three behaviours (i.e. adaptive behaviour, functional ability and autonomy), which we subsequently refer to as pro-ageing behaviours (i.e. behaviours that protect or support health). The specific objectives are to (1) formulate a theoretical framework on which our proposed approach is based and (2) map the core action plans of the Decade of Healthy Ageing onto health promotion activities across a continuum of societal groups.

This chapter comprises eight sections. The first section sets the background and aim of the chapter, and the second section summarises the key attributes of the Decade of Healthy Ageing. A theoretical framework that validates our health promotion approach and sets the foundation for mapping the core action plans is propounded in the third section. In the fourth section, a life course approach to health promotion is discussed. The action plans are then mapped onto our proposed health promotion activities in the fifth section. Implications of our framework for healthy ageing are delineated in the sixth section, whereas limitations and future research directions are identified in the seventh section. Concluding remarks are presented in the eighth section.

7.2 Overview of the Decade of Healthy Ageing

The Decade of Healthy Ageing 2016–2020 initiative replaced WHO's active ageing programme and was renewed into the Decade of Healthy Ageing 2021–2030 in a bid to realise some healthy ageing targets by 2030 (Keating, 2022; Rudnicka et al., 2020). These targets are tied to four action plans, which are to (1) alter the way people think, feel and act towards older adults and ageing, (2) enable older adults to maintain abilities (e.g. functional ability) as they age, (3) support older adults to maintain access to quality person-centred, integrated and primary care and (4) provide access to long-term care for older adults (Keating, 2022). These four action plans are the core of ten priorities.

A priority related to the first action plan is to undertake a global campaign to combat ageism (Keating, 2022), ensuring that society thinks and acts positively towards older adults. Another priority is to enhance the global network of Age-Friendly Communities and Cities (AFCCs), which is in harmony with the plan to support older adults in maintaining their abilities. The global network of AFCCs was launched in 2010 and now includes more than 1000 communities and cities (Rudnicka et al., 2020), and stakeholders aim to enlarge this network in a bid to transform as many neighbourhoods as possible into age-friendly places. Related to the fourth action plan is fostering human resources necessary for integrated care, which focuses on coordinated forms of health and social care delivery across relevant stakeholders (Hughes et al., 2020). The four action plans serve as a lens for understanding key attributes of our health promotion approach.

Driving the Decade of Healthy Ageing agenda is stakeholders' interest in improving the "abilities" by which people maintain health in the ageing process (Keating, 2022). Such abilities are implicit in functional ability that individuals need to remain engaged with life through participation in social, economic and physical activities in their communities. Examples of these activities are social participation, physical activity and participation in the labour market. The literature suggests that people are supported to maintain these abilities through health promotion (Asiamah et al., 2023a, b, c, d, e; Bauer et al., 2020; Menassa et al., 2023), which is the process of enabling individuals to have control over and improve their health (Green & Raeburn, 1988; Smith et al., 2006). In gerontology, health promotion interventions follow a "health promotion model of healthy ageing" (Menassa et al., 2023) intended to prevent disease and disability by encouraging prophylactic behaviours (i.e. physical activity, healthcare utilisation and healthy eating habits).

Our health promotion perspective on healthy ageing does not only draw on the "health promotion model of healthy ageing" but also applies elements of an integrative model formulated recently (Asiamah, 2023). Founded on the Decade of Healthy Ageing initiative, this model comprises thematic pathways to healthy ageing, including a "health promotion pathway" characterised by interdisciplinary efforts to prevent disease and disability across the lifespan. This integrative model is superior to the more expensive pathway aimed at supporting and caring for frail and morbid older adults. The superiority of this pathway has the following theoretical foundation.

7.3 Theoretical Framework

Our proposed health promotion approach to healthy ageing assumes that older adults can avoid disease and delay the ageing process by relishing the pro-ageing behaviours, especially functional ability, across the lifespan. Functional ability is the capacity to perform physical and social tasks (e.g. toileting, bathing and attending a meeting) independently (Asiamah et al., 2023a) and is necessary for a normal and enjoyable life. According to the Activity Theory of Ageing (ATA) developed by Robert James Havighurst, people without physical disabilities can maintain social and physical activities implicit in functional ability across the lifespan. This argument is supported by the Continuity Theory of Ageing (CTA) (Atchley, 1989) and empirical research (Sulander et al., 2012; Welstead et al., 2021).

Both the ATA and CTA posit that ageing people can maintain a lifelong trajectory of social and physical ability through conscious adaptation of previous experiences. Adaptation of previous experiences was referred to as "adaptive behaviour" (Asiamah et al., 2023b, c), which is about leveraging previous experiences, networks and resources to maintain functioning ability. For instance, an ageing person can utilise health information from previous social networks to overcome the barriers to lifelong physical activity participation.

The above argument of the ATA and CTA is, nevertheless, opposed by the Disengagement Theory of Ageing (DTA). The DTA argues that people lose functional ability and pro-health resources (e.g. social networks) as they age, which limits their autonomy in later life. Ageing people may become frail and lose the ability to draw on experiences and resources. Though the DTA and ATA are at odds with each other, both are valid in different contexts (Asiamah, 2017). The ATA is valid in a situation where people can maintain access to pro-health neighbourhood attributes (e.g. parks, sidewalks and services) and social networks, whereas DTA is valid in contexts where these resources and support for health are not available. Thus, people can maintain prophylactic behaviours that protect health over the life course if resourced and supported. Health promotion models of healthy ageing (Menassa et al., 2023) suggest that stakeholders can provide some of the needed resources and support through health promotion programmes. These models advocate sustained disease and disability prevention in ways that provide lifelong autonomy rather than pathways focused on treating diseases.

Autonomy is both a requirement and an outcome of functional ability. Independent participation in activities is a dignified way to enjoy life and maintain health. From this standpoint, autonomy is a requirement for healthy longevity and the maintenance of functional ability. Alternatively, people preserve autonomy when they maintain health through lifelong physical functioning. Suffice it to say that people are more likely to lose their autonomy if they become frail and unhealthy, possibly for failing to adapt previous experiences and resources to maintain health-seeking behaviours. Older adults in this situation would need assistance to visit places and perform activities of daily living such as toileting and bathing. Research suggests that older adults are unhappy about their dependence on others to perform daily activities (Cooper et al., 2011; Sofia Campos, 2018; Treas & Mazumdar, 2002), a feeling that can catalyse mental health declines and the ageing process. Thus, sustained autonomy is necessary for healthy longevity and optimal functional ability in later life.

The Socioemotional Selectivity Theory (SST) (Cleveland & Agbeke, 2019) implies that autonomy and functional ability can fall as the individual ages owing to age-related changes in life goals. As people age, their goals and interests may change, which would necessitate one's withdrawal from some social networks and activities. SST posits that people become selective of their daily activities (i.e. selectivity) in response to age-related changes in goals, interests and other personal circumstances. A person who used to participate in neighbourhood social activities may decide later in life to spend more time with grandchildren and other loved ones at home. Such an individual would be physically fit and healthy but may choose to withdraw from the wider society to care for grandchildren.

Selectivity is not necessarily a negative or harmful behaviour because new choices made by the individual can improve or maintain pro-ageing behaviours (Asiamah et al., 2023b). To illustrate, people may decide to avoid previously useful neighbourhood social networks that have become unsupportive or even harmful. This decision would require avoiding social and physical activities previously performed with such networks and focusing on proximal networks rich in trust and reciprocity. A withdrawal from unsupportive or harmful networks as well as activities linked to them is often necessary, given that the value of social networks changes with time (Kyeremeh & Schafer, 2024).

We argue that changes in life goals and decisions that support one's pro-ageing behaviours require health literacy rooted in "informed life experiences." We define "informed life experiences" as knowledge and skills obtained over the life course that enable the individual to identify health risks (including irrelevant social networks and activities) and make life changes to avoid these risks. These skills and knowledge are inherently part of the experiences adapted by the individual in the ageing process (Asiamah et al., 2023c). They come from multiple sources (e.g. health education, being in an affluent family and employment) experienced in life. A noteworthy source is health education or any process that improves people's health literacy over the life course. The literature recognises this source as a core salutogenic driver of health (Greenhalgh, 2015; Lindström & Eriksson, 2011).

The Theory of Salutogenesis is a positive paradigm of health credited to Aaron Antonovsky (Becker et al., 2010; Hewis, 2023). It argues in agreement with the ATA that people's view of themselves and life experiences shape their health. The model also recognises the use of collective and individual resources as a basis for avoiding disease. Collective resources include a workplace or national programme aimed at enabling people to maintain physical activity, whereas individual resources encompass income and physical abilities for performing pro-health activities. A specific example of a collective resource is the WHO's regional physical activity programme intended to enable individuals to maintain health (Okely et al., 2021). We argue that this and related collective resources must complement personal resources to encourage prophylactic behaviour towards healthy ageing. They are the foundation of "informed life experiences" with which ageing people can make good decisions to maintain pro-ageing behaviours. Informed life experiences partly come from health promotion programmes aimed at enhancing the health literacy of the population.

In summary, life experiences are a collective resource for healthy longevity, which is implicit in the ability to maintain pro-ageing behaviours across the lifespan. As the Theory of Salutogenesis suggests, these experiences should be "informed" or ideally enriched with health literacy and the ability to make good decisions to avoid disease across the lifespan. Without health literacy, people cannot make good decisions to maintain healthy adaptive behaviours and health. Our health promotion (salutogenic) approach advocates the empowerment of people to make good decisions about their health and maintain lifelong health-seeking behaviours. As the next section indicates, this approach is best implemented over the life course.

7.4 Life Course Approach to Health Promotion

Our health promotion perspective prioritises support for everyone to maintain health over the life course, which is consistent with the health promotion model of healthy ageing. It may involve specialised support for older adults in harmony with the

Decade of Healthy Ageing (Keating, 2022), but disease prevention in all segments of the population is at its core. A recent review (Asiamah, 2023) suggests that support is provided (1) through policy-oriented campaigns to encourage lifelong prophylactic behaviours, (2) an introduction of health promotion curricula at all educational levels, (3) research to test the effectiveness of longitudinal health promotion interventions and (4) the use of the mass media to improve awareness about health risks and healthy behaviours.

The infusion of health promotion in curricula at all educational levels is a powerful way to improve the health literacy of people earlier in their lives. Access to the media has improved dramatically in the past decade (Cho et al., 2024; Vinoi et al., 2024); hence, policy-driven campaigns facilitated with media to create awareness about health risks and the importance of health-seeking behaviours are relevant to our health promotion approach. One of the priorities of the Decade of Healthy Ageing is enhancing research evidence needed for action (Rudnicka et al., 2020), which endorses investment in research evaluating the long-term effect of population-based health promotion programmes, including those aimed at improving health literacy in the general population.

We argue, based on the ATA and CTA, that every segment of the population can maintain health across the lifespan. This viewpoint is supported by researchers (Asiamah et al., 2023b) who found in their review that both younger and older adults can maintain active transportation behaviour (a form of healthy behaviour) over the life course. Another review acknowledges the possibility of older adults maintaining physical functioning, especially in contexts where there are resources and support for social and physical activities (Herold et al., 2024). We reason that health promotion programmes that provide support for performing pro-health behaviours over the life course can maximise the ability of individuals in the general population to maintain health. The general population is part of a macro system of social, cultural and environmental attributes encapsulated in Fig. 7.1.

Our model (see Fig. 7.1) draws on the Ecological Systems Theory developed by Urie Bronfenbrenner (Asiamah et al., 2023b; Yang, 2021). The macro system of this model is analogous to the larger society characterised by a social, physical and cultural environment where people cohabit. The outer layer of our model (i.e. national and regional) includes governmental institutions, civil society and the policies influenced or developed by them. Depending on the geographical coverage of policies developed by these institutions, the influence of the macro layer can span countries and regions. Thus, this layer can operate at the national, regional or global level. The WHO with its Decade of Healthy Ageing initiative operates at this level in a global context and seizes the opportunity to influence smaller levels (i.e. Province and Community).

By the "Province and Community" layer, we suggest that public health interventions within communities and provinces are influenced by policies and guidelines developed at the macro level. To illustrate, healthcare within communities and provinces is based on national frameworks developed by the government (Hedayatipour et al., 2024; Palmers et al., 2024) or international standards from the International Standards Organisation (ISO). Similarly, physical activity promotion programmes

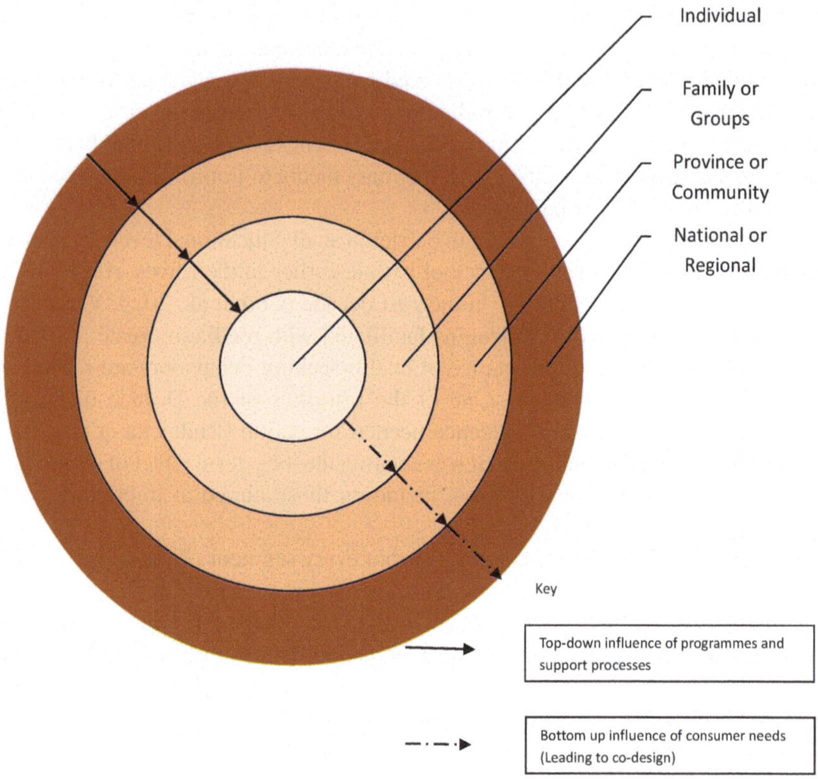

Fig. 7.1 Authors' conceptual framework of the potential influence of health promotion efforts on four societal layers

in a State of the United States are influenced by national frameworks or guidelines from the WHO (Thornton et al., 2016). These examples signify that the influence of national or international health policies trickles from the macro to the community or provincial environment where groups (e.g. families, churches and businesses) are expected to thrive.

Within the community or province are families and groups such as businesses. As demonstrated by the intersecting arrows pointing towards the centre of the model (see Fig. 7.1), practices at the "Province and Community" level are influenced by national or international policies and guidelines. Families and groups (e.g. exercise groups) function within this layer and may act in harmony with community, provincial and national culture. Reviews and adaptions of the Ecological Systems Theory (Asiamah et al., 2023b; Yang, 2021) suggest that whatever families and groups do in this sphere generally follows guidelines, policies and culture implicit in the macro system. Children often learn from their families and communities, which are subject to national norms. As such, whatever children do as they age can be determined by norms shared in the community and country. This view unfolds the significance of the smallest part of our framework (i.e. individual) where people make choices. The

Ecological Systems Theory recognises this layer as the smallest unit of society where the individual begins to learn and develop (Asiamah et al., 2023b; Yang, 2021).

The unbroken arrows in Fig. 7.1 illustrate the potential influence of national health promotion activities for healthy ageing. A national physical activity guideline, for example, can positively modify behaviours across all layers of society, but a similar guideline developed for a community is unlikely to influence the general population. A key attribute of a life course approach to healthy ageing is empowering everyone (not only older adults) to maintain pro-ageing behaviours, so guidelines and policies limited to communities are inferior to those having a top-down influence on the population. Yet, as evidenced in a study based on women (Evans et al., 2019), policies and guidelines ought to be developed based on "consumer needs" (i.e. the needs of individuals and groups) in the inner spheres of the model. This necessity is demonstrated with the broken arrows pointing towards the outer sphere (i.e. the bottom-up influence of needs).

Researchers (Maher et al., 2017; Slattery et al., 2020) agree that guidelines and policies are more effective when co-produced with the beneficiary population. Co-production means developing guidelines and policies with beneficiaries or those whose behaviours are being influenced (Maher et al., 2017). With this approach, guidelines and policies are more likely to meet the needs, expectations and diverse circumstances of the target population. If so, top-down health promotion activities should ultimately be based on a bottom-up influence of needs as mirrored in Fig. 7.1. The following section, nonetheless, focuses on how the top-down approach can be applied to the Decade of Healthy Ageing initiative and employed as a macro-level process towards healthy ageing.

7.5 Achieving Healthy Ageing Through the "Decade of Healthy Ageing"

To reiterate, the core action plans of the Decade of Healthy Ageing initiative are relevant to the realisation of healthy ageing, but these action plans would yield the best outcomes if rolled out to prevent disease and disability from a life course perspective. This reasoning is congruent with the import of the health promotion model of healthy ageing (Cardoso et al., 2022; Menassa et al., 2023), which emphasises a salutogenic approach to ageing. Stakeholders (e.g. governments) would maximise the economic worth of human capital and reduce the burden of disease if they enable ageing people to remain healthy and productive across the lifespan through the health promotion pathway. In this section, we draw on our theoretical framework to relate the four action plans (see Table 7.1) of the Decade of Healthy Ageing to some disease and disability prevention activities that stakeholders may employ. The activities are mapped onto our four societal layers through which stakeholders should influence the population with health promotion programmes (e.g. measures to create awareness, improve health literacy and encourage prophylactic behaviours) to engender healthy longevity.

Table 7.1 Authors' mapping of health-promoting activities onto action plans of the Decade of Healthy Ageing and the four societal layers

	Proposed health promotion activities within societal layers			
Action plan	National or regional	Provincial or community	Family or groups	Individual
Combating ageism	Adopting a policy to enforce zero-tolerance for ageism and abuse of older people. Rolling out national interventions to prevent social isolation, and mental health problems (e.g. depression and anxiety) resulting from ageism and abuse. National campaigns creating awareness[a] about the consequences of ageism must be rolled out.	Every community should have a surveillance system to detect and report ageism (including self-ageism[c]). The negative impact of ageism on social inclusion must be avoided. Communities must eschew violence and discrimination and foster social cohesion where altruistic behaviour is upheld as a norm.	Families and groups should protect their members from ageism and abuse. Families and groups must ensure that ageism does not discourage social engagement and negatively affect the mental health of their members.	The individual should: Be trained or supported to identify different forms of ageism. Be able to report ageist stereotypes experienced. Take steps in compliance with national campaigns to avoid ageism. Overcome self-ageism by seeking support.
Fostering the abilities of older people in the community	Adopting national policies enforcing investment in age-friendly ecosystems and interventions. Governments should create awareness of prophylactic behaviours through which diseases can be avoided. Adopting policies encouraging and supporting research on the effect of population-level health promotion interventions on healthy ageing	Every community or province ought to attain an "age-friendly neighbourhood status"[d]. Social and built environmental resources (e.g. social support and parks) should be developed to support prophylactic behaviours. Every community should be equipped to join the global network of AFCCs.	Families and groups should adopt healthy behaviours (e.g. regular physical activity, healthy diet and healthcare utilisation) as a norm. Families and groups should support members to perform healthy behaviours. Families and groups should enhance their cohesiveness.	Maintain physical activity and social engagement over the life course. Eat a healthy diet based on campaigns and research evidence. Utilise healthcare to detect or prevent diseases or disabilities. Make use of other neighbourhood resources (e.g. parks) in physical and social activities.

Delivering person-centred, integrated care in response to needs	A national integrated care system that prevents disease and disability should be established. Integrated and person-centred care can be used to educate people to maintain health-seeking behaviours. Adopting a policy supporting research on the feasibility of providing health education on person-centred care.	Every community must have enough facilities to provide person-centred and integrated services in response to current and evolving needs. Services within communities should educate residents to pursue health-seeking behaviours.	Families and groups should be equipped to support their older adults to access integrated care. Group and family members should be supported (e.g. financial support) to access person-centred care.	Regularly utilise person-centred care. Ask nagging questions about health and health-seeking behaviours in person-centred care. Live by professionals' prescriptions in person-centred care.
Provide access to long-term care for older adults in need of it	A policy-oriented long-term care system should be developed to meet the needs of older adults. The system should be implemented to prevent disease or limit the development of age-related diseases and disability	Every community must have enough facilities that provide curative and "preventive care"[b]. Preventive care should focus on encouraging regular physical activity and a healthy diet.	Families and groups should be equipped to support their older adults to access long-term care. Group and family members should be supported (e.g. financial support) to access long-term care.	Ask nagging questions about health and health-seeking behaviours in long-term care. Live by professionals' prescriptions (about diet and exercise) in long-term care.

Note: AFCCs—Age-Friendly Cities and Communities
[a]Awareness is created by teaching about ageism and the importance of prophylactic behaviour in schools across all levels of formal education
[b]Preventive care refers to utilising healthcare, not to treat diseases, but to avoid disease and disability
[c]self-ageism refers to negative attitudes and perceptions about one's ageing or old age
[d]Age-friendly neighbourhood status is the stage where a neighbourhood provides access to all psychosocial (e.g. trust and social support) and built environment (e.g. streets and parks) resources necessary for prophylactic behaviours

As our theoretical framework suggests, healthy ageing requires the maintenance of the pro-ageing behaviours, which are easy to perform in age-friendly environments where there is empowerment (e.g. through health promotion programmes) and resources necessary for participating in social, economic and physical activities. The effective use of resources and empowerment programmes in such contexts is, nevertheless, impossible without neighbourhood safety (Asiamah et al., 2023c; Wahl & Gerstorf, 2018). A deviant behaviour that threatens safety is ageism (Jacobson, 2006; Vale et al., 2020), which is why the first action plan of the Decade of Healthy Ageing aimed at discouraging ageism is important.

Ageism increases older adults' sense of unsafety and is a risk factor for mental health problems such as depression and anxiety (Jacobson, 2006; Vale et al., 2020). As such, older adults experiencing it may be more vulnerable to cognitive and neurodegenerative disorders. Our health promotion pathway, therefore, proposes national policies that prevent ageism as a macro-level (i.e. regional and national) effort that indirectly prevent disease and disability. The prevention of ageism through macro-level policies would foster communities where families and individuals can avoid ageism and its mental health risks. Table 7.1 shows specific steps for preventing ageism across the four societal layers. One of these steps is creating awareness about different types of ageism (e.g. self-ageism), how to identify them and how they affect health. Policy-driven national campaigns against ageism, education educational curricula through which ageism is taught as a health risk and the use of the mass media to create awareness about ageism can protect population health.

Many victims of ageism are unable to report their experiences to authorities, and the social welfare system poorly identifies and prosecutes culprits of ageist stereotypes (Chang et al., 2020; Phelan, 2008). This problem creates a need for communities and provinces to provide surveillance systems with which ageism can be detected and reported. Ageism is bred or facilitated by violence as well as social discrimination and segregation; hence, communities can avoid it by fostering social cohesion, peace and a shared identity. Yet, a shared identity and social cohesion require bonding within and between families and groups that provide a social system for battling ageism and abuse. Finally, individuals can report their experiences of ageism if their families and communities are cohesive and trustworthy.

Regarding the second action plan in Table 7.1, a macro-level strategy is to implement policies intended to improve the age-friendliness of communities since pro-ageing behaviours are best maintained in such places (Asiamah et al., 2023c, d; Wahl & Gerstorf, 2018). A community-level effort is to ensure that the national policy allows every community to attain a desired "age-friendly status," which we define as the stage where a neighbourhood sufficiently offers psychosocial conditions (e.g. safety and social cohesion) for maintaining pro-ageing behaviours. This status is the third stage of the neighbourhood development continuum (Asiamah et al., 2023e) and includes a community's recognition as a member of the global network of AFCCs. Families and groups are more likely to, as a norm, instil health-seeking behaviours into their members in such contexts, especially if awareness is created about the relevance of these behaviours to health. Individuals would achieve targets in physical activity, healthy diet and health over the life course if made aware of health risks and the importance of prophylactic behaviour through health promotion programmes.

The third and fourth action plans focus on the improvement of access to health and social care services. In the context of our health promotion pathway, the population must be equipped with health literacy in health and social care settings where professionals' prescriptions and recommendations are followed by patients. To enhance health literacy at the macro-level, stakeholders need to introduce policies for the regular provision of health promotion activities in primary, person-centred and long-term care. An example of such policies being enforced in many countries (e.g. the United States, Germany and Canada) is physical activity promotion in primary care (Thornton et al., 2016). Given that this policy can be effective at delaying age-related disabilities and declines in health (Lion et al., 2019; Thornton et al., 2016), all countries are encouraged to adopt and implement it. Similar policy-informed programmes promoting a healthy diet and prophylactic healthcare utilisation are also needed in every country. This effort would yield desired outcomes within communities, groups and individuals as reported in Table 7.1.

7.6 Implications for the "Decade of Healthy Ageing"

Our framework has implications for the implementation of the Decade of Healthy Ageing campaign, the first of which is a need to execute the campaign's action plans with a health promotion model. As our theoretical model (see Fig. 7.1) suggests, healthy ageing occurs as a lifelong process in which the pro-ageing behaviours are maintained. The ability of people to perform these behaviours throughout their lives depends on how well they avoid disability and disease. There is a consensus among researchers (Lindström & Eriksson, 2011; Menassa et al., 2023) that health promotion intended to improve health literacy and prophylactic behaviours lends significant support to this ability. As such, health promotion efforts intended to influence all segments of the population over the life course should take precedence over action plans aimed at supporting only older adults.

The support intended by stakeholders of the Decade of Healthy Ageing initiative is appreciably inclusive in the sense that it is targeted at not only older adults but also their families and communities (Keating, 2022). Action plans to provide this support offer an opportunity to positively influence all age groups over the life course with health promotion programmes. This influence takes the form of the adoption of prophylactic behaviours within communities by groups, families and individuals across the lifespan. As our framework demonstrates, this influence stems from a top-down flow of health information across four layers of society in policy-oriented health promotion. The trickling of health information across a continuum of societal layers is necessary since everyone goes through the ageing process and healthy children may become unnecessarily sick and frail later in life if not informed and supported to maintain health.

Our framework also upholds the importance of co-designing health promotion programmes and support processes with members of the population. Co-designed programmes are more effective than programmes not involving target beneficiaries (Maher et al., 2017), which demonstrates the significance of the bottom-up influence of consumer needs on the creation of support processes and health promotion programmes (see Fig. 7.1). Co-design of programmes and support processes should take cognisance of different needs within each segment of the population. Worth noting are differences in the needs of different age groups that must be understood and incorporated into the co-design process. For example, health promotion programmes that work for older adults may not work for children and young adults. What is unclear, nonetheless, is whether a health promotion approach targeted at the population is economically worthwhile.

Researchers agree that health promotion models intended to prevent disease and disability may be cost-intensive in the short term but are more economically rewarding in the long term than models focused on the treatment of diseases (Crealey et al., 2024; Wei et al., 2024). A systematic review (Duplaga et al., 2016) suggests that most of the evidence supporting this consensus comes from programmes tested on smaller samples and groups. Our framework proposes co-designed programmes targeted at the wider society, so their expenditure and outcomes may be different. We, therefore, call for future research investigating the economic worth and feasibility of macro-level health promotion models, given that the sustainability of investments in interventions is a priority of the Decade of Healthy Ageing initiative (Rudnicka et al., 2020). In any case, there should be no trade-off between healthy longevity and national wealth since health is priceless at any stage of life.

7.7 Limitations and Future Research

Our health promotion pathway encompasses many salutogenic efforts towards healthy longevity, but this chapter has not considered all these efforts. The recommendations in Table 7.1 are inexhaustive, and their significance and implementation would differ across contexts with different socio-economic statuses. Future research may, therefore, provide a more exhaustive framework and develop related models suited for different socio-economic profiles. This chapter does not provide a detailed analysis of different health-promoting activities by which the top-down influence across the four societal layers can be made. Our assumption that healthy longevity is implicit in the maintenance of pro-ageing behaviours may not apply to all populations and individuals. For example, people born with disabilities may not be able to exercise and maintain these behaviours as they age, which means they may live with disability and poor health even earlier in their lives. We call for future models and evidence addressing this and related nuances to build or improve upon our proposed health promotion approach to the implementation of the Decade of Healthy Ageing initiative.

7.8 Conclusion

The Decade of Healthy Ageing is a timely campaign aimed at fostering healthy ageing by supporting older adults, their families and the communities where they live. By seeking to support older adults and their families in their socio-environmental context, this initiative recognises the necessary roles of communities and families in the well-being of older adults. This recognition provides insight into the inclusive support needed by older adults to navigate challenges unique to late life. Yet, the campaign's support ought to be delivered over the life course through a salutogenic approach to healthy ageing. This approach supports everyone, emphasises disease and disability prevention and thrives on policy-driven health promotion. Through health promotion, individuals are informed to practice prophylactic behaviours over the life course, enabling them to delay age-related disability and health problems. It works best in situations where health promotion programmes informed by the needs of the population produce a top-down influence across four societal layers (i.e. national, community, family or groups and individuals). This influence is in the form of acquired healthy lifestyles. This chapter suggests that action plans for the Decade of Healthy Ageing campaign should be implemented through the foregoing salutogenic approach.

Review Questions

1. Why is the Decade of Healthy Ageing campaign a suitable framework for rolling out a salutogenic approach to healthy ageing?
2. Briefly explain the role of a top-down influence of health promotion programmes on four societal layers in healthy ageing efforts.
3. Why is a bottom-up influence of needs on health promotion programmes necessary, and how can this influence be realised?
4. Define "informed life experiences" and identify its primary source. How can health promotion shape individuals' "informed life experiences"?
5. Discuss some other ways in which the four action plans of the Decade of Healthy Ageing can be implemented with our proposed health promotion approach.

References

Asiamah, N. (2017). Social engagement and physical activity: Commentary on why the activity and disengagement theories of ageing may both be valid. *Cogent Medicine, 4*(1), 1289664. https://doi.org/10.1080/2331205x.2017.1289664

Asiamah, N. (2023). 'Sustainable ageing' in a world of crises. In N. Asiamah, H. T. A. Khan, P. Villalobos Dintrans, M. J. Koohsari, E. Mogaji, E. R. Vieira, R. Lowry, & H. K. Mensah (Eds.), *Sustainable neighbourhoods for ageing in place* (pp. 217–236). Springer Nature. https://doi.org/10.1007/978-3-031-41594-4_12

Asiamah, N., Agyemang, S. M., Vieira, E. R., Khan, H. T. A., & Gasana, J. (2023a). Sedentary behaviour among older adults residing in flat and hilly neighbourhoods and its association with frailty and chronic disease status. *BMC Public Health, 23*(1), 1–11. https://doi.org/10.1186/s12889-023-17029-0

Asiamah, N., Awuviry-Newton, K., Nesser, W., & Alvarez, E. N. (2023b). Carbon footprints of active and non-active transport modes: Hierarchy and intergenerational narrative analyses. *Sustainability (Switzerland), 15*(17), 1–16. https://doi.org/10.3390/su151712795

Asiamah, N., Bateman, A., Hjorth, P., Khan, H. T. A., & Danquah, E. (2023c). Socially active neighborhoods: Construct operationalization for aging in place, health promotion and psychometric testing. *Health Promotion International, 38*(1), 1–10.

Asiamah, N., Kanekar, A., Khan, H. T. A., & Dintrans, P. V. (2023d). Neighbourhood services and ageing in place: An extreme industrialisation perspective. In N. Asiamah, H. T. A. Khan, P. Villalobos Dintrans, M. J. Koohsari, E. Mogaji, E. R. Vieira, R. Lowry, & H. K. Mensah (Eds.), *Sustainable neighbourhoods for ageing in place* (pp. 91–110). Springer Nature. https://doi.org/10.1007/978-3-031-41594-4_6

Asiamah, N., Koohsari, M. J., & Lowry, R. (2023e). Ageing in place: The present and future social and health threats. In N. Asiamah, H. T. A. Khan, P. Villalobos Dintrans, M. J. Koohsari, E. Mogaji, E. R. Vieira, R. Lowry, & H. K. Mensah (Eds.), *Sustainable neighbourhoods for ageing in place* (pp. 15–35). Springer Nature. https://doi.org/10.1007/978-3-031-41594-4_2

Atchley, R. C. (1989). A continuity theory of normal aging. *Gerontologist, 29*(2), 183–190. https://doi.org/10.1093/geront/29.2.183

Baird, J., Jacob, C., Barker, M., Fall, C. H. D., Hanson, M., Harvey, N. C., Inskip, H. M., Kumaran, K., & Cooper, C. (2017). Developmental origins of health and disease: A lifecourse approach to the prevention of non-communicable diseases. *Healthcare (Switzerland), 5*(1). https://doi.org/10.3390/healthcare5010014

Bauer, G. F., Roy, M., Bakibinga, P., Contu, P., Downe, S., Eriksson, M., Espnes, G. A., Jensen, B. B., Juvinya Canal, D., Lindström, B., Mana, A., Mittelmark, M. B., Morgan, A. R., Pelikan, J. M., Saboga-Nunes, L., Sagy, S., Shorey, S., Vaandrager, L., & Vinje, H. F. (2020). Future directions for the concept of salutogenesis: A position article. *Health Promotion International, 35*(2), 187–195. https://doi.org/10.1093/HEAPRO/DAZ057

Becker, C. M., Glascoff, M. A., & Felts, W. M. (2010). Salutogenesis 30 years later: Where do we go from here? Origins of salutogenesis. *International Electronic Journal of Health Education, 13*, 25–32. http://files.eric.ed.gov/fulltext/EJ895721.pdf

Cardoso, R. B., Caldas, C. P., Brandão, M. A. G., de Souza, P. A., & Santana, R. F. (2022). Healthy aging promotion model referenced in Nola Pender's theory. *Revista Brasileira de Enfermagem, 75*(1), 1–9. https://doi.org/10.1590/0034-7167-2020-0373

Chang, A. Y., Skirbekk, V. F., Tyrovolas, S., Kassebaum, N. J., & Dieleman, J. L. (2019). Measuring population ageing: An analysis of the global burden of disease study 2017. *The Lancet Public Health, 4*(3), e159–e167. https://doi.org/10.1016/S2468-2667(19)30019-2

Chang, E. S., Kannoth, S., Levy, S., Wang, S. Y., Lee, J. E., & Levy, B. R. (2020). Global reach of ageism on older persons' health: A systematic review. *PLoS One, 15*(1), 1–24. https://doi.org/10.1371/journal.pone.0220857

Cho, H., Cannon, J., Lopez, R., & Li, W. (2024). Social media literacy: A conceptual framework. *New Media and Society, 26*(2), 941–960. https://doi.org/10.1177/14614448211068530

Cleveland, J. N., & Agbeke, D. V. (2019). Socioemotional selectivity theory lifespan perspectives on job performance, performance appraisal/management and creative performance. 2009.

Cooper, C., Bebbington, P., King, M., Jenkins, R., Farrell, M., Brugha, T., McManus, S., Stewart, R., & Livingston, G. (2011). Happiness across age groups: Results from the 2007 National Psychiatric Morbidity Survey. *International Journal of Geriatric Psychiatry, 26*(6), 608–614. https://doi.org/10.1002/gps.2570

Crealey, G. E., Hickey, G., & McGilloway, S. (2024). A cost-effectiveness analysis of a universal, preventative-focused, parent and infant programme. *BMC Health Services Research, 24*(1), 1–13. https://doi.org/10.1186/s12913-023-10492-w

Duplaga, M., Grysztar, M., Rodzinka, M., & Kopec, A. (2016). Scoping review of health promotion and disease prevention interventions addressed to elderly people. *BMC Health Services Research, 16*(Suppl 5). https://doi.org/10.1186/s12913-016-1521-4

Evans, E. A., Tennenbaum, D. L., Washington, D. L., & Hamilton, A. B. (2019). Why women veterans do not use VA-provided health and social services: Implications for health care design and delivery. *Journal of Humanistic Psychology, 2019*, 1–30. https://doi.org/10.1177/0022167819847328

Green, L. W., & Raeburn, J. M. (1988). Health promotion. What is it? What will it become? *Health Promotion International, 3*(2), 151–159. https://doi.org/10.1093/heapro/3.2.151

Greenhalgh, T. (2015, February). Health literacy: Towards system level solutions. *BMJ (Online), 350*, 24–25. https://doi.org/10.1136/bmj.h1026

Hedayatipour, M., Etemadi, S., Hekmat, S. N., & Moosavi, A. (2024). Challenges of using evidence in managerial decision-making of the primary health care system. *BMC Health Services Research, 24*(1), 1–14. https://doi.org/10.1186/s12913-023-10409-7

Herold, F., Theobald, P., Gronwald, T., Kaushal, N., Zou, L., de Bruin, E. D., Bherer, L., & Müller, N. G. (2024). Alexa, let's train now! — A systematic review and classification approach to digital and home-based physical training interventions aiming to support healthy cognitive aging. *Journal of Sport and Health Science, 13*(1), 30–46. https://doi.org/10.1016/j.jshs.2023.01.004

Hewis, J. (2023). A salutogenic approach: Changing the paradigm. *Journal of Medical Imaging and Radiation Sciences, 54*(2), S17–S21. https://doi.org/10.1016/j.jmir.2023.02.004

Hughes, G., Shaw, S. E., & Greenhalgh, T. (2020). Rethinking integrated care: A systematic hermeneutic review of the literature on integrated care strategies and concepts. *Milbank Quarterly, 98*(2), 446–492. https://doi.org/10.1111/1468-0009.12459

Jacobson, T. A. (2006). Overcoming "ageism" bias in the treatment of hypercholesterolaemia: A review of safety issues with statins in the elderly. *Drug Safety, 29*(5), 421–448. https://doi.org/10.2165/00002018-200629050-00005

Keating, N. (2022). A research framework for the United Nations decade of healthy ageing (2021–2030). *European Journal of Ageing, 19*(3), 775–787. https://doi.org/10.1007/s10433-021-00679-7

Kuruvilla, S., Sadana, R., Montesinos, E. V., Beard, J., Vasdeki, J. F., De Carvalho, I. A., Thomas, R. B., Drisse, M. N. B., Daelmans, B., Goodman, T., Koller, T., Officer, A., Vogel, J., Valentine, N., Wootton, E., Banerjee, A., Magar, V., Neira, M., Bele, J. M. O., et al. (2018). A life-course approach to health: Synergy with sustainable development goals. *Bulletin of the World Health Organization, 96*(1), 42–50. https://doi.org/10.2471/BLT.17.198358

Kyeremeh, E., & Schafer, M. H. (2024, August). Keep around, drop, or revise? Exploring what becomes of difficult ties in personal networks. *Social Networks, 76*, 22–33. https://doi.org/10.1016/j.socnet.2023.06.001

Lindström, B., & Eriksson, M. (2011). From health education to healthy learning: Implementing salutogenesis in educational science. *Scandinavian Journal of Public Health, 39*(1), 85–92. https://doi.org/10.1177/1403494810393560

Lion, A., Vuillemin, A., Thornton, J. S., Theisen, D., Stranges, S., & Ward, M. (2019). Physical activity promotion in primary care: A utopian quest? *Health Promotion International, 34*(4), 877–886. https://doi.org/10.1093/heapro/day038

Maher, L. M., Hayward, B., Hayward, P., & Walsh, C. (2017). Increasing sustainability in co-design projects: A qualitative evaluation of a co-design programme in New Zealand. *Patient Experience Journal, 4*(2), 44–52. https://doi.org/10.35680/2372-0247.1150

Menassa, M., Stronks, K., Khatmi, F., Roa Díaz, Z. M., Espinola, O. P., Gamba, M., Itodo, O. A., Buttia, C., Wehrli, F., Minder, B., Velarde, M. R., & Franco, O. H. (2023). Concepts and definitions of healthy ageing: A systematic review and synthesis of theoretical models. *EClinicalMedicine, 56*, 101821. https://doi.org/10.1016/j.eclinm.2022.101821

Muszyńska, M. M., & Rau, R. (2012). The old-age healthy dependency ratio in Europe. *Journal of Population Ageing, 5*(3), 151–162. https://doi.org/10.1007/s12062-012-9068-6

Okely, A. D., Kontsevaya, A., Ng, J., & Abdeta, C. (2021). 2020 WHO guidelines on physical activity and sedentary behavior. *Sports Medicine and Health Science, 3*(2), 115–118. https://doi.org/10.1016/j.smhs.2021.05.001

Palmers, E. E., De Almeida Mello, J., Janssens, L., De Visschere, L., Declerck, D., & Duyck, J. (2024). Implementing an oral health policy in long-term care facilities for older adults in Flanders, Belgium: The Oral Health Care Track. *Gerodontology, 41*(1), 149–158. https://doi.org/10.1111/ger.12693

Peel, N., Bartlett, H., & McClure, R. (2004). Healthy ageing: How is it defined and measured? *Australasian Journal on Ageing, 23*(3), 115–119. https://doi.org/10.1111/j.1741-6612.2004.00035.x

Phelan, A. (2008). Elder abuse, ageism, human rights and citizenship: Implications for nursing discourse. *Nursing Inquiry, 15*(4), 320–329. https://doi.org/10.1111/j.1440-1800.2008.00423.x

Rudnicka, E., Napierała, P., Podfigurna, A., Męczekalski, B., Smolarczyk, R., & Grymowicz, M. (2020, February). The World Health Organization (WHO) approach to healthy ageing. *Maturitas, 139*, 6–11. https://doi.org/10.1016/j.maturitas.2020.05.018

Slattery, P., Saeri, A. K., & Bragge, P. (2020). Research co-design in health: A rapid overview of reviews. *Health Research Policy and Systems, 18*(1), 1–13. https://doi.org/10.1186/s12961-020-0528-9

Smith, B. J., Tang, K. C., & Nutbeam, D. (2006). WHO health promotion glossary: New terms. *Health Promotion International, 21*(4), 340–345. https://doi.org/10.1093/heapro/dal033

Sofia Campos. (2018). Social & behavioural sciences icH & Hpsy 2018 4 th international conference on health and health psychology parental practices: IMPACT on child behavior. *The European Proceedings of Social & Behavioural Sciences*, 8.

Sulander, T., Heinonen, H., Pajunen, T., Karisto, A., Pohjolainen, P., & Fogelholm, M. (2012). Longitudinal changes in functional capacity: Effects of socio-economic position among ageing adults. *International Journal for Equity in Health, 11*(1), 1–7. https://doi.org/10.1186/1475-9276-11-78

Thornton, J. S., Frémont, P., Khan, K., Poirier, P., Fowles, J., Wells, G. D., & Frankovich, R. J. (2016). Physical activity prescription: A critical opportunity to address a modifiable risk factor for the prevention and management of chronic disease: A position statement by the Canadian Academy of Sport and Exercise Medicine. *British Journal of Sports Medicine, 50*, 1109–1114. https://doi.org/10.1136/bjsports-2016-096291

Treas, J., & Mazumdar, S. (2002). Older people in America's immigrant families dilemmas of dependence, integration, and isolation. *Journal of Aging Studies, 16*(3), 243–258. https://doi.org/10.1016/S0890-4065(02)00048-8

Vale, M. T., Stanley, J. T., Houston, M. L., Villalba, A. A., & Turner, J. R. (2020). Ageism and behavior change during a health pandemic: A preregistered study. *Frontiers in Psychology, 11*(November), 1–12. https://doi.org/10.3389/fpsyg.2020.587911

Vinoi, N., Shankar, A., Khalil, A., Mehrotra, A., & Kumar, J. (2024). Holding on to your memories: Factors influencing social media hoarding behaviour. *Journal of Retailing and Consumer Services, 76*(November 2023), 103617. https://doi.org/10.1016/j.jretconser.2023.103617

Wahl, H. W., & Gerstorf, D. (2018). A conceptual framework for studying COntext Dynamics in Aging (CODA). *Developmental Review, 50*(August), 155–176. https://doi.org/10.1016/j.dr.2018.09.003

Wei, X., Sun, L., Slade, E., Fierheller, C. T., Oxley, S., Kalra, A., Sia, J., Sideris, M., McCluggage, W. G., Bromham, N., Dworzynski, K., Rosenthal, A. N., Brentnall, A., Duffy, S., Evans, D. G., Yang, L., Legood, R., & Manchanda, R. (2024). Cost-effectiveness of gene-specific prevention strategies for ovarian and breast cancer. *JAMA Network Open, 7*(2), 1–17. https://doi.org/10.1001/jamanetworkopen.2023.55324

Welstead, M., Jenkins, N. D., Russ, T. C., Luciano, M., & Muniz-Terrera, G. (2021). A systematic review of frailty trajectories: Their shape and influencing factors. *Gerontologist, 61*(8), E463–E475. https://doi.org/10.1093/geront/gnaa061

Yang, C. (2021). Moral education in mainland China today: A bio-ecological systems analysis. *Journal of Moral Education, 50*(4), 529–543. https://doi.org/10.1080/03057240.2020.1847054

Chapter 8
Climate Change Adaptation for Healthy Ageing

Faith Hope Muhonja, Simon Mawulorm Agyemang, Reginald Arthur-Mensah, and Sarra Sghaier

Acronyms and Abbreviations

AC	Adaptive capacity
AI	Artificial intelligence
ATA	Activity theory of ageing
BA	Behavioural adaptation
CCA	Climate change adaptation
COVID-19	Coronavirus Disease 2019
DNA	Deoxyribonucleic acid
HA	Healthy ageing
NCDs	Non-communicable diseases
PA	Physiological adaptation
SARS	Severe acute respiratory syndrome

F. H. Muhonja (✉)
Department of Community Health, School of Public Health, Amref International University, Nairobi, Kenya
e-mail: faith.muhonja@amref.ac.ke

S. M. Agyemang
Department of Science/Health, Physical Education, and Sports, Abetifi Presbyterian College of Education, Abetifi, Ghana
e-mail: simonagyemang340@gmail.com

R. Arthur-Mensah
School of Nursing and Midwifery, Pentecost University, Kaneshie, Greater Accra Region, Ghana
e-mail: Ramensah@pentvars.edu.gh

S. Sghaier
Department of Gerontology and Geriatrics, Africa Centre for Epidemiology, Accra North, Accra, Ghana
e-mail: sarra.sgh@hotmail.com

N. Asiamah et al. (eds.), *Sustainable Ageing*,
https://doi.org/10.1007/978-3-031-69475-2_8

STA Structural adaptation
UN United Nations
WHO World Health Organization

8.1 Introduction

Climate change refers to any change in average weather conditions that lasts for a long period of time (Gutterman, 2022). Climate change events, which include heat waves, floods, and famine, are a threat to health and longevity. Older adults are more vulnerable to these events owing to their physiological limitations and underlying health problems (Gutterman, 2022). Because elderly people are more likely to experience heat stroke and dehydration, the rising incidence of climate change presents a serious concern. Furthermore, climate change and poor ventilation can contribute to chronic disorders like pulmonary and cardiac malfunctions (Hajat et al., 2010). Moreover, elderly people are more likely to be injured or die during extreme weather events because of their decreased mobility and physical fragility (Thompson et al., 2018).

According to Gardner (2023), climate change is the "perfect moral storm" since it is planetary in scope, has lasting consequences across generations, and lacks the political muscle needed to address its social, economic, and environmental threats. In the absence of considerable efforts to minimise emissions of greenhouse gases (GHG), climate change can be expected to have an increasing adverse impact on humans, especially older adults. Although there is currently a concerted effort to achieve net-zero emissions due to the declared goals of numerous companies and the laws of some governments, climate change remains a global problem.

While promoting sustainable ageing, WHO (2020) maintains that, in spite of societal and climate-related changes, older people should be able to continue to enjoy an adequate level of well-being as they age. In doing so, issues related to social inclusion, health, economic security, and environmental sustainability must be addressed (Ouyang et al., 2022). Unfortunately, older individuals' unique needs and functional capabilities are frequently disregarded by current adaptation policies and practices (Arigoni, 2023). A comprehensive grasp of the risks and functional capabilities of this population is necessary for effective climate change adaptation for sustainable ageing (Zalon, 2019). Asiamah et al. (2023) defines sustainable ageing as the maintenance of the functional capacity necessary for well-being in old age in contexts experiencing crises such as climate change and war. In such contexts, access to basic needs, including health services, may be limited. Furthermore, elderly people (including those with restricted access to food and water) might give away their meagre resources to family members in a climate emergency (Zalon, 2019).

The role of climate change adaptation in sustainable ageing is critical and needs to be recognised by policymakers. As populations age, there is a growing need for strategies that not only mitigate the impacts of climate change but also ensure the well-being and resilience of older adults. The implementation of these strategies requires an integrated approach that encompasses efforts from professionals in healthcare, social care and welfare, urban planning, and disaster preparedness (Rudnicka et al., 2020). The goal of this chapter is to conceptualise human adaptation as a behavioural requirement for ageing well in contexts experiencing climate change. Key concepts on adaptation are highlighted to frame what we refer to as "climate change adaptation", an individual behaviour necessary for sustainable ageing. By means of this discourse, we delineate postulates for future research and identify implications for policy. This chapter, for the first time, offers insights into the role of adaptive behaviour in sustainable ageing. Thoughts presented can play a role in the successful implementation of existing and emerging health ageing initiatives such as the United Nations' Decade of Healthy Ageing 2021–2030 campaign.

The first section of this chapter identifies the aim and significance of our discourse, setting the foundation for Sect. 8.2 where we have a summary of key initiatives against climate change. In Sect. 8.3, the role of climate change adaptation in healthy ageing is proffered and postulates about levels of adaptation are analysed. Theoretical perspectives on climate change adaptation and its role in healthy ageing are then provided in Sect. 8.4, clarifying postulates presented in the preceding section. In Sect. 8.5, the dimensions of climate change adaptation are discussed, allowing us to analyse implications of our thoughts for practice in the Sect. 8.6. Concluding remarks are presented in Sect. 8.7.

8.2 Initiatives Against Climate Change

Climate change and its potential challenges have been discussed for a period of approximately four decades. The discussions have been centred around the global address of the impending impact of climate change through mitigation measures. Various frameworks, approaches, and strategies have been proposed and implemented with partial success. Some include the United Nations publication of the Brundtland Report, on the role of information and communication Technology for Sustainable Development (ICTD) (Andersson & Hatakka, 2023). Another pivotal approach for sustainable development was Our Common Future: Report of the World Commission on Environment and Development, Geneva (Zangerolame Taroco & Sabbá Colares, 2020).

The Sustainable Development Goals (SDGs) are another universal call to action signed by 193 countries in 2015 as part of the 2030 agenda. One of the goals is to protect the planet and improve lives (Suárez Giri & Sánchez Chaparro, 2023). Most of the SDGs contribute to climate change. They include SGD 11, 13, 14, and 15 (sustainable cities and communities, take urgent action to combat climate change and its impacts, conserve and sustainably use the oceans, seas, and marine resources for sustainable development, and protect, restore, and promote sustainable use of terrestrial ecosystems, combat desertification, and halt biodiversity loss, respectively) (Cordonier Segger, 2016).

Another milestone in the fight against climate change is the Paris global legally binding international agreement on climate change. The treaty was adopted by 196 countries at the UN Climate Change Conference (COP21), which took place in Paris, France, on 12 December 2015. The binding agreement is to cut emissions of greenhouse gases to foster economic, social, and environmental concerns in the twenty-first century (Cozier, 2015; Gouvernement de la République Française, 2015; Semenov & Oganesyan, 2023). These agreements are pivotal in the climate change agenda for a better and healthy planet. To realise the goals of these agreements and initiatives, individuals and communities must perform adaptive behaviour, hereby referred to as adaptation, in the face of climate change events such as extreme weather.

8.3 The Role of Climate Change Adaptation in Healthy Ageing

Adaptation to evade extinction is imperative for any living organism, man included (Rainbow, 2011). It is paramount to adjust to align with the current prevailing changes in ecological and socio-economic systems. This change could be a response to actual or expected stimuli (climate change) and the potential resultant effects (Jamal, 2022). Adaptation is the process by which an organism changes as a result of the dictates of the prevailing or anticipated adverse effects of climate to maximise its survival. It can be a temporary or permanent change, depending on the context and sustainability of the adopted change, or the intermittent or continuous presence of the trigger and its impact on healthy ageing.

Ageing is chronological, biological, or psychological. Chronological age is the amount of time that has elapsed from birth to a given date. Thus, chronological ageing is getting older over time, which results in physiological changes such as wrinkling of the skin. Biological ageing is changes in the mass of tissues, muscles, and bones over time (Asiamah et al., 2023). Psychological ageing is how old one feels, acts, and behaves (Chow & Bai, 2011; Kocyigit, 2023). Thus, psychological ageing is a gradual change in the way people behave, act, and feel owing experiences over the life course. Since feelings about ageing ideally originate from the individual's body, psychological ageing and chronological ageing are outcomes of biological ageing.

Studies have reported the concept of ageing as multifactorial (López-Otín et al., 2023) with various dimensions including changes in cellular senescence, telomere attrition, deregulated nutrient sensing, genomic instability, loss of proteostasis, epigenetic alterations, disabled macroautophagy, mitochondrial dysfunction, stem cell exhaustion, and altered intercellular communication, which increases vulnerability to diseases and reduces ability to adapt to climate change (Saul & Kosinsky, 2021; Schmauck-Medina et al., 2022).

The ability to adapt to climate change, referred to as climate change adaptation, occurs at four key levels, namely process, behavioural, structural, and physiological levels (Raskov et al., 2023). At the process level, individuals or organisms perform relevant activities to achieve a goal or set of goals such as coping with extreme temperatures. Actions are performed in view of the prevailing socio-economic and ecologic circumstances geared towards achieving sustainable adaptation to climate change for healthy ageing. The second level of climate change adaptation is at the practice or behavioural level, which occurs when an organism shades off some mannerism to cope with or overcome the current problem for survival. To illustrate, social distancing during the coronavirus disease (COVID-19) pandemic was necessary for the survival of many individuals (Ayalon & Roy, 2023a, b), especially those with chronic diseases. The third level of adaptation is at the structural (natural and built) level, such as the shedding of excess fur during the hot season by an animal (Eisenhauer, 2016). Lastly, the fourth level of adaptation to change can occur at the physiology or functional level, which can result from a cellular deoxyribonucleic acid (DNA) mutation (López-Otín et al., 2023) or exposure to adverse events such as non-communicable diseases like cancer and diabetes, which alter the normal functioning of the body (Raskov et al., 2023). Table 8.1 shows a summary of attributes of the four levels of adaptation.

Adaptation to climate change is aimed at mitigating potential damages from unfavourable events or maximising the individual's potential to overcome these events to age well (Gardner, 2023). Adaptation to climate change as a strategy for healthy ageing has gained momentum over the past few decades (Bukvic et al., 2018). This is due to the drastic change in climatic conditions and their resultant negative impact on humans and the environment (Enríquez-de-Salamanca et al., 2017; Liu et al., 2019; Nalau & Verrall, 2021).

The devastating impact of climate change has been reported to be a precursor to adaptation to climate change among the ageing population. Studies have reported adaptation as either free will or coercion; however, most of the studies reported adaptation to climate change as the ability of an organism to adapt to the environment over time as a requirement for its survival (Jamal, 2022). Information in Table 8.1 substantiates this thought with examples of how the phases of adaptation can benefit the individual.

The summary in Table 8.1 suggests that the four levels of adaptation are an essential component of human behaviour that would facilitate survival amidst crises such as climate change events. Survival from this perspective can foster well-being and longevity, an idea that has a theoretical basis with a long history.

8.4 Theoretical Perspectives on Adaptation and Its Role in Healthy Ageing

Global drastic changes in climatic conditions, which threaten the survival of human species in the twenty-first century, has rekindled the Darwinian debate of "survival of the fittest" anchored on human variation, heredity, and the origin of races between

Table 8.1 Authors' summary of key attributes of the four levels of adaptation

Adaptation level	Description	Examples/key elements
Process	Series of actions undertaken to achieve a set goal or desired change (adaptation to climate change). The components of a process include its design, tools or instruments, and the inputs required for successful adaptation to climate change.	(1) Minimum resources, including money and social networks, needed for the climate change adaptation. (2) The outcome of the process concurs with the set goal of adaptation to climate change. (3) The process of adaptation to climate change should be able to withstand any intensity of climatic events.
Behaviour	The way an organism (person) acts in response to external stimuli (climate change) or its anticipated adverse effects on healthy ageing	(1) Visible actions like migrating or moving away from disaster risk zones to safer zones, having insurance cover as a precautionary measure, and social distancing. (2) Internal dialogue, thinking, imagination, and perceptions towards climate change and its potential negative impact.
Structural	Arrangement of parts of an organism where its components work together for its survival. It can be natural living organisms or an entity orchestrating deliberate measures to promote climate change adaptation.	(1) Transition from fossil fuels to renewable energy to reduce greenhouse gas emissions. (2) Some changes may be seen in animals, like excessive growth of fur in bears, shedding of leaves by plants during drought, and secretion of high melanin pigmentation by humans amidst heat waves.
Physiological adaptation	Refers to internal change by organisms for their own survival. It includes the metabolism and function of the body in an organism to regulate metabolism activities and maintain body metabolism.	For instance, if exposed to toxic substances, the body releases the toxic substance. Also, if there are extreme weather patterns, like cold or hot, the body regulates the temperature for the survival of the organism.

1790 and 1835 (Ariew, 2007; Gardner, 2023; Jenkins, 2020; Rainbow, 2011). At the backdrop of the COVID-19 pandemic, other life-threatening infections like Ebola and severe acute respiratory syndrome (SARS), and non-communicable diseases like cancer, it is evident that there is a need for adaptation for survival, especially for the ageing population (Mendonça et al., 2023; Mukhra et al., 2021; Raskov et al., 2023).

Charles Darwin's theory provides a foundational understanding of life on earth and importance of adaptive behaviour. The theory posits the need for species to naturally adapt to survive. This theory has been emphasised by Neo-Darwinism's Gregory Mendel and Modern Synthesis Theory, which have integrated genetics and natural selection and their role in adaptation (Hemminger, 2021; Ibaca León, 2019). Similarly, the Activity Theory of Ageing (ATA) developed by Robert Havighurst in

1961 recognises the role of adaptive behaviour in maintaining health and achieving healthy longevity (Asiamah et al., 2023). It posits that ageing people can maintain functional ability and well-being in later life by adapting past experiences to maintain social and physical activities. The ATA adds that whether people will age well depends on their ability to overcome barriers to successful ageing such as a loss of muscle and bone mass.

Deductively, organisms or individuals who are not able to adapt as they experience unfavourable conditions may not survive or maintain health (Jenkins, 2020). The goal of healthy ageing is to maintain health and functional ability, but climate change events may make it daunting for ageing people to avoid disability and disease. Amidst the current climate crises, adaptation as proposed by Charles Darwin would involve moving to safer communities (Ayalon et al., 2021; Ayalon & Roy, 2023a). The possibility of people relocating to other places to avoid danger in times of crisis was recently acknowledged as a protective behaviour (Asiamah et al., 2023).

Additionally, mitigative actions towards climate change are dependent on the perceived threats and benefits of adapting to change, including socio-economic and political consequences (Osberghaus, 2017). Thus, older adults experiencing life difficulties due to climate change would act to preserve their health and lives. The fact that crises can be harmful and result in disability, diseases, or death may motivate individuals to take mitigative action. As mentioned earlier, relocating to a safer place or seeking support from social network members can be an effective way to avoid harms from a climatic event. These examples recall the different components of adaptation to climate change, which are discussed in the next section.

8.5 Components of Climate Change Adaptation for an Ageing Population

8.5.1 Adaptive Capacity

The ability of the ageing population to adapt to crises that threaten their well-being is paramount in the execution of change. As the ATA illustrates, adaptive behaviour is necessary to overcome the barriers to healthy ageing. For this reason, individuals and policymakers ought to recognise climate change events and other crises as new barriers to healthy ageing. This attitude may enable them to prepare mentally and physically to achieve resilience when faced with crises. The ability to migrate to safer zones when crises occur is part of adaptive behaviour that may lead to the preservation of health, functional ability, and possibly personal resources. Structural and physiological changes, where a personal walks away from violence to promote good health, are dependent on physical and socio-economic capacity. Yet, this capacity may be low in older adults and may, therefore, limit their ability to overcome climate change events, which are rampant and unpredictable (Malmquist et al., 2022; Serdeczny et al., 2024).

8.5.2 Adaptive Vulnerability

The ageing process introduces an individual to a double morbidity burden of both non-communicable diseases and infectious diseases. The degeneration of the body defence system increases the susceptibility of a person to infectious diseases, especially among older adults. Despite emerging and rising episodes of pandemics, older adults may not have the necessary immunity to avoid infectious diseases. No doubt, infectious diseases may threaten the ability of older adults to overcome climate change events and other crises, especially among older adults with disability. Suffice it to say that infectious diseases may limit older adults' ability to sustain adaptation (Carter et al., 2016; Rhoades et al., 2018; Smorenberg et al., 2021).

8.5.3 Adaptive Resilience

The ability of the elderly population to bounce back to normalcy after a disaster like flood, hurricane, or disease pandemic is faced with a myriad of challenges. Displacement from their physical and social networks leads to disorientation and mental disorders like anxiety and depression. This compounds the inability to make sound independent decisions to sustain adaptive behaviour in response to climate change events. Forming new social networks and maintaining existing ones can be difficult for older adults experiencing the adverse effects of climate change. Yet, these networks are always needed for exercising resilience. When older adults experience crises in or near their social networks, they are more likely to receive encouragement for coping. It can, therefore, be inferred that the preservation of social networks during crises can play a role in adaptive behaviour and resilience. This fact was echoed by researchers who have acknowledged the need for resilience to be maintained by victims of crises (Fontes & Neri, 2019; Meléndez et al., 2015; Vannini et al., 2021).

8.5.4 Adaptive Strategies

Deliberate development of adaptation strategies or coping mechanisms may empower individuals to maintain healthy behaviours and well-being. The climate crises are universal and are felt by everyone, but older adults are affected more strongly by them owing to their physiological limitations. The older population is less likely to adjust to drastic climate change owing to their low functional and cognitive capacity. For these reasons, having clear projections of climate change events may forewarn individuals to take protective action. Prompt action against crises may enable individuals, especially older adults, to be successful in their adaptation. Finally, measures intended to help vulnerable groups to evacuate their homes or cities in response to climate change events can promote healthy ageing (Fontes & Neri, 2019).

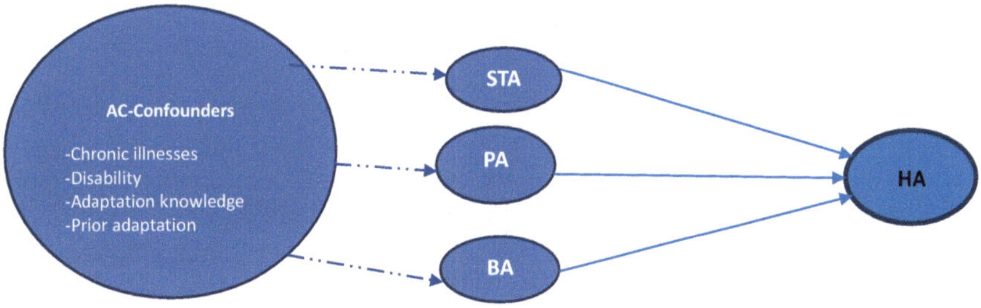

Fig. 8.1 Authors' conceptualisation of the link between adaptation to climate change and healthy ageing. *Note*: Adaptive capacity (AC), structural adaptation (STA), physiological adaptation (PA), behavioural adaptation (BA), healthy ageing (HA)

8.5.5 Adopting an Adaptation-Mitigation Approach

Adaptation to climate change would not necessarily eliminate the impacts of its events. Adaptation is only a reactionary process in which the individual may minimise impact or preserve potentials, resources, and well-being (Gietel-Basten, 2021). As Fig. 8.1 illustrates, the ability of the elderly population to maintain well-being over the life course depends on successful adaptation. The model (see Fig. 8.1) suggests that there exists an interplay between four key constructs, namely adaptive capacity (AC), structural adaptation (STA), physiological adaptation (PA), and behavioural adaptation (BA), which together influences healthy ageing (HA). The interplay is confounded by individual characteristics such as income, age, and place of residence. For instance, the ability to achieve adaptive capacity may depend on whether the individual has money to secure services outside their neighbourhood where a crisis is being experienced.

Morbidity status is another personal factor that may serve as a confounder since existing chronic conditions can limit the ability to adapt well to climate change. Older adults with underlying chronic conditions experience a double burden in confronting climate change and thus needs extraordinary support and resilience to cope with unfavourable events. Such individuals are often saddened by being too dependent on their health care providers, families, and friends, which degrades their sense of autonomy (Chebib et al., 2021; Smorenberg et al., 2021; Vannini et al., 2021).

Autonomy in one's response to climate change can also be confounded by the knowledge of the need to adapt. Knowledge of early warning signs of disasters and how to respond to them is key. Most of the elderly population is caught off-guard by the challenges of climate change and hence fails to respond on time and effectively. An effective and timely response to climate change adaptation can also be confounded by prior experience with the specific disaster. This could either positively or negatively influence the adaptation to change. If the experience was beneficial, life-threatening, or led to severe consequences, it will be used as a term of reference for decision-making. This and other thoughts shared have implications for policy as discussed below.

8.6 Implications for Practice and Policy

All sectors are affected in one way or the other by climate change events, so collective action against the climate crisis is imperative. Isolated approaches are less likely to yield the expected outcome for healthy ageing since interdisciplinary efforts are necessary for fostering healthy longevity (Rudnicka et al., 2020). We, therefore, call for the involvement of all stakeholders in enabling individuals to adapt to climate change. The key players include the United Nations, governments, traditional leaders of communities, civil society organisations, and beneficiaries (e.g. older adults) of interventions against climate change for healthy ageing. The United Nations, through the WHO, is already championing initiatives such as the Decade of Healthy Ageing 2021–2030. It is incumbent on other stakeholders to support these initiatives. A key step that can be taken in response to climate change is town or city planning and infrastructural development to ensure resilient and climate change-sensitive built environment. The planners should incorporate mitigative and early warning systems with bias in the type of disaster within the local context and recovery mechanisms like insurance covers.

The trade, transport, and communication sectors should also contribute to measures such as pro-climate change adaptation policies and guidelines. The health sector and disaster management agencies may take similar actions to ensure safety or achieve a swift recovery of communities from disasters. Having a robust health care infrastructure is necessary for a timely response to crises, especially in older populations. Governments, for political good will, must mitigate the impact of climate change on macro-economies and call for or roll out new policies and guidelines. Governments are responsible for the development of climate change adaptation and transition policies and allocating resources for implementing these policies both at the local and national levels.

Non-governmental organisations are also key stakeholders in climate change adaptation for accountability, equality, and sustainability. Their presence motivates and encourages governments and other agencies to act responsibly in the interest of society. Also, having philanthropic foundations such as the Bill and Melinda Gates Foundations and Rocker Fellow Foundations can be transformative, given the role they played in response to the COVID-19 pandemic. In addition, higher learning institutions ought to be part and parcel of the debate for an evidence-based approach to adaptation to an ageing population.

Financial institutions have a role to play in the fight against climate change in ways that foster healthy ageing. The World Bank and the Africa Development Bank are noteworthy financial institutions that can provide sustained financial resources for implementing interventions against climate change and for healthy ageing. The Decade of Healthy Ageing 2021–2030, for example, needs sustained funding to yield expected results. Stakeholders should leverage the existing potential of communities in different contexts, for instance, in Africa, where the population is young. Provision of public education aimed at creating awareness about climate change and measures against it can prepare the minds of younger generations in Africa to contribute to interventions against the climate crisis.

Technological innovation can also be leveraged to predict climate change events or unfavourable weather conditions. More research focused on exploring artificial intelligence, robotics, and other innovations may open doors to the use of intelligent technological systems to predict climate change events and empower people to act in response to these events. Integration of climate change adaptation into national planning and budgeting for sustained funding of anti-climate change projects is imperative. In developing countries, this step would eliminate over-dependence on aid in addressing climate change problems and make it possible for older adults to be supported locally. In a situation where countries enhance their financial agility and avoid excessive dependence on foreign aid, a reasonable budget can be dedicated to not only climate change interventions but also healthy ageing initiatives, especially by member states supporting the Decade of Healthy Ageing 2021–2030.

8.7 Conclusion

Climate change and other crises are a strong force against healthy ageing as they pose threats that prevent ageing people from maintaining health-seeking behaviours and well-being. Their global presence requires skills such as resilience, coping ability, and adaptive behaviour. This chapter, therefore, provides insights into the role of adaptation in navigating the challenges posed by climate change. The chapter proposes a multi-level framework of climate change adaptation, where adaptive behaviour against climatic threats can occur at the global, national, community, and individual levels. Effective adaptation requires collaborative efforts aimed at preventing climate crises or empowering individuals and communities to maintain health-seeking behaviours and well-being amidst these crises

Review Questions

1. Why is adaptation necessary for healthy ageing amidst climate change and other crises?
2. What can stakeholders do to enable individuals to succeed in climate change adaptation?
3. Discuss five stakeholders and their respective roles in climate change adaptation for healthy ageing.
4. Explain the four levels of adaptation to climate change. Why are these levels significant for healthy ageing?

References

Ariew, A. (2007). Under the influence of Malthus's law of population growth: Darwin eschews the statistical techniques of Aldolphe Quetelet. *Studies in History and Philosophy of Biological and Biomedical Sciences, 38*(1), 1. https://doi.org/10.1016/j.shpsc.2006.12.002

Arigoni, D. (2023). *Climate resilience for an aging nation*. Island Press.

Asiamah, N., Koohsari, M. J., & Lowry, R. (2023). Ageing in place: The present and future social and health threats. In *Sustainable neighbourhoods for ageing in place* (pp. 15–35). Springer Nature Switzerland. https://doi.org/10.1007/978-3-031-41594-4_2

Ayalon, L., & Roy, S. (2023a). The role of ageism in climate change worries and willingness to act. *Journal of Applied Gerontology, 42*(6), 1305. https://doi.org/10.1177/07334648221130323

Ayalon, L., & Roy, S. (2023b, June 6). The role of chronological age in climate change attitudes, feelings, and behavioral intentions: The case of null results. *PLoS One, 18*. https://doi.org/10.1371/journal.pone.0286901.

Ayalon, L., Keating, N., Pillemer, K., & Rabheru, K. (2021). Climate change and mental health of older persons: A human rights imperative. *American Journal of Geriatric Psychiatry, 29*(10), 1038. https://doi.org/10.1016/j.jagp.2021.06.015

Bukvic, A., Gohlke, J., Borate, A., & Suggs, J. (2018). Aging in flood-prone coastal areas: Discerning the health and well-being risk for older residents. *International Journal of Environmental Research and Public Health, 15*(12). https://doi.org/10.3390/ijerph15122900

Carr, E. R., & Nalau, J. (2023). Adaptation rationales and benefits: A foundation for understanding adaptation impact. In *Climate risk management* (Vol. 39). https://doi.org/10.1016/j.crm.2023.100479

Carter, T. R., Fronzek, S., Inkinen, A., Lahtinen, I., Lahtinen, M., Mela, H., O'Brien, K. L., Rosentrater, L. D., Ruuhela, R., Simonsson, L., & Terama, E. (2016). Characterising vulnerability of the elderly to climate change in the Nordic region. *Regional Environmental Change, 16*(1), 43. https://doi.org/10.1007/s10113-014-0688-7

Chebib, N., Cuvelier, C., Malézieux-Picard, A., Parent, T., Roux, X., Fassier, T., Müller, F., & Prendki, V. (2021). Pneumonia prevention in the elderly patients: the other sides. In *Aging Clinical and Experimental Research* (Vol. 33, Issue 4). https://doi.org/10.1007/s40520-019-01437-7

Cordonier Segger, M. C. (2016). Advancing the paris agreement on climate change for sustainable development. *Cambridge International Law Journal, 5*(2). https://doi.org/10.4337/cilj.2016.02.03

Cozier, M. (2015). The un COP21 Climate Change Conference and the role of CCS. *Greenhouse Gases: Science and Technology, 5*(6). https://doi.org/10.1002/ghg.1577 Gouvernement de la République Française. (2015). Paris 2015 UN Climate Change Conference COP21. Paris Agreement Short Glossary, August 2002.

Chow, N., & Bai, X. (2011). The effects of sociodemographic characteristics on Chinese elders' perception of the image of ageing. *International Journal of Population Research, 2011*. https://doi.org/10.1155/2011/642874

Eisenhauer, D. C. (2016). Pathways to climate change adaptation: Making climate change action political. *Geography Compass, 10*(5), 207. https://doi.org/10.1111/gec3.12263

Enríquez-de-Salamanca, Á., Díaz-Sierra, R., Martín-Aranda, R. M., & Santos, M. J. (2017). Environmental impacts of climate change adaptation. *Environmental Impact Assessment Review, 64*, 87. https://doi.org/10.1016/j.eiar.2017.03.005

Fontes, A. P., & Neri, A. L. (2019). Coping strategies as indicators of resilience in elderly subjects: A methodological study. *Ciencia e Saude Coletiva, 24*(4), 1265. https://doi.org/10.1590/1413-81232018244.05502017

Gardner, A. (2023). The rarer-sex effect. *Philosophical Transactions of the Royal Society B: Biological Sciences, 378*(1876), 20210500. https://doi.org/10.1098/rstb.2021.0500

Gietel-Basten, S. (2021). Adopting an adaptation-mitigation-resilience framework to ageing. *Age and Ageing, 50*(3). https://doi.org/10.1093/ageing/afaa282

Gutterman, A. (2022). *Impacts of climate change on older persons.*

Hajat, S., O'Connor, M., & Kosatsky, T. (2010). Health effects of hot weather: From awareness of risk factors to effective health protection. *The Lancet, 375*(9717), 856–863. https://doi.org/10.1016/S0140-6736(09)61711-6

Hemminger, H. (2021). Evolution: The modern synthesis. In *New Approaches to the Scientific Study of Religion* (Vol. 10). https://doi.org/10.1007/978-3-030-70408-7_5

Ibaca León, J. M. (2019). Acerca de la biología evolutiva como una ciencia normal. *Cuadernos de Filosofía, 37*(37).

IPCC, 2021*: Climate change 2021—The Physical Science basis* | *Interaction.* (n.d.). Retrieved May 22, 2024, from https://search.informit.org/doi/abs/10.3316/informit.315096509383738

Jamal, S. (2022). Adaptation to climate change in Africa. *Global Journal of Ecology, 7*(2). https://doi.org/10.17352/gje.000058

Jenkins, B. (2020). Race before Darwin: Variation, adaptation and the natural history of man in post-Enlightenment Edinburgh, 1790-1835. *British Journal for the History of Science, 53*(3). https://doi.org/10.1017/S0007087420000217

Kocyigit, E. (2023). BODY image in aging. *Anti-Aging Eastern Europe, 2*(1), 23. https://doi.org/10.56543/aaeeu.2023.2.1.04

Liu, T., Ren, Z., Zhang, Y., Feng, B., Lin, H., Xiao, J., Zeng, W., Li, X., Li, Z., Rutherford, S., Xu, Y., Lin, S., Nasca, P. C., Du, Y., Wang, J., Huang, C., Jia, P., & Ma, W. (2019). Modification effects of population expansion, ageing, and adaptation on heat-related mortality risks under different climate change scenarios in Guangzhou, China. *International Journal of Environmental Research and Public Health, 16*(3). https://doi.org/10.3390/ijerph16030376

López-Otín, C., Blasco, M. A., Partridge, L., Serrano, M., & Kroemer, G. (2023). Hallmarks of aging: An expanding universe. *Cell, 186*(2). https://doi.org/10.1016/j.cell.2022.11.001

Malmquist, A., Hjerpe, M., Glaas, E., Karlsson, H., & Lassi, T. (2022). Elderly people's perceptions of heat stress and adaptation to heat: An interview study. *International Journal of Environmental Research and Public Health, 19*(7). https://doi.org/10.3390/ijerph19073775

Meléndez, J. C., Fortuna, F. B., Sales, A., & Mayordomo, T. (2015). The effects of instrumental reminiscence on resilience and coping in elderly. *Archives of Gerontology and Geriatrics, 60*(2). https://doi.org/10.1016/j.archger.2014.12.001

Mendonça, A. A., de Pinto-Neto, W. P., da Paixão, G. A., da Santos, D. S., De Morais, M. A., & De Souza, R. B. (2023). Journey of the probiotic bacteria: Survival of the fittest. *Microorganisms, 11*(1). https://doi.org/10.3390/microorganisms11010095

Mukhra, R., Krishan, K., & Kanchan, T. (2021). COVID-19 pandemic and "survival of the fittest". *Journal of Infection in Developing Countries, 15*(10). https://doi.org/10.3855/jidc.13490

Nalau, J., & Verrall, B. (2021). Mapping the evolution and current trends in climate change adaptation science. *Climate Risk Management, 32*, 100290. https://doi.org/10.1016/j.crm.2021.100290

Osberghaus, D. (2017). Prospect theory, mitigation and adaptation to climate change. *Journal of Risk Research, 20*(7), 909. https://doi.org/10.1080/13669877.2015.1121907

Ouyang, H., Tang, X., Kumar, R., Zhang, R., Brasseur, G., Churchill, B., Alam, M., Kan, H., Liao, H., Zhu, T., Chan, E. Y. Y., Sokhi, R., Yuan, J., Baklanov, A., Chen, J., & Patdu, M. K. (2022). Toward better and healthier air quality: Implementation of WHO 2021 global air quality guidelines in Asia. *Bulletin of the American Meteorological Society, 103*(7), E1696–E1703. https://doi.org/10.1175/BAMS-D-22-0040.1

Rainbow, P. S. (2011). Charles Darwin and marine biology. *Marine Ecology, 32*(Suppl. 1), 130. https://doi.org/10.1111/j.1439-0485.2010.00421.x

Raskov, H., Gaggar, S., Tajik, A., Orhan, A., & Gögenur, I. (2023). Metabolic switch in cancer—Survival of the fittest. *European Journal of Cancer, 180*, 30. https://doi.org/10.1016/j.ejca.2022.11.025

Rhoades, J. L., Gruber, J. S., & Horton, B. (2018). Developing an In-depth understanding of Elderly Adult's vulnerability to Climate Change. *Gerontologist, 58*(3), 567. https://doi.org/10.1093/geront/gnw167

Rudnicka, E., Napierała, P., Podfigurna, A., Męczekalski, B., Smolarczyk, R., & Grymowicz, M. (2020, February). The World Health Organization (WHO) approach to healthy ageing. *Maturitas, 139*, 6–11. https://doi.org/10.1016/j.maturitas.2020.05.018

Saul, D., & Kosinsky, R. L. (2021). Epigenetics of aging and aging-associated diseases. *International Journal of Molecular Sciences, 22*(1). https://doi.org/10.3390/ijms22010401

Schmauck-Medina, T., Molière, A., Lautrup, S., Zhang, J., Chlopicki, S., Madsen, H. B., Cao, S., Soendenbroe, C., Mansell, E., Vestergaard, M. B., Li, Z., Shiloh, Y., Opresko, P. L., Egly, J. M., Kirkwood, T., Verdin, E., Bohr, V. A., Cox, L. S., Stevnsner, T., et al. (2022). New hallmarks of ageing: A 2022 Copenhagen ageing meeting summary. *Aging, 14*(16), 6829. https://doi.org/10.18632/aging.204248

Semenov, A., & Oganesyan, E. (2023). Carbon footprint: IPCC targets vs. building and social standards. E3S Webof Conferences, 403. https://doi.org/10.1051/e3sconf/202340302011

Serdeczny, O., Andrijevic, M., Fyson, C., Lissner, T., Menke, I., Schleussner, C. F., Theokritoff, E., & Thomas, A. (2024). Climatic risks to adaptive capacity. *Mitigation and Adaptation Strategies for Global Change, 29*(1). https://doi.org/10.1007/s11027-023-10103-3

Smorenberg, A., Peters, E. J., van Daele, P. L. A., Nossent, E. J., & Muller, M. (2021). How does SARS-CoV-2 targets the elderly patients? A review on potential mechanisms increasing disease severity. In. *European Journal of Internal Medicine, 83*, 1. https://doi.org/10.1016/j.ejim.2020.11.024

Suárez Giri, F., & Sánchez Chaparro, T. (2023). Measuring business impacts on the SDGs: a systematic literature review: Measuring business impact on the SDGs. *Sustainable Technology and Entrepreneurship, 2*(3). https://doi.org/10.1016/j.stae.2023.100044

Thompson, R., Hornigold, R., Page, L., & Waite, T. (2018). Associations between high ambient temperatures and heat waves with mental health outcomes: A systematic review. *Public Health, 161*, 171–191. https://doi.org/10.1016/j.puhe.2018.06.008

Vannini, P., Gagliardi, G. P., Kuppe, M., Dossett, M. L., Donovan, N. J., Gatchel, J. R., Quiroz, Y. T., Premnath, P. Y., Amariglio, R., Sperling, R. A., & Marshall, G. A. (2021). Stress, resilience, and coping strategies in a sample of community-dwelling older adults during COVID-19. *Journal of Psychiatric Research, 138*. https://doi.org/10.1016/j.jpsychires.2021.03.050

Wardhana, D. H. A., & Prawira, M. R. (2024). The analysis of Indonesia's climate change policies in response to the 2021 Intergovernmental Panel on Climate Change (IPCC) assessment report/AR6 Group 1 (2021–2023). *Proirofonic, 1*(1), Article 1.

WHO. (2020). *UN Decade of Healthy Ageing (2021—2030)*. Decade of Healthy Ageing. https://www.google.com/search

Zalon, M. L. (2019). Preparing older citizens for global climate change: Collaborate and advocate to meet patient needs' and' implement policy change. *American Nurse Today, 14*(2), 5–10.

Zangerolame Taroco, L. S., & Sabbá Colares, A. C. (2020). The UN Framework Convention on Climate Change and the Paris Agreement: Challenges of the Conference of the Parties. *Prolegómenos, 22*(43). https://doi.org/10.18359/prole.3449

Part III
Data and Research for Healthy Ageing

Chapter 9
Research-Practice Gap: Impact on Campaigns and Mitigation Strategies

Evelyn N. Alvarez, Alexys Garcia, Patricia Amoroto, and Marlene Huerta

Acronyms and Abbreviations

LACDPH	Los Angeles County Department of Public Health
RTP	Research to practice
SES	Socio-economic status
UN	United Nations

9.1 Introduction

As climate change continues to pose significant threats to healthy aging in Los Angeles County and elsewhere in the world, developing resiliency strategies is key. One way to encourage adoption of a resiliency strategy is by launching campaigns, specifically campaigns that can offer co-benefits: (1) relief from climate change–related events such as heat waves, and (2) promotion of healthy aging in the context of a warming world. The United Nations (UN) has named the period of 2021–2030 as The Decade of Healthy Aging, and one of the domains it has sought to prioritize

E. N. Alvarez (✉) · P. Amoroto
Department of Public Health, California State University, Los Angeles, Los Angeles, CA, USA
e-mail: evelyna@calstatela.edu; PAmoroto@ph.lacounty.gov

A. Garcia
Los Angeles County Department of Department of Health Services, Torrance, CA, USA
e-mail: agarcia230adc@dhs.lacounty.gov

M. Huerta
Molina Healthcare of California, Long Beach, CA, USA
e-mail: Marlene.Huerta@molinahealthcare.com

N. Asiamah et al. (eds.), *Sustainable Ageing*,
https://doi.org/10.1007/978-3-031-69475-2_9

as a research area is that of climate change at the intersection of aging in place. Aging in place is generally defined as the ability of older adults to maintain physical activity, good health, and independence, thus allowing them to thrive in their communities and homes (Pani-Harreman et al., 2021). In this chapter, the authors aim to connect this priority area of research with a campaign that aims to address climate change vulnerability in older adults.

The Los Angeles County Department of Public Health (LACDPH) has put forth its Cooling Centers campaign as a response to the demand for greater climate change resiliency strategies. However, there is a lack of research that has been done regarding Cooling Centers in Los Angeles County as well as on the effectiveness of the LACDPH campaign. This chapter aims to highlight previous research that has been done on Cooling Centers in Los Angeles County and in other major cities in the United States to further inform how future strategies and recommendations can be implemented in Cooling Centers in Los Angeles County and other counties aiming to utilize Cooling Centers as a climate change resiliency strategy that could promote aging in place.

This chapter first provides an overview on how Cooling Centers can be utilized as resiliency strategies and their implementation in major cities in the United States. The methods highlight the five main themes found in the literature concerning Cooling Centers and adjacent topics as well as the categorization of different types of Cooling Centers. The dearth in the literature regarding Cooling Centers leads to the proposition of a theoretical framework, the Cornell RTP Consensus Workshop model, as a strategy to bridge the gap between aging research and practice.

9.2 An Overview of Cooling Centers as a Climate Change Resiliency Campaign

Cooling Centers, areas identified by LACDPH, offer an air-conditioned place for residents to escape the heat during extreme heat events. Cooling Centers are largely composed of air-conditioned public libraries but also include air-conditioned recreational centers where community members can seek relief from extreme heat events. The utilization of Cooling Centers is not well understood; however, preliminary data suggest they are underutilized, and in one key example in New York State, 38% of counties reported that Cooling Centers are not a priority for them and neither do they promote them (Nayak et al., 2017). Furthermore, there is a dearth of research in the literature that examines their uptake. Only recently, a study examining smartphone location and Cooling Center usage found that only about 20% of the population utilize Cooling Centers in Los Angeles County (Derakhskan et al., 2023). Given the certainty of continued extreme heat events as a consequence of climate change (IPCC, 2022), it is essential to assess the coverage of Cooling Centers in the literature.

Cooling Centers are places that have been designated as areas that can provide shade and air conditioning to community members during extreme heat events. They were originally developed in response to the climate change crisis. Public areas with air conditioning accessibility, such as libraries, community centers, senior centers, churches, temples, synagogues, mosques, police stations, and schools, and others are selected by city and county officials and promoted as a cost-effective intervention to provide much-needed relief and protection during heat waves (Widerynski et al., 2017). Some of these cooling centers have also been utilized as places where medical services can be provided, in addition to fans and potable water, which are highly critical elements during heat waves, thereby revealing their potential public health co-benefits (Widerynski et al., 2017).

There has been some interest in investigating the methods by which Cooling Centers are placed in specific community areas. In one particular study regarding Cooling Centers, cities at higher latitudes were more prepared (as measured by cooling center population coverage) than cities at lower latitudes (Adams et al., 2023; Kim et al., 2021). There have been studies that have examined obstacles to accessing Cooling Centers to better gauge how to effectively promote their usage (Sampson et al., 2013; White-Newsome et al., 2014), but few have quantified the actual uptake of Cooling Centers in major US cities, such as Los Angeles. One notable aforementioned study has examined the utilization of Cooling Centers in New York City (Nayak et al., 2017). Over one-third of counties in New York State did not have Cooling Centers nor plans to designate Cooling Centers because they did not deem extreme heat events to be a threat in their area.

9.3 Methods

Using Cooling Centers, areas identified by local county health departments in the United States as places that offer an air-conditioned place for residents to escape the heat during extreme heat events as a case study, PubMed, Google Scholar, and OneSearch were searched for research articles regarding Cooling Centers and aging populations. The prevalent categories of Cooling Centers and themes related to aging in place helped to inform a framework that best illustrates this research-practice gap.

A preliminary search, utilizing the terms in Table 9.1, focused on Cooling Centers in Los Angeles County. This was done to capture both primary and secondary research concerning Cooling Centers specific to the Los Angeles County region. When the preliminary search indicated that there was a dearth of knowledge concerning this topic, a second search was then performed utilizing the terms in Table 9.2. The second search focused on Cooling Centers around the United States and globally in order to garner a better understanding of current and past literature surrounding Cooling Centers. The period that was covered for these searches was from February 2023 to February 2024. The authors anticipated a dearth of article coverage on the topic of Cooling Centers; therefore, inclusion criteria were flexible enough to include reports, review papers, and original research articles. All articles had to discuss Cooling Centers to some extent and those that did not were excluded if they were reflected in a search. The authors did not set any a priori themes, so Table 9.5 reflects themes that were observed after assessing each article.

Table 9.1 Overview of the search term combinations utilized regarding Cooling Centers in Los Angeles County

Cooling Centers in Los Angeles County Search Terms	Database
Cooling Center, Los Angeles	Onesearch
Cooling Centers in Los Angeles County	Onesearch
Scholarly articles on cooling Centers in Los Angeles	Google-UCLA
Cooling Centers in Los Angeles	Google Scholar
Electricity demand, extreme heat, climate change	Google Scholar

Table 9.2 Overview of the search term combinations utilized regarding Cooling Centers around the United States and globally

Cooling Centers General Search Terms	Database
Cooling Center	PubMed
Cooling Center utilization	PubMed
US cities, cooling center	Onesearch
Staying cool, heat events	Onesearch
Cooling Centers, heat event	Onesearch
Use of Cooling Centers	Onesearch
Cooling Center, public health	Onesearch
Cooling Center, heat wave	Onesearch
Cooling shelter	Onesearch
Cooling Center, heat wave	Onesearch
Cooling Center, extreme heat	Onesearch
Evidence based strategies, air conditioning, effective cooling solutions	PubMed

The Cornell Research-to-Practice (RTP) Consensus Workshop Model was examined in four articles that the program features in its advertisements (Pillemer et al., 2011a, b, 2015; Sabir et al., 2009). We used findings from Tables 9.3, 9.4, and 9.5 to inform an adapted model that aims to address the research-practice gap in Cooling Center utilization by older adults.

9.4 Findings

Figure 9.1 demonstrates the main themes found in the literature related to Cooling Centers in Los Angeles County and Cooling Centers in the United States and globally based on the data of Table 9.3. We identified five main coverage topics: Cooling Centers in Los Angeles County, Greenspace and Urban Planning, Comparison of Cooling Center Locations, Cooling Centers in other States, and Cooling Centers Globally. Most of the articles found corresponded to the categories, "Greenspace and Urban Planning" and "Cooling Centers in Other States," followed by "Los Angeles County Cooling Centers" and "Comparison of Cooling Center Locations,"

Table 9.3 The authors' compilation of primary topics of Cooling Centers in Los Angeles as depicted in the literature

Explicitly Mention LA County	Chu et al. (2021); Fraser et al. (2016, 2018); Hulley et al. (2019); Kalkstein et al. (2022); Derakhskan et al. (2023)
Comparison of major US cities	Kim et al. (2021); Jin and Sanders (2022); Sampson et al. (2013); Widerynski et al. (2017)
Green space/urban planning to combat adverse heat in the United States	Jin and Sanders (2022); Sampson et al. (2013); Widerynski et al. (2017); Sanchez and Reames (2019); Kalkstein et al. (2022); Shafiei Shiva et al. (2022); Jay et al. (2021)
Studies done in other countries	Woo et al. (2021); Yoon et al. (2022); Shafiei Shiva et al. (2022)
Cooling centers in other states	Berisha et al. (2017); Nayak et al. (2019); Mallen et al. (2022); Nayak et al. (2017); Voelkel et al. (2018); Hayden et al. (2017); Sanchez and Reames (2019)

Table 9.4 The authors' compilation of categories of Cooling Center types

Formal Cooling Centers	Derakhskan et al. (2023); Fraser et al. (2018); Woo et al. (2021); Yoon et al. (2022); Berisha et al. (2017); Kim et al. (2021); Jin and Sanders (2022); Nayak et al. (2019); Nayak et al. (2017); Mallen et al. (2022); Sanchez and Reames (2019); Voelkel et al. (2018); Hayden et al. (2017)
Informal cooling centers	Derakhskan et al. (2023); Woo et al. (2021); Yoon et al. (2022); Berisha et al. (2017); Kim et al. (2021); Jin and Sanders (2022); Sanchez and Reames (2019); Nayak et al. (2017); Nayak et al. (2019); Voelkel et al. (2018); Hayden et al. (2017)
Residential air conditioning	Fraser et al. (2016); Chu et al. (2021); Fraser et al. (2018); Jay et al. (2021); Berisha et al. (2017); Kim et al. (2021); Jin and Sanders (2022); Sampson et al. (2013); Sanchez and Reames (2019); Sanchez and Reames (2019); Mallen et al. (2022); Voelkel et al. (2018); Hayden et al. (2017)
Air-conditioned public space	Fraser et al. (2016); Woo et al. (2021); Yoon et al. (2022); Fraser et al. (2016); Hulley et al. (2019); Kalkstein et al. (2022)

Table 9.5 Article coverage of Cooling Centers and healthy aging (by common themes)

Accessibility	Fraser et al. (2016, 2018); Hulley et al. (2019); Woo et al. (2021); Yoon et al. (2022); Berisha et al. (2017); Kim et al. (2021); Jin and Sanders (2022); Sampson et al. (2013); Widerynski et al. (2017); Sanchez and Reames (2019); Nayak et al. (2017); Nayak et al. (2019); Mallen et al. (2022); Voelkel et al. (2018)
Dissemination of information	Chu et al. (2021); Jin and Sanders (2022); Widerynski et al. (2017); Sampson et al. (2013); Sampson et al. (2013); Nayak et al. (2017); Voelkel et al. (2018)
Equity	Chu et al. (2021); Kim et al. (2021); Sanchez and Reames (2019)
Urban green spaces	Chu et al. (2021); Hulley et al. (2019); Kalkstein et al. (2022); Shafiei Shiva et al. (2022); Jay et al. (2021); Jin and Sanders (2022); Widerynski et al. (2017); Sanchez and Reames (2019)

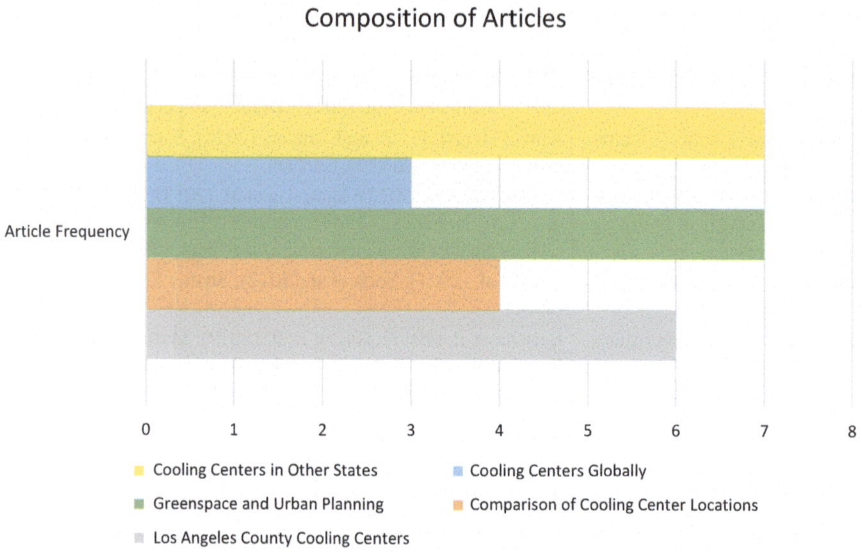

Fig. 9.1 Chart depicting themes and frequency found in the 23 articles

with the fewest in the category of "Greenspace and Urban Planning." Figure 9.1 is a visual representation of Table 9.3, which includes the authors' compilation of primary topics of Cooling Centers in Los Angeles as found in the literature.

Table 9.4 includes the authors' compilation of categories of Cooling Center types based on the literature. Most articles reviewed focused on *formal Cooling Centers*, such as specific public buildings designated as official city Cooling Centers (e.g., libraries, recreational centers, parks) and made some reference to *residential air conditioning* (air conditioning found in a home and not in a public space). *Informal Cooling Centers* (areas that are not officially recognized as Cooling Centers but are recommended as places to seek relief during extreme heat events) was the third most common category of Cooling Center, followed by *air-conditioned public spaces* (this is a category that could encapsulate *informal* and *formal Cooling Centers*).

Table 9.5 highlights article coverage of Cooling Centers and healthy aging (by common themes). The most common theme related to healthy aging was "accessibility" of Cooling Centers, followed by "urban green spaces," "dissemination of information," and "equity."

Figure 9.2 depicts a schematic where authors suggest Cooling Center planning should explicitly include discussion of older adults, in addition to ethnic minorities and low-socioeconomic (SES) populations.

Oftentimes, older adults are grouped in the category of "heat-vulnerable" populations without mention specifically of "older adults" who may have different needs than ethnic minorities and low-socioeconomic (SES) populations (and may overlap across categories). The language of campaigns such as that of Cooling Centers

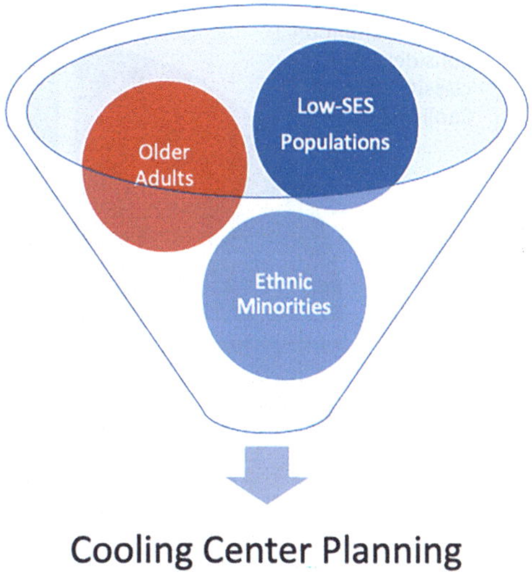

Fig. 9.2 The author's proposed emphasis of older adults as a priority population in Cooling Center planning

should reflect this. The authors' emphasis is to center older adults as a priority population in Cooling Center planning through the disaggregation of older adults apart from the larger category of heat-vulnerable populations. Distinctly recognizing older adults as a priority population with unique and heightened vulnerabilities at times of extreme heat is critical if intentional outreach and interventions are to be done (Benmarhnia et al., 2015). The language of campaigns such as that of Cooling Centers should reflect this, by way of tailoring and reframing messaging that emphasizes specialized support and accommodations based on age-related challenges that can be both physical and cognitive. Moreover, the authors also push to integrate older adults as main collaborators in Cooling Center Planning as consideration to the population's self-perceived vulnerability and what defines their needs in extreme heat events. Ultimately, the goal is to facilitate knowledge sharing between research entities, local governance, and older adult participants in proposing better Cooling Center planning frameworks and processes.

9.5 Integration of Theoretical Framework

The RTP Consensus Workshop Model integrates a theoretical framework by fostering interdisciplinary discussions between aging researchers and clinicians, facilitating the translation of research findings into effective practices to improve care for older adults. With the threat of climate change continuing to pose disproportionate public health challenges to the notion of aging in place, it is imperative that evidence is translated into practice. The sustainability of healthy aging research and its funding in contexts addressing crises depend on bridging the gap between research and practice. The RTP Consensus Workshop Model helps us better understand the

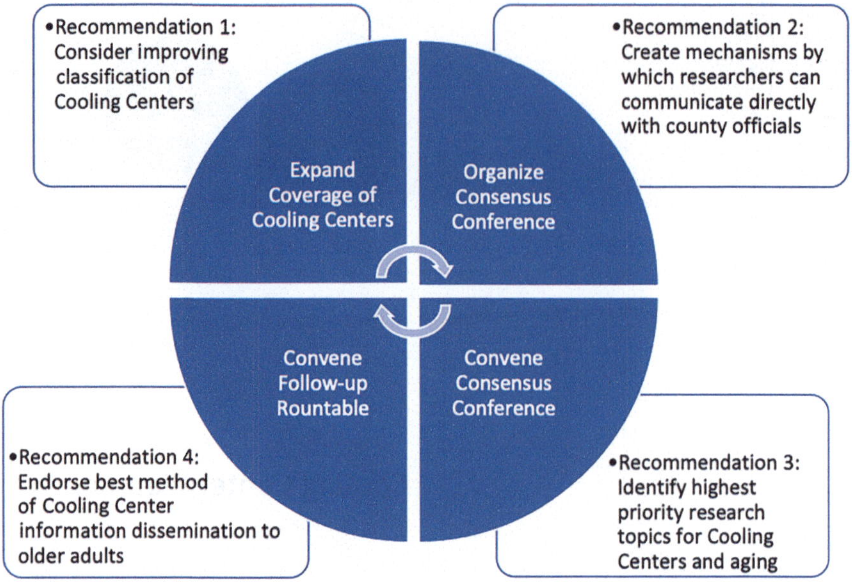

Fig. 9.3 The author's proposed application of the Cornell RTP Consensus Workshop Model to the Cooling Centers campaign case study

obstacles and solutions related to aging and climate change. By using this model, we can gain valuable insights into which barriers and strategies should be given priority and focus. It works mainly by facilitating learning about the challenges of a given topic, in this case aging and climate change, and enables participants to gain insights into the barriers and information surrounding both issues.

The RTP Consensus Workshop Model is a proposed strategy to bridge the gap between aging research and practice by promoting a conference or workshop environment to ignite discussions between researchers and clinicians in the area of aging (Black et al., 1999; Brownson et al., 2023). To date, the model has been applied to a wide range of aging topics of interest including older adult mistreatment and palliative care (Pillemer et al., 2011a, 2015). Figure 9.3 illustrates our adaptation of the RTP Consensus Workshop Model within the context of Cooling Centers and aging in place. We used Tables 9.3, 9.4, and 9.5 to inform which categories and common themes to prioritize. We chose to showcase "dissemination" of Cooling Center information because although "equity" is the least covered theme in regard to Cooling Centers and healthy aging, its amorphous aspect does not make it immediately actionable and rendering of a deliverable. Instead, we included "dissemination" because it is a concrete, measurable outcome. This model offers valuable insights into prioritizing barriers and strategies, as evidenced by its application to research on Cooling Centers and healthy aging, where the emphasis on "dissemination" was selected for its tangible and quantifiable attributes. The model also contributes to sustainability in this research by providing a structured framework for identifying and addressing barriers and strategies in an iterative fashion. Its application in studying Cooling Centers and healthy aging, particularly focusing on "dissemination," underscores the importance of viewing sustainability through measurable outcomes, ensuring that the insights gained can be implemented and evaluated over time to support ongoing efforts in promoting healthy aging initiatives.

Recommendation 1 Since our search revealed a dearth of research on Cooling Centers, and more specifically on Cooling Centers and healthy aging, it is imperative that counties expand their classification of Cooling Centers, which would result in more of them being available. This recommendation is born from the finding that only 20% of the population in Los Angeles County use Cooling Centers. Counties should explore converting emptier air-conditioned public buildings to Cooling Centers or partnering with other air-conditioned businesses to offer those sites as Cooling Center options during the off-time.

Recommendation 2 Across all four articles on the RTP Consensus Workshop Model we examined, creating mechanisms by which researchers and practitioners could communicate was critical. In adapting the model, we suggest counties create mechanisms by which researchers and county officials can directly communicate. This can be achieved by organizing consensus workshops where both parties can discuss how best to address the research-practice gap between Cooling Centers research and their utilization.

Recommendation 3 To identify the most important priority research topic areas for Cooling Centers and healthy aging, it is recommended to convene a consensus conference so county officials, researchers, and older adults can come together to discuss.

Recommendation 4 After a consensus conference, it is recommended to convene a follow-up roundtable that focuses on one key priority area that is identified during the consensus conference. In this example, we use our findings from Table 9.5. This proposed framework adaptation can be easily adopted by counties to address and improve Cooling Center utilization by older adults.

In the circle, each wedge represents a way that a county can address each recommendation. The arrows indicate the directionality of each "way" to address each recommendation. The RTP model emphasizes community-based participatory research critique and review of an issue critical to a particular community (Sabir et al., 2009). The author's proposed application of the RTP Model to the Cooling Centers campaign case study emphasizes mutual learning and translational science. The aim is to inform Cooling Center policy and practice by way of interdisciplinary collaboration. The RTP model builds on collaborative problem solving and knowledge exchange with critical recommendations carefully compartmentalized in wedges. It follows a structured timeline and process, each building upon the other, synthesizing ideas and perspectives through convening and consensus building of critical stakeholders involved: researchers, LA County officials, and older adults. The RTP model, as adapted here, focuses on dialogue and deliberation with all parties involved. It coalesces the collaborative capacities of key players with corresponding research exemplifying an iterative process and feedback loop that can eventually be used to evaluate outcomes. The authors believe that through this, Cooling Centers, as social infrastructures, can better uphold extreme heat resilience for older adults and thus support aging in place.

9.6 Recommendations for Increasing Accessibility in Cooling Centers

There has been a significant increase in the number of older adults that utilize wheelchairs in the United States (Nie et al., 2024). Therefore, wheelchair accessibility in Cooling Centers is integral for the aging population. Research done on Cooling Centers in New York City found that 22% of the Senior Centers that are utilized as Cooling Centers did not have wheelchair access (Bureau of Policy and Research, 2022). Simply ensuring that Cooling Centers are wheelchair accessible will enable the aging population to access these facilities during adverse heat events. An additional recommendation could be made to ensure that bathrooms in places that are designated as Cooling Centers have appropriate hand rails and spaces for increased wheelchair accessibility given the older populations that are intended to make use of them.

9.7 Future Research

Due to climate change, extreme heat events in Los Angeles County will be common occurrences. Therefore, future research on accessibility and designation of Cooling Centers is pertinent to the health of heat-vulnerable populations, including low-income minorities living inland and older adults who may have co-morbidities and lack access to air-conditioning in their homes. Similar research has been done in the state of New York and can pose as a framework for future research regarding Cooling Centers in Los Angeles County (Nayak et al., 2019). If Cooling Centers are to be provided as a cost-effective, city-wide intervention during extreme heat-related events, their accessibility and utility must be critically examined in the literature.

A new, promising area of interest is the promotion of urban green spaces. This could offer an additional type of unofficial Cooling Center to be launched as a campaign targeted at older adults. Urban green spaces have been proven to significantly affect temperatures and spaces in urban heat islands (Aram et al., 2019). Understanding that Cooling Centers require energy, staff, and facilities, heat mitigation strategies such as green space innovations can more naturally serve to keep Los Angeles County residents cool during heat waves by minimizing heat in residential homes and outdoor areas. Furthermore, green spaces have co-benefits in that they provide heat relief and shade in addition to aesthetic value.

9.8 Implications for Aging and Policy

At the local, state, and federal levels, the government has developed measures to help protect individuals at high risk of exposure to heat. The government works to see who is at risk of exposure during extreme heat waves. Some criteria are taken into account to protect vulnerable individuals at the local level. Strategic planning efforts take place by the government to provide Cooling Centers as resources to support high-risk populations and minimize heat-related illnesses, but the efforts are not specifically tailored to older adults' needs, which presents a missed opportunity in this decade of healthy aging.

Accessibility to Cooling Centers is not the most significant barrier faced by high-risk, vulnerable populations like older adults. How the local government disseminates information on Cooling Centers can affect accessibility and utilization among at-risk populations, which is why we decided to include dissemination of information in our proposed application of the RTP Model. Navigating Cooling Centers can be difficult for individuals aged 65 or older based on their census tract vulnerability (Kim et al., 2021). The dissemination of information regarding Cooling Centers must be increased to bring awareness to vulnerable communities (e.g., aged 65 or older) during extreme heat waves. This will allow for a decrease in hospitalization and deaths among vulnerable communities. There also needs to be more funding and improvement in media and outreach on how to access these Cooling Centers in low-income communities.

9.9 Limitations

There is limited data on how many individuals access Cooling Centers each year. There is a notable lack of literature assessing the uptake and effectiveness of Cooling Centers. There needs to be more transparency of data related to Cooling Centers to evaluate and improve them for high-risk populations' accessibility (such as older adults) and utilization in Los Angeles County and beyond. Additionally, an evaluation effort can enhance the operation of Cooling Centers in Los Angeles County by assessing what is working well and addressing what is not.

Additional limitations include not capturing all potential surrogate terms for Cooling Centers as well as using a theoretical framework application as reported in the literature without enrolling in the program (subject to fees). As such, we relied on peer-reviewed articles to learn how to apply and subsequently adapt it for our Cooling Centers case study. Many of the studies that utilize the RTP model need to provide more specificity and details around the framework so that the scientific community can better understand this tool. Relying on the dearth of details reported in the literature hindered us from being able to apply the model to our case study in more complex ways. Our lists in Tables 9.3, 9.4, and 9.5 may not fully represent an exhaustive list as Web of Science and Scopus were omitted from our search. Lastly, this chapter did not follow a rigorous protocol such as the Joanna Briggs Institute checklist tool; therefore, as more research on Cooling Centers is published, it is imperative to use such robust tools to evaluate this growing body of research.

9.10 Conclusions

We conducted a search in the literature for multiple combinations of terms related to Cooling Centers and aging and examined the literature for commonalities in Cooling Centers categories and common themes that incorporated healthy aging. We then used those findings in applying the strengths of the Cornell RTP Consensus Workshop Model, as depicted in the literature, to the case study of Cooling Centers as a climate change resiliency strategy. This chapter provides an adapted framework application that counties can leverage when discussing best practices to connect older adults with public health campaigns, such as those related to Cooling Centers.

A model for bridging this gap is novel and timely given the urgency to continue healthy aging research as existing crises such as climate change are exacerbated by emerging threats like pandemics. A community that embodies healthy aging is a community that does so in the face of climate change. By capturing and synthesizing evidence-based recommendations in the area of Cooling Centers and connecting them to their subsequent practice or lack thereof, we make a critical contribution to the goals of aging in place research. Furthermore, this is also a call to action to ensure that the promotion and creation of Cooling Centers are in concert with evidence-based actions. Ultimately, if our universal goal is to promote healthy aging in times of crises such as climate change, campaigns and interventions like Cooling Centers must be implemented in concert with evidence-based practices. Additionally, the research loop must also be closed by subsequently evaluating their effectiveness. Given how Cooling Centers can be a critical tool for aging populations in times of climate change and how older adults are at higher risk of heatwave morbidity and mortality, it is imperative that the research-practice gap is addressed and that steps are taken to mitigate the disproportionate public health impacts of climate change on aging populations.

Review Questions

1. In what ways does climate change impact healthy aging?
2. What are Cooling Centers and how do they relate to climate change?
3. How do Cooling Centers campaigns and climate change relate to the United Nations Decade of Healthy Ageing (2021–2030)?
4. Describe how Cooling Centers campaigns can be leveraged to promote healthy aging.

5. Describe the two most dominant topics of Cooling Centers specifically addressing Los Angeles County.

References

Adams, Q. H., Chan, E. M. G., Spangler, K. R., Weinberger, K. R., Lane, K. J., Errett, N. A., et al. (2023). Examining the optimal placement of cooling centers to serve populations at high risk of extreme heat exposure in 81 US cities. *Public Health Reports, 333549221148174*, 955. https://doi.org/10.1177/00333549221148174

Aram, F., Higueras García, E., Solgi, E., & Mansournia, S. (2019). Urban green space cooling effect in cities. *Heliyon, 5*(4), e01339. https://doi.org/10.1016/j.heliyon.2019.e01339

Benmarhnia, T., Deguen, S., Kaufman, J. S., & Smargiassi, A. (2015). Review article: Vulnerability to heat-related mortality: A systematic review, meta-analysis, and meta-regression analysis. *Epidemiology, 26*(6), 781–793. https://doi.org/10.1097/EDE.0000000000000375

Berisha, V., Hondula, D., Roach, M., White, J. R., McKinney, B., Bentz, D., et al. (2017). Assessing adaptation strategies for extreme heat: A public health evaluation of cooling centers in Maricopa County, Arizona. *Weather, Climate, and Society, 9*(1), 71–80. https://doi.org/10.1175/WCAS-D-16-0033.1

Black, N., Murphy, M., Lamping, D., McKee, M., Sanderson, C., Askham, J., & Marteau, T. (1999). Consensus development methods: A review of best practice in creating clinical guidelines. *Journal of Health Services Research & Policy, 4*(4), 236–248. https://doi.org/10.1177/135581969900400410

Brownson, R. C., Colditz, G. A., & Proctor, E. K. (2023). *Dissemination and implementation research in health : Translating science to practice* (3rd ed.). Oxford University Press.

Bureau of Policy and Research. (2022). *Overheated, underserved: Expanding cooling center access*. https://comptroller.nyc.gov/reports/overheated-underserved/

Chu, H., Adams, J., Li, J., & Goldmuntz, S. (2021). *Equity-focused heat adaptation strategies for Los Angeles County*. L. A. C. O. o. E. M. UCLA Luskin Center for Innovation. https://innovation.luskin.ucla.edu/wp-content/uploads/2021/06/Equity-Focused-Heat-Adaptation-Strategies-for-LA-County.pdf

Derakhskan, S., Bautista, T. N., Bouwman, M., Huang, L., Lee, L., Tarczynski, J., et al. (2023). Smartphones reveal patterns of cooling center use as a heat mitigation strategy. *Applied Geography, 150*, 102821. https://doi.org/10.1016/j.apgeog.2022.102821

Fraser, A. M., Chester, M. V., Eisenman, D., Hondula, D. M., Pincetl, S. S., English, P., & Bondank, E. (2016). Household accessibility to heat refuges: Residential air conditioning, public cooled space, and walkability. *Environment and Planning B: Urban Analytics and City Science, 44*(6), 1036–1055. https://doi.org/10.1177/0265813516657342

Fraser, A. M., Chester, M. V., & Eisenman, D. (2018). Strategic locating of refuges for extreme heat events (or heat waves). *Urban Climate, 25*, 109–119. https://doi.org/10.1016/j.uclim.2018.04.009

Hayden, M. H., Wilhelmi, O. V., Banerjee, D., Greasby, T., Cavanaugh, J. L., Nepal, V., et al. (2017). Adaptive capacity to extreme heat: Results from a household survey in Houston, Texas. *Weather, Climate, and Society, 9*(4), 787–799. https://doi.org/10.1175/WCAS-D-16-0125.1

Hulley, G., Shivers, S., Wetherley, E., & Cudd, R. (2019). New ECOSTRESS and MODIS land surface temperature data reveal fine-scale heat vulnerability in cities: A case study for Los Angeles County, California. *Remote Sensing, 11*(18) https://www.mdpi.com/2072-4292/11/18/2136

IPCC. (2022). In H.-O. Pörtner, D. C. Roberts, M. Tignor, E. S. Poloczanska, K. Mintenbeck, A. Alegría, M. Craig, S. Langsdorf, S. Löschke, V. Möller, A. Okem, & B. Rama (Eds.), *Climate change 2022: Impacts, adaptation, and vulnerability. Contribution of Working Group II to the Sixth Assessment Report of the Intergovernmental Panel on Climate Change*. Cambridge University Press. https://doi.org/10.1017/9781009325844

Jay, O., Capon, A., Berry, P., Broderick, C., de Dear, R., Havenith, G., et al. (2021). Reducing the health effects of hot weather and heat extremes: From personal cooling strategies to green cities. *The Lancet, 398*(10301), 709–724. https://doi.org/10.1016/S0140-6736(21)01209-5

Jin, A. S., & Sanders, K. T. (2022). Analyzing changes to U.S. municipal heat response plans during the COVID-19 pandemic. *Environmental Science & Policy, 128*, 347–358. https://doi.org/10.1016/j.envsci.2021.11.022

Kalkstein, L. S., Eisenman, D. P., de Guzman, E. B., & Sailor, D. J. (2022). Increasing trees and high-albedo surfaces decreases heat impacts and mortality in Los Angeles, CA. *International Journal of Biometeorology, 66*(5), 911–925. https://doi.org/10.1007/s00484-022-02248-8

Kim, K., Jung, J., Schollaert, C., & Spector, J. T. (2021). A comparative assessment of cooling center preparedness across twenty-five U.S. Cities. *International Journal of Environmental Research and Public Health, 18*(9). https://doi.org/10.3390/ijerph18094801

Mallen, E., Roach, M., Fox, L., Gillespie, E., Watkins, L., Hondula, D. M., et al. (2022, 2022/06/17/). Extreme heat exposure: Access and Barriers to Cooling Centers–Maricopa and Yuma Counties, Arizona, 2010-2020. *Morbidity and Mortality Weekly Report*, 781+. https://link-gale-com.mimas.calstatela.edu/apps/doc/A708169780/AONE?u=calstate&sid=bookmark-AONE&xid=a6bd6225

Nayak, S. G., Lin, S., Sheridan, S. C., Lu, Y., Graber, N., Primeau, M., et al. (2017). Surveying local health departments and county emergency management offices on cooling centers as a heat adaptation resource in New York State. *Journal of Community Health, 42*(1), 43–50. https://doi.org/10.1007/s10900-016-0224-4

Nayak, S. G., Shrestha, S., Sheridan, S. C., Hsu, W.-H., Muscatiello, N. A., Pantea, C. I., et al. (2019). Accessibility of cooling centers to heat-vulnerable populations in New York State. *Journal of Transport & Health, 14*, 100563. https://doi.org/10.1016/j.jth.2019.05.002

Nie, Q., Rice, L. A., Sosnoff, J. J., Shen, S., & Rogers, W. A. (2024). Understanding wheelchair use in older adults from the National Health and aging trends study. *Archives of Physical Medicine and Rehabilitation, 105*(3), 514–524. https://doi.org/10.1016/j.apmr.2023.09.006

Pani-Harreman, K. E., Bours, G. J. J. W., Zander, I., Kempen, G. I. J. M., & van Duren, J. M. A. (2021). Definitions, key themes and aspects of 'ageing in place': A scoping review. *Ageing and Society, 41*(9), 2026–2059. https://doi.org/10.1017/S0144686X20000094

Pillemer, K., Breckman, R., Sweeney, C. D., Brownell, P., Fulmer, T., Berman, J., et al. (2011a). Practitioners' views on elder mistreatment research priorities: Recommendations from a research-to-practice consensus conference. *Journal of Elder Abuse & Neglect, 23*(2), 115–126. https://doi.org/10.1080/08946566.2011.558777

Pillemer, K., Wells, N. M., Wagenet, L. P., Meador, R. H., & Parise, J. T. (2011b). Environmental sustainability in an aging society: A research agenda. *Journal of Aging and Health, 23*(3), 433–453. https://doi.org/10.1177/0898264310381278

Pillemer, K., Chen, E. K., Riffin, C., Prigerson, H., & Reid, M. C. (2015). Practice-based research priorities for palliative care: Results from a research-to-practice consensus workshop. *American Journal of Public Health, 105*(11), 2237–2244. https://doi.org/10.2105/AJPH.2015.302675

Sabir, M., Wethington, E., Breckman, R., Meador, R., Reid, M. C., & Pillemer, K. (2009). A community-based participatory critique of social isolation intervention research for community-dwelling older adults. *Journal of Applied Gerontology, 28*(2), 218–234. https://doi.org/10.1177/0733464808326004

Sampson, N. R., Gronlund, C. J., Buxton, M. A., Catalano, L., White-Newsome, J. L., Conlon, K. C., et al. (2013). Staying cool in a changing climate: Reaching vulnerable populations during heat events. *Global Environmental Change, 23*(2), 475–484. https://doi.org/10.1016/j.gloenvcha.2012.12.011

Sanchez, L., & Reames, T. G. (2019). Cooling Detroit: A socio-spatial analysis of equity in green roofs as an urban heat Island mitigation strategy. *Urban Forestry & Urban Greening, 44*, 126331. https://doi.org/10.1016/j.ufug.2019.04.014

Shafiei Shiva, J., Chandler, D. G., & Kunkel, K. E. (2022). Mapping heat wave Hazard in urban areas: A novel multi-criteria decision making approach. *Atmosphere, 13*(7) https://www.mdpi.com/2073-4433/13/7/1037

Voelkel, J., Hellman, D., Sakuma, R., & Shandas, V. (2018). Assessing vulnerability to urban heat: A study of disproportionate heat exposure and access to refuge by socio-demographic status in Portland, Oregon. *International Journal of Environmental Research and Public Health, 15*(4) https://www.mdpi.com/1660-4601/15/4/640

White-Newsome, J. L., McCormick, S., Sampson, N., Buxton, M. A., O'Neill, M. S., Gronlund, C. J., et al. (2014). Strategies to reduce the harmful effects of extreme heat events: A four-city study. *International Journal of Environmental Research and Public Health, 11*(2), 1960–1988. https://doi.org/10.3390/ijerph110201960

Widerynski, S., Schramm, P., Conlon, K., Noe, R., Grossman, E., Hawkins, M., et al. (2017). *The use of cooling centers to prevent heat-related illness: Summary of evidence and strategies for implementation climate and health technical report series climate and health program*. Centers for Disease Control and Prevention. https://doi.org/10.13140/RG.2.2.32267.59688

Woo, S., Yoon, S., Kim, J., Hwang, S. W., & Kweon, S. J. (2021). Optimal cooling shelter assignment during heat waves using real-time mobile-based floating population data. *Urban Climate, 38*, 100874. https://doi.org/10.1016/j.uclim.2021.100874

Yoon, S., Woo, S., Kim, J., Hwang, S. W., & Kweon, S. J. (2022). The location routing problem for cooling shelters during heat waves. *Urban Climate, 44*, 101138. https://doi.org/10.1016/j.uclim.2022.101138

Chapter 10
An Evaluation of the Financing of Healthy Aging Through the Lens of Social Welfare: Healthy Aging Index

Özge Kutlu and Mehmet Öçal

Acronyms and Abbreviations

EU	European Union
GDP	Gross Domestic Product
HAI	Healthy Aging Index
PPS	Purchasing Power Standard
SDG	Sustainable Development Goals
UN	United Nations
WHO	World Health Organization

10.1 Introduction

Discussions about the aging demographic structure have increased in recent years. These discussions address issues such as how the aging population affects the demographic structure and how social services and health systems can adapt to this change (Fried & Rowe, 2020). As the world population ages rapidly, it brings with it the need for social transformation at many levels regarding health, retirement, migration, and social services (Lee et al., 2023). However, the effects of global

Ö. Kutlu (✉)
Elderly Care Program, Çavdır Vocational School, Burdur Mehmet Akif Ersoy University, Burdur, Türkiye
e-mail: okutlu@mehmetakif.edu.tr

M. Öçal
Department of Social Work, Faculty of Economics and Administrative Sciences, Burdur Mehmet Akif Ersoy University, Burdur, Türkiye
e-mail: mocal@mehmetakif.edu.tr

N. Asiamah et al. (eds.), *Sustainable Ageing*,
https://doi.org/10.1007/978-3-031-69475-2_10

crises such as pandemics, migrations, and climate change on older people population are attracting increasing attention (Carmody et al., 2021). International organizations such as the United Nations (UN) undertake policy-making and guidance roles on these issues. In particular, fundamental problems such as exclusion, discrimination, and inequality are among the issues that need to be addressed in the international arena (Hallegatte & Rozenberg, 2017). Older adults often face discrimination in various situations due to their age, such as in the workplace, where they may be overlooked for promotions, in healthcare settings, where their medical needs are frequently underestimated, and in social services, where they may receive less support compared to younger individuals.

Studies have shown that older adults face significant age discrimination, as evidenced by their reduced employment opportunities and lower quality of healthcare services, leading to poorer health outcomes compared to younger age groups. This widespread discrimination not only marginalizes older adults but also has broader societal impacts, including increased healthcare costs and underutilization of a potentially active workforce (Nelson, 2017; Molina-Luque et al., 2022; Rippon et al., 2013; Pak et al., 2022; Dobrowolska et al., 2019). The UN and other international organizations strive to develop policy recommendations and frameworks to solve problems shaped by discrimination. The aim of this effort made by international organizations is to ensure that the aging population lives a positive and healthy life, to protect the rights of elderly individuals and to minimize the effects of the aging process on societies. The United Nations' Decade of Healthy Ageing 2021–2030 is one of the international efforts to highlight the importance of aging and call for action. The aim of this program is to increase the social and individual importance of aging, create urgency for the development of aging-related policies and practices, and create change to turn population aging into an opportunity rather than a challenge (WHO, 2020).

The concept of healthy aging includes a lifestyle in which people of all ages can be healthy, safe, and socially active, and also has a holistic view focusing on a productive aging process (Demirtaş et al., 2017). The concept of healthy aging, which emphasizes the participation of older people in social life, is based on a balanced and healthy diet during old age, physical and social activity, avoiding addictions, regular treatment of diseases, correct use of medications, and protecting older people from loneliness and stress by supporting them socially. Supporting older people so that they do not lose their social functionality is among the goals of the approach. As a matter of fact, the participation of older adults in life in socio-economic, cultural, and political areas is possible with healthy aging (Öz, 2002). The World Health Organization (WHO) has defined healthy aging as the process of maintaining functional ability to ensure well-being in older ages (WHO, 2020; Rudnicka et al., 2020). As understood from this definition, well-being is one of the basic elements of healthy aging. Factors that increase well-being, such as education, economic security, and social support systems, are essential because they help individuals protect and improve their health (Livingston et al., 2022). For instance, higher levels of education correlate with better health literacy, enabling individuals to make informed decisions about their healthcare and lifestyle (Van den Broucke & Renwart, 2014).

Additionally, economic security provides the necessary resources for accessing quality healthcare services and maintaining a healthy diet (Vaudin et al., 2022). Social support systems offer not only emotional reassurance but also practical help in managing health challenges, which can significantly alleviate stress and improve overall well-being (Panayiotou & Karekla, 2013). Collectively, these factors contribute to a healthier, more resilient society. The concept of well-being is equated with "good life" and is defined as the total universe of human living spaces (WHO, 2015). Ensuring well-being includes the social, emotional, and mental needs of older adults in addition to their physical health. Meeting these needs is important to increase the participation of older adults in society, prevent social isolation, improve quality of life, and make older people feel valuable and active. Because of its positioning as an outcome of healthy aging, well-being becomes central to determining the success of the Decade of Healthy Ageing actions (Keating, 2022).

Although the Decade of Healthy Ageing actions serves as a global guide for the healthy aging of the aging population, population aging varies in different regions of the world. Different demographic aging rates in different regions affect economic systems, especially in developed countries, where faster population aging increases retirement costs and causes difficulties in labor markets. Regions with more elderly populations require more long-term care services, which put pressure on healthcare systems and family structures. The aging population also affects consumption habits and market demands. In addition, the aging population has a significant impact on the planning of health systems and the provision of health services. Another area affected by the aging of the population is the labor market. The aging population affects labor force participation rates and changes the balance of demand and supply in labor markets. Differences in aging rates in different parts of the world can have various effects in economic, social, cultural, and health areas. In this context, it is a fact that the world is aging, but this aging shows contextual differences. At this point, it is important to understand to what extent healthy aging can be achieved in different contexts of the world in order for the Decade of Healthy Ageing actions to become functional as a global guide. As a matter of fact, one of the four main action areas specified in the Decade of Healthy Ageing Program is the development of measurement tools for healthy aging and obtaining comparable data across countries (WHO, 2020). The lack of any reference criteria to measure and evaluate healthy aging makes it difficult to compare research and studies on aging (Lara et al., 2015; Michel & Sadana, 2017).

In this chapter, the "Healthy Aging Index" (HAI) has been developed based on the parameters related to healthy aging. The aim of the developed index is to develop a new set of healthy aging indicators in which global data are integrated. The Healthy Aging Index can be used to better understand the effects of aging on health and well-being and to monitor the aging process in different geographic regions, different socioeconomic groups, and different age groups. The developed index is an important step toward advancing research and policy development in the field of healthy aging. As a matter of fact, developing healthy aging indicators and increasing their availability contribute to improving the health and well-being of older adults and reducing the effects of the aging process on societies.

This book chapter discusses in detail the process of population aging and the evaluation of the financing of the concept of healthy aging in terms of social welfare. The introduction section focuses on the importance of healthy aging and the reasons for examining this subject. In the first part, the demographic dynamics of the aging population and the concept of healthy aging are explained comprehensively. In the methodology section, details of how the Healthy Aging Index was created and what statistical analyses were used are presented. While the results section includes analysis of the data obtained, the discussion section focuses on what these results mean, ways to measure healthy aging, and how healthy aging may vary in different contexts. The chapter concludes by evaluating the limitations and strengths of the research and emphasizing the broader significance of the findings. This chapter provides information that may influence the funding and policy-making processes of studies on healthy aging, thereby guiding readers in developing strategies to improve the well-being of older people.

10.2 Population Aging and the Concept of Healthy Aging

Population aging is a global phenomenon. One of the theories used to explain how changes in the population structure of societies affect their social and economic structures is the theory of demographic transformation. The theory of demographic transformation, put forward in the 1970s, refers to the transformation of high fertility and death rates into low fertility and death rates (Timonen, 2008). According to this theory, demographic transformation begins as a result of decreasing death rates and increasing life expectancy worldwide. According to World Population Prospects (2022), the proportion of people aged 65 and over is projected to increase globally between 2022 and 2050. In 2022, approximately 10% of people in the world will be 65 years or older. It is estimated that the proportion of elderly people in the world will reach approximately 12% in 2030 and 16% in 2050. Projections show that by 2050, one in four people in Europe and North America could be aged 65 or over (United Nations, 2022). Table 10.1 shows the population rate and projections of people aged 65 or older for the world and the Sustainable Development Goals (SDG) regions (United Nations, 2022).

Table 10.1 Percentage of population aged 65 years or over for the World and SDG regions

Region	2022	2030	2050
World	**9.7**	**11.7**	**16.4**
Sub-Saharan Africa	3.0	3.3	4.7
Northern Africa and Western Asia	5.5	7.0	12.5
Central and Southern Asia	6.4	8.1	13.4
Eastern and South-Eastern Asia	12.7	16.3	25.7
Latin America and the Caribbean	9.1	11.5	18.8
Australia/New Zealand	16.6	19.4	23.7
Oceania (excluding Australia and New Zealand)	3.9	5.1	8.2
Europe and Northern America	18.7	22.0	26.9

Current demographic trends in the world show that global population growth is accelerating in various countries and older people population constitutes the largest part of this increase (Alexandre et al., 2005; WHO, 2020). In response to these dramatic changes in demographics, the United Nations has declared 2021–2030 as the "Decade of Healthy Ageing." This initiative, supported by the United Nations and the World Health Organization, works to enhance the health and well-being of older populations globally. International efforts during this decade have focused on developing aging-related policies and improving health services to enhance the quality of life for older people. During this decade, reports addressing various issues related to aging are published, events are held, and policy recommendations are presented. The Decade of Healthy Ageing aims to promote collaboration between societies, governments, non-governmental organizations, and other stakeholders to improve the health and well-being of older people population (World Health Organization, 2020). This initiative focuses on intersectoral collaboration to ensure that older individuals maintain optimal functionality throughout their lives, regardless of their gender and socioeconomic status (Rugel et al., 2022).

Population aging affects every aspect of society, from health to social security, education, job opportunities, and family life. Nowadays, policies and programs regarding aging focus on improving quality of life and general health. Organizing sustainable policies for older people for healthy and active older adults in society, taking measures in health and social security systems that take into account demographic changes in the population, and adapting education and employment policies to these changes are the elements that national and international organizations have made a focal point in response to the aging population. The concept of active aging was adopted by the World Health Organization after the 1990s (Malderen et al., 2013; Mendes, 2013). The World Health Organization has defined active aging as the process of maximizing people's opportunities for health, participation, and safety to improve their quality of life as they age (WHO, 2002). Active aging enables individuals to realize their physical, social, and mental well-being potential throughout life from an early age and to participate in society, while providing them with adequate protection, security, and care when they need it. After the active aging policies developed in 2002, the concept of healthy aging became the focus of aging studies for the years 2015–2030 and replaced active aging. Healthy aging, like active aging, emphasizes the ability of older individuals to be active in a way that enables them to contribute to their families, societies, and economies.

Although most definitions of healthy aging focus on preserving individual capacities by reducing risky behaviors and supporting chronic disease management, built (Tuckett et al., 2018; Garin et al., 2014), natural (de Kaijzer et al., 2020; Kabisch et al., 2017), and social environments (Clarke & Nieuwenhuijsen, 2009) all play an important role in healthy aging. The World Health Organization defines healthy aging as "the process of developing and maintaining functions that ensure well-being in later ages" (WHO, 2015; Michel & Sadana, 2017;Fallon & Karlawish, 2019). Functioning refers to the abilities that enable individuals to do the things they value and live as independently as possible. These abilities include being able to meet basic needs, decision-making ability, mobility, establishing and maintaining relationships, and contributing to society (Beard et al., 2016). In other words, functionality consists of the individual's internal capacity, environmental characteristics, and the interactions between them (Beard et al., 2017). Intrinsic capacity includes the mental and physical capacities of the individual, while environmental characteristics relate to the home, community, and society in general. These interactions enable individuals to function healthily and maintain their quality of life during old age. Living in environments that support and protect internal capacity and functionality is the key to healthy aging (WHO, 2015).

10.3 Methods

The main research question is "can welfare regimes be categorised within the framework of social protection for older people?" In order to find an answer to this question, the Healthy Aging Index was developed within the scope of the research. Healthy aging is a process caused by many factors. An individual's living standards are among the most important components of healthy aging. Individual's living standards are closely related to the social state and social policy. The social state and its foundation, social policy, play a pivotal role in humanizing capitalism's perspective on people by providing a framework that prioritizes social welfare and equity. In essence, they serve as the cornerstone of a system where the well-being and dignity of individuals are upheld alongside economic interests. The social state, based on social policy described as a humanitarian quest, provides a guarantor for a life worthy of human dignity for all individuals. In fact, the social state is a shield that protects individuals from the market. The negative impact of the capitalist market on human welfare is tried to be limited by the social policies put forward by the social state. The social state draws "red lines" on the market and tries to prevent going beyond these lines with a corporatist style of action. These red lines appear as prohibitions, obligations, and incentives in every field that concerns human welfare. For example, in working life, minimum wage refers to the lowest wage that can be given to an employee and prohibits paying lower wages. In addition, the employment obligation of disabled and ex-convict individuals can be cited as an example of encouraging social inclusion (Öçal & Kutlu, 2023; Alcock et al., 2011).

Healthy aging is one of the most important social policy actions of States that define themselves as a social state and have accepted to compromise for the well-being and welfare of individuals. Achieving healthy aging, which has a significant impact on social welfare, is today defined as a basic social state duty. Although promoting healthy aging is considered a fundamental responsibility of the social state, variations in welfare regime typologies lead to differences in the degree, intensity, and scope of social policies among States. Differences in the political, economic, and socio-cultural values and traditions of States differentiate the social policies implemented by States. Although the actions implemented are essentially implemented for human welfare and are described as social policies, the levels of these social policies vary due to the emphasized variables. In short, the social policies implemented by States regarding healthy aging vary. There is no clear indication as to which state attaches importance to healthy aging and what level of social protection it provides to older adults (Esping-Andersen, 1991; Titmuss, 1968).

Within the scope of this chapter, an index for healthy aging was developed. With this index, different values that can be considered as indicators of healthy aging were analyzed by relating them to each other. A Healthy Aging Index was calculated for each country, and in line with this index, it was determined which country was more age-friendly. Within the scope of the developed index, Min–Max Normalization, also known as Feature Scalin, was used.

10.4 Construction of the Healthy Aging Index

Healthy Aging Index was created by standardizing and analyzing the parameters given in Fig. 10.1.

Healthy aging undoubtedly has many factors and variables. However, data on these variables are not available for every country. Within the scope of this study, the Healthy Aging Index was developed based on the parameters given in Fig. 10.1 in order to determine which country is more "age friendly." In this context, social policies implemented by the state for healthy aging are divided into two: social protection and social security. Parameters regarding the resources and intensity of protection transferred to older people are included in social protection actions. In other words, healthy aging actions that indirectly affect older people are included. In the field of social security, parameters that directly affect older people through pensions are taken into account. Individual factors are included in the index as average life and healthy life expectancy.

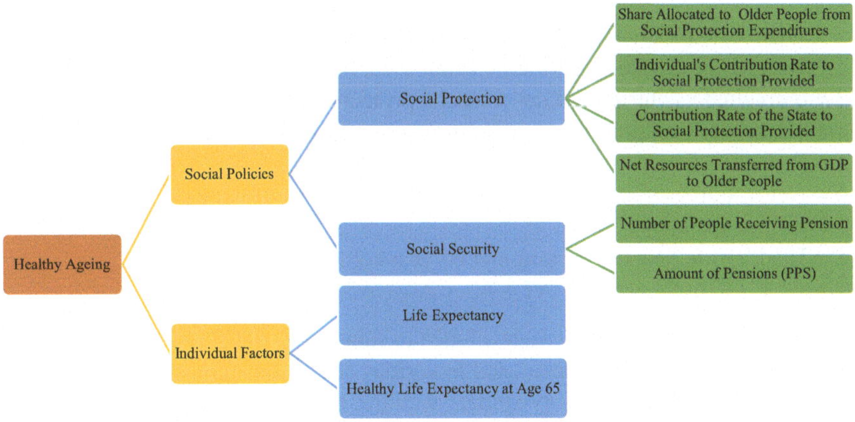

Fig. 10.1 Authors' construction of the parameters affecting healthy aging

The index reveals the Healthy Aging Index Coefficient based on the scope and intensity of social policies implemented by welfare regimes toward older people. With this coefficient, countries are placed in the "age-friendly" ranking. On the other hand, with the developed index, the healthy aging policies of today's welfare regimes become more clear.

10.4.1 Statistical Analyses

Within the scope of the Healthy Aging Index, the normalization method was used to correlate and evaluate very different data. Within the scope of the developed index, Min–Max Normalization, also known as Feature Scalin, was used. Feature Scalin is a statistical formula that is used and its validity is accepted, especially in classifying data of different quality and quantity by reducing them to a single data, in other words, in distinguishing the data class called the target set from all other possible objects called outliers (Yıldırım, 2014; Anorim et al., 2023). The method is a scaling process, also called standardized and normalized, in its most commonly used definition. This standardization process converts different data into a value between 0 and 1. In this way, comparability of different data is ensured (Juszczak et al., 2002).

Feature Scalin can be used with two different equations depending on the nature of the data to be analyzed. These are benefit and cost equations. The benefit equation is $x' = (x–\min(x)) / (\max(x)–\min(x))$ while the cost equation is $x' = (\min(x) – x' / (\max(x)–\min(x))$. Two different equations are used depending on the direction of the effect of the data on the analysis (Han et al., 2012).

The Healthy Aging Index is based on the social policies implemented by welfare regimes toward older people that directly and indirectly affect them and the impact of these policies on the lifespan/health of individuals. At this point, the HAI's components are listed below:

A1 = Share of GDP transferred to higher education (%).
A2 = Number of people receiving pension.
A3 = Individual's contribution rate to social protection provided (%) (cost equation).
A4 = State's contribution rate to social protection provided (%).
A5 = Pension amount ($).
A6 = Net resources transferred to older people (million Euros).
A7 = Life expectancy (years).
A8 = Healthy life years expectation at 65 years old (years).
Healthy Aging Index = (A1 + A2 + A3 + A4 + A5 + A6 + A7 + A8)/8.

The HAI formula, which was developed to standardize data of different qualities and analyze them, has also been used in various academic studies. Accordingly, in a study conducted on university student welfare, the "University Student Friendly Index" was developed based on the Feature Scalin method, and the same formula used in the study was used in the developed index (Öçal, 2022). Similarly, it can be said that another study used the same formula and index method and classified human social communication skills and emotions in line with Electroencephalogram (EEG) signals (Akbulut, 2020).

The benefit equation of the relevant normalization was used for A1, A2, A4, A5, A6, A7, and A8, and the cost equation was used for A3. The increase in the A3 value, which is expressed as the contribution of individuals to the social protection provided, creates a cost-oriented rather than a benefit-oriented effect on the individual, unlike other parameters.

10.5 Results

The Healthy Aging Index determines the degree of "age friendly" of a country by classifying countries based on the content and type of social policies implemented for healthy aging. The scope of the index is the European Union countries and the countries that are candidate countries for membership. In addition, the United Kingdom, which left the union with the Brexit process, and some selected Balkan countries were included in the study. In this context, the panel data set used in the analysis was accessed through EUROSTAT, and the obtained data was subjected to normalization analysis with the Statistical Package for the Social Science, version 25. Considering that most of the countries included in the index are classified in different welfare regime typologies, it is thought that sufficient coverage has been achieved for the classification.

As a result of the analysis performed by normalizing the data on healthy aging of selected countries, a Healthy Aging Index between 0 and 1 was obtained for each country. Subsequently, these values were classified and the "age-friendly country" ranking was revealed. Figure 10.2 shows the authors' ranking of countries with respect to age-friendliness.

In Table 10.2, where the Healthy Aging Index is shown, the minimum value of the index is Bosnia, everyone with 0.322772, while the highest value is France with 0.936502. The average "Healthy Aging Index" of 37 countries was calculated as 0.568032. Turkey's index value is 0.589915. The distinctions between welfare typologies also emerge in the analysis carried out. In fact, the countries in which the analysis was carried out are divided into at least four typologies as liberal, social democratic, conservative, and Southern European typologies, according to the classifications made by Esping-Andersen (1991) and Leibfried (1993). When the range of the index is examined, this distinction clearly stands out. In particular, the distribution of pensions according to purchasing power parity and the monetary value of the resources transferred from Gross Domestic Product to elderly individuals have been decisive in determining how age friendly the analyzed countries are. All countries examined within the scope of the index are countries that implement social policies for older people. Although all the countries evaluated at this point are "age friendly," three degrees were revealed when they were classified according to the intensity of the policies they implemented. The social transfers to be evaluated in the index developed by us, the degree of importance of social transfers, or the new

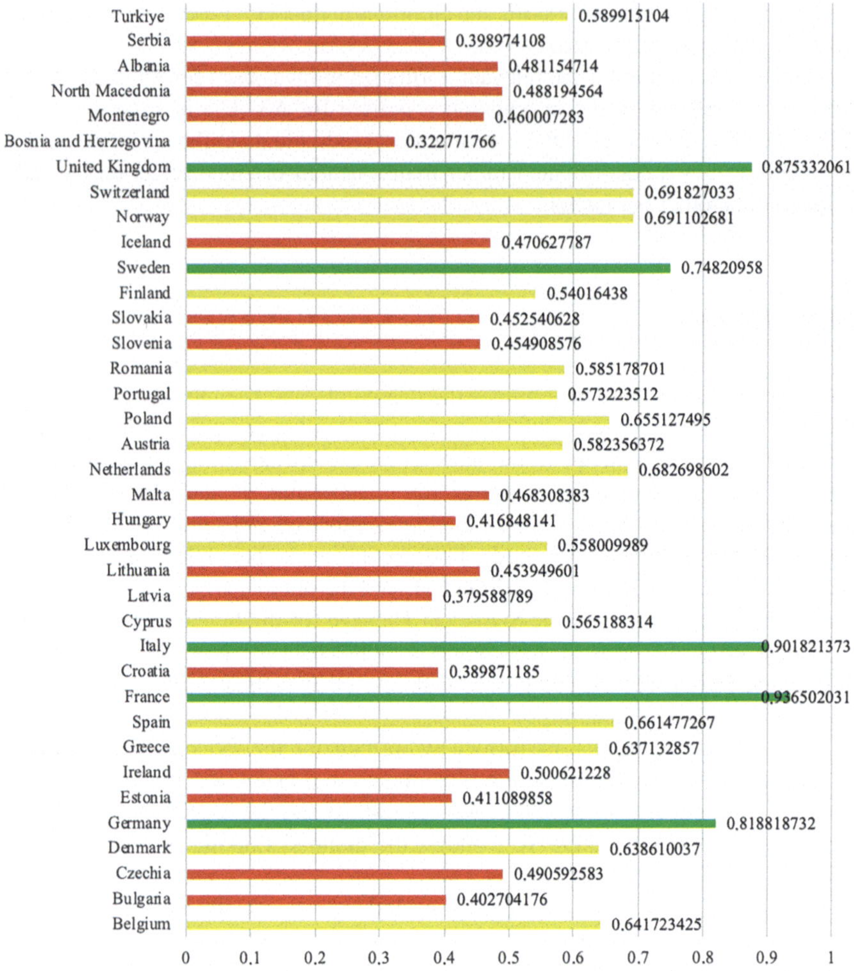

Fig. 10.2 Authors' ranking of age-friendly countries according to healthy aging index (The age-friendly country ranking was reached as a result of the classification of the HAI according to percentile analysis. Countries in red are called low age-friendly countries, countries in yellow are called moderately age-friendly countries, and countries in green are called age-friendly countries)

countries to be added may cause differences in this rating (Esping-Andersen, 1991; Leibfried, 1993).

Healthy Aging Index data were classified according to the percentile method. With this classification (EUROSTAT, 2023a, b, c) the "age-friendly" status of countries has been reached. Accordingly, France, Germany, Italy, Sweden, and England can be considered as "age-friendly countries" in the green category. While 14 countries, including Turkey, are positioned as "medium age-friendly countries," 17 countries can be described as "low age-friendly countries." It is seen that the distribution of age-friendly countries is similar to welfare regime typologies. Accordingly, it has

Table 10.2 Analysis of social policies implemented by selected countries for older people according to the Healthy Aging Index

Country	A1	A2	A3	A4	A5	A6	A7	A8	Healthy aging index
Belgium	0.485841	0.128022	0.537815	0.462185	0.74595	0.171561	0.75	0.568966	0.641723425
Bulgaria	0.683252	0.08385	0.663866	0.336134	0.167972	0.015633	0	0.465517	0.402704176
Czechia	0.55178	0.121955	0.605042	0.394958	0.453815	0.067957	0.377358	0.37069	0.490592583
Denmark	0.427184	0.059667	0.781513	0.218487	0.797507	0.102767	0.806604	0.637931	0.638610037
Germany	0.322411	1	0.184874	0.815126	0.813501	1	0.113208	0.663793	0.818818732
Estonia	0.517799	0.014763	1	0	0.200092	0.005681	0.54717	0.181034	0.411089858
Ireland	0.014968	0.042574	0.87395	0.12605	0.397251	0.045682	0.787736	0.715517	0.500621228
Greece	1	0.099187	0.478992	0.521008	0.55272	0.077527	0.783019	0.310345	0.637132857
Spain	0.463188	0.42118	0.756303	0.243697	0.48421	0.404613	0.669811	0.525862	0.661477267
France	0.439725	0.884469	0.546218	0.453782	0.936803	0.985373	0.872642	0.5	0.936502031
Croatia	0.269822	0.048816	0.403361	0.596639	0.163912	0.013314	0.783019	0.060345	0.389871185
Italy	0.80178	0.662067	0.630252	0.369748	0.715151	0.714689	1	0.517241	0.901821373
Cyprus	0.499191	0.003806	0.588235	0.411765	0.359665	0.005045	0.971698	0.551724	0.565188314
Latvia	0.492314	0.020807	0.789916	0.210084	0.253961	0.006547	0.495283	0.008621	0.379588789
Lithuania	0.363269	0.03551	0.445378	0.554622	0.295618	0.011571	0.90566	0.112069	0.453949601
Luxembourg	0.235841	0.005509	0.537815	0.462185	0.875528	0.013062	0.830189	0.387931	0.558009989
Hungary	0.599919	0.085844	0.563025	0.436975	0.222786	0.034961	0.367925	0.189655	0.416848141
Malta	0.373382	0.000749	0.915966	0.084034	0.281797	0.002165	0.410377	0.741379	0.468308383
Netherlands	0.420307	0.182862	0.184874	0.815126	0.866235	0.225844	0.900943	0.5	0.682698602
Austria	0.618932	0.10444	0.336134	0.663866	1	0.157721	0.311321	0.301724	0.582356372
Poland	0.669498	0.440849	0.647059	0.352941	0.422751	0.149619	0.877358	0.37069	0.655127495
Portugal	0.755259	0.119085	0.630252	0.369748	0.507142	0.075096	0.75	0.232759	0.573223512
Romania	0.93123	0.210569	0.12605	0.87395	0.362645	0.062094	0.806604	0.137931	0.585178701
Slovenia	0.438916	0.024782	0.176471	0.823529	0.429192	0.015319	0.476415	0.344828	0.454908576
Slovakia	0.524272	0.073065	0.504202	0.495798	0.230082	0.024617	0.863208	0	0.452540628

(continued)

Table 10.2 (continued)

Country	A1	A2	A3	A4	A5	A6	A7	A8	Healthy aging index
Finland	0.606796	0.065318	0.613445	0.386555	0.841995	0.091386	0.221698	0.413793	0.54016438
Sweden	0.662621	0.113871	0.789916	0.210084	0.73603	0.174849	0.801887	1	0.74820958
Iceland	0	0	0.831933	0.168067	0.562122	0.003349	0.396226	0.862069	0.470627787
Norway	0.377832	0.058202	0.689076	0.310924	0.755534	0.109733	0.90566	0.939655	0.691102681
Switzerland	0.536812	0.129985	0	1	0.904316	0.205581	0.891509	0.482759	0.691827033
United Kingdom[a]	0.664644	0.663852	0.747899	0.252101	0.597758	0.869168	0.896226	0.560345	0.875332061
Bosnia and Herzegovina	0.238673	0.025782	0	1	0	0.003177	0.160377	0.508621	0.322771766
Montenegro	0.284385	0.001911	0.344538	0.655462	0.075895	0	0.915094	0.482759	0.460007283
North Macedonia[b]	0.522654	0.010203	0.319328	0.680672	0.01395	0.000773	0.976415	0.405172	0.488194564
Albania	0.967638	0.025506	0.756303	0.243697	0.000612	−0.0011	0.273585	0.62069	0.481154714
Serbia	0.633091	0.065544	0.361345	0.638655	0.1231	0.01388	0.075472	0.482759	0.398974108
Turkey	0.730987	0.617149	0.731092	0.268908	0.101324	0.130532	0.330189	0.62931	0.589915104

A7 and A8 data were compiled from the World Health Organization (WHO) 2019 data, and other data were compiled from the European Union (EU) Statistical Institute 2021 data (EUROSTAT). The analyzed data are the latest updated data announced by the relevant institutions (EUROSTAT, 2024a, b, c; WHO, 2024a, b).

[a]Due to the Brexit process, the data compiled for the United Kingdom is dated 2019

[b]The last updated data for North Macedonia in the EUROSTAT database is dated 2017

been observed that the welfare regimes defined as age-friendly countries in the green category are strong social States classified as conservative and social democratic welfare regimes. However, it stands out that the middle and low age-friendly countries are countries that can implement palliative social policies, although they define themselves as a social state, referred to as the Southern European welfare regime type. The classification of age-friendly countries, which was created based on the Healthy Aging Index, enabled an inter-country comparison to be made based on the social policies implemented by selected countries toward elderly individuals. It is thought that the developed index and ranking, in this form, will make a significant contribution to eliminating the deficiency in inter-country comparisons regarding healthy aging, which is emphasized in the Decade of Healthy Ageing Baseline Report put forward by the United Nations.

10.6 Discussion

10.6.1 Measuring Healthy Aging

In order for societies to support healthy aging, they must first measure healthy aging. For this measurement, a definition of healthy aging is undoubtedly needed. However, it is very difficult to find a uniform definition of healthy aging. The concept of healthy aging has gone through a long historical process and turned into an ideal that includes a successful, healthy, productive, and active life (Behr et al., 2023). Establishing a consistent definition of this concept is important for international comparability, because the aging process and health conditions may differ in different countries. However, the development of standardized measures will help objectively assess healthy aging and develop effective health policies and programs (Daskalopoulou et al., 2017; Lara et al., 2013).

A systematic literature review identifying 74 studies and reviews on definitions and concepts of healthy aging showed that many parallel concepts are frequently used in research. Healthy, successful, active, and productive aging all describe similar and partially intertwined concepts of operationalizing and measuring the process of aging well (Behr et al., 2023). In the study by Cosco et al. (2014), in which they examined 84 studies, five basic aspects of the concept of healthy aging are emphasized, such as physiological structures, participation structures, well-being structures, personal resources, and external factors. These key aspects highlight the multifaceted nature of healthy aging. Michel and Sadana's (2017) classification States that healthy and active aging is related to health outcomes. There are four markers for healthy aging, which include health and well-being; symptom-oriented measures of illness or morbidity; performing roles, activities, and functions; and adaptation to or coping with limitations. In addition to these markers, external conditions, especially wars, crises, welfare level, and environmental effects, affect the aging process of the individual. These factors have a significant impact on the health, well-being, and quality of life of individuals in old age. For example, wars and crises negatively affect the safety, nutritional status, and access to health services of older individuals. This causes increased health problems and decreased quality of life in old age (Sadana & Thiyagarajan, 2019).

Although there are studies in the literature that created a healthy aging score, only 5.9% of the studies used a score, scale, or index to evaluate healthy aging (Behr et al., 2023). The most frequently evaluated categories in the studies were demographic characteristics and individual aspects of health (82%) (Behr et al., 2023). Hospitalization, functional decline, morbidity, and mortality are indicators focused on studies on healthy aging (Mount et al., 2016; O'Caoimh et al., 2015). One of the scales on healthy aging in the literature was developed by Charlson et al. (2022) and focuses on vitality. Physiologic Index of Comorbidity, developed by Newman et al. (2008), takes vitality and cognition as criteria. The Healthy Aging Indexes, developed by McCabe et al. (2016) and Wu et al. (2017), focus on vitality and cognition, similar to the Physiologic Index of Comorbidity. Another index on the subject is the Active Aging Index, which includes cognition, mobility, relationships, and contribution to society as domains (European Centre Vienna, 2013). The criteria addressed by the Selfie Aging Index developed by Goncalves et al. (2017) are vitality, cognition, making decisions, mobility, relationships, and contributing to society. Based on this, it is possible to say that in index studies, the individual and biological aspects of health are emphasized and the social and environmental aspects are ignored (Mount et al., 2016).

10.6.2 Contextual Differences in Healthy Aging

Changes in population structure have significant effects on economic and social policies. In particular, an aging population brings with it a number of new requirements. These requirements demand new measures to be taken in the field of social policy. Factors such as the aging trend in developed countries, the decrease in the working age population, and the increase in older people population make policy changes in areas such as retirement systems, health services, long-term care, and support for older people necessary.

The classification of countries as "age-friendly countries," "medium age-friendly countries," and "low age-friendly countries" according to the Healthy Aging Index was obtained by weighting and comparing the HAI scores of the countries. As a result of the comparison of HAI scores, age-friendly countries are colored green, medium-level age-friendly countries are colored yellow, and low-level age-friendly countries are colored red. Thanks to the weighting and coloring of the scores, countries could be compared easily and understandable tables were presented.

According to the Healthy Aging Index, France, Germany, Italy, Sweden, and the United Kingdom are considered age-friendly countries in the green category. Germany is known as the pioneer of conservative welfare States (Taşçı, 2010). With the emergence of social insurance practices by Otto von Bismarck in 1883, Germany became an important country in terms of social policy (Kalkan, 2020). In Germany, the care insurance system is among the compulsory insurances. It aims to cover a large part of the society and is a premium system. The scope of care insurance includes home care, long-term care, medical care, retirement homes and nursing homes, elderly care rehabilitation centers, and some other services such as social care services (Kocabaş & Kol, 2020). One of the age-friendly countries with a social democratic welfare regime is Sweden. Social democratic welfare state is generally defined as a type of state that tries to ensure that its citizens are socially well and tries to create minimum living standards for individuals (Toprak, 2015). Elderly care, a social right in Sweden, has been an important municipal duty for many years and is regulated by the Swedish Social Services Act.

Elderly care services are provided through 290 local municipalities, and costs are mainly based on local taxes (Edebalk, 2010). Sweden constitutes a fundamental place in Europe in terms of elderly care services. This is not only due to good data, but also because Sweden has long been the prototype of welfare States (Sundström & Johansson, 2005). Another country in the green category is England, which is a country with a liberal welfare regime. The liberal welfare state emphasizes more individualism regarding benefits and emphasizes the need not to interfere with market gains (Tamkoç, 2020). The first attempts to provide basic care services to elderly individuals by England date back to the Poverty Law of 1834 (Çadır, 2017). Like Germany, Denmark, and the Netherlands, the United Kingdom allocates approximately 1% of its general budget for long-term care of older people. In England, there are friendship services, legal services, an advice line to ask questions about old age, and help older people to avoid loneliness, have social harmony, live without being excluded from society, and help them know their rights (Bağcı Torun, 2019).

10.7 Limitations and Strengths

The Healthy Aging Index created is a tool used to measure the health and welfare of older adults through the social welfare policies of countries. This index was created by combining individual indicators of healthy aging and social policy indicators. The parameters chosen when creating HAI do not cover all indicators of healthy aging, but is based only on the data available for EU countries. This is one of the main limitations of the study. Collecting and keeping up-to-date data required for HAI can be time-consuming, and in some regions or countries, this data may be missing or not up-to-date, which may affect the accuracy of the index. In addition to these limitations, HAI makes it possible to evaluate the well-being of older people from both individual and social policy perspectives, addresses the concept of healthy aging by including biopsychosocial aspects, and provides a holistic view. The Healthy Aging Index can be used in the development and evaluation of aging-related policies and programs. This index can also serve as a guide to identify the needs of older individuals and produce appropriate solutions. The Healthy Aging Index, which makes data on aging comparable across countries, can help raise public awareness about the health and well-being of older people.

10.8 Conclusions

Our study highlights the comprehensive framework of healthy aging defined by the World Health Organization, encompassing physical health, cognitive, emotional, and social well-being, along with environmental factors. It underscores the importance of considering both individual and environmental aspects in promoting healthy aging effectively. Amid global crises like pandemics, migrations, and climate change, societies are rapidly transforming. Hence, recognizing the value of aging populations becomes crucial. Instead of perceiving them as a burden, societies should appreciate older adults as valuable assets capable of significant contributions to social cohesion and intergenerational knowledge transfer. Our primary recommendation is to enhance societal awareness and appreciation of older adults' contributions. By valuing their experiences and wisdom, societies can leverage the potential of aging populations for more inclusive and fulfilling environments. This involves reimagining societal structures and policies to better support healthy aging and ensure older adults' well-being amid evolving challenges. In conclusion, our study underscores the importance of reshaping perceptions of aging and implementing policies that empower older adults to lead meaningful lives in changing societies.

Review Questions

1. How does the Healthy Aging Index reflect health and well-being inequalities across different contexts?
2. How do social welfare factors affect the healthy aging process?
3. What is the role of the Healthy Aging Index in planning social policies?
4. How can the impact of social welfare policies on the health and well-being of older adults be assessed?

References

Akbulut, O. (2020). Feature normalization effect in emotion classification based on EEG Signals. *Sakarya University Journal of Science, 24*(1), 60–66.

Alcock, P., Mayi, M., & Rowlingson, R. (2011). *Sosyal Politika: Kuramlar ve Uygulamalar*. Siyasal Kitabevi.

Alexandre, D., Cordeiro, C., & Ramos, L. (2005). Factors associated with the successful aging of the socially-active elderly in the metropolitan region of porto alegre. *Brazilian Journal of Psychiatry*, 613–621.

Anorim, L., Cavalcanti, G., & Cruz, R. (2023). The choice of scaling technique matters for classification performance. *Applied Soft Computing*, 2–37.

Bağcı Torun, T. (2019). *Türkiye'de Yaşlılara Yönelik Sosyal Politikalar*. Bolu Abant İzzet Baysal University.

Beard, J., Officer, A., Carvalho, I., Sadana, R., Pot, A., Michel, J., et al. (2016). The World report on ageing and health: A policy framework for healthy ageing. *The Lancet, 387*, 2145–2154.

Beard, J., de Carvalho, I., Sumi, Y., Officer, A., & Thiyagarajan, J. (2017). Healthy ageing: Moving forward. *Bulletin of the World Health Organization, 95*, 730–730A.

Behr, L., Simm, A., Kluttig, A., & Grosskopf, A. (2023). 60 years of healthy aging: On definitions, biomarkers, scores and challenges. *Ageing Research Reviews, 88*, 1–14.

Çadır, M. (2017). İngiltere'de Yaşlılara Yönelik Sosyal Hizmetlerin Dönüşümü: Huzurevi Sektörüne Genel Bir Bakış. *Sosyal Politika Çalışmaları Dergisi, 17*, 9–32.

Carmody, P., McCann, G., Colleran, C., & O'Halloran, C. (2021). *Covid19 in the Global South: Impacts and responses*. Bristol University.

Charlson, M., Carrozzino, D., Guidi, J., & Patierno, C. (2022). Charlson comorbidity index: A critical review of clinimetric properties. *Psychiatry and Psychology, 91*, 8–35.

Clarke, P., & Nieuwenhuijsen, E. (2009). Environments for healthy ageing: A critical review. *Maturitas, 64*, 14–19.

Cosco, T., Prina, A., Perales, J., Stephan, B., & Brayne, C. (2014). Operational definitions of successful aging: A systematic review. *International Psychogeriatrics, 26*, 373–381.

Daskalopoulou, C., Stubbs, B., Kralj, C., Koukounari, A., Prince, M., & Prina, A. (2017). Physical activity and healthy ageing: A systematic review and meta-analysis of longitudinal cohort studies. *Ageing Research Reviews, 38*, 6–17.

de Kaijzer, C., Bauwelinck, M., & Dadvand, P. (2020). Long-term exposure to residential greenspace and healthy ageing: A systematic review. *Current Environmental Health Reports, 7*, 65–88.

Demirtaş, Ş., Güngör, C., & Demirtaş, R. (2017). Sağlıklı Yaşlanma ve Fiziksel Aktivite: Bireysel, Psikososyal ve Çevresel Özelliklerin Buna Katkısı. *Osmangazi Tıp Dergisi, 39*, 100–108.

Dobrowolska, B., Jędrzejkiewicz, B., Pilewska-Kozak, A., Zarzycka, D., Ślusarska, B., Deluga, A., et al. (2019). Age discrimination in healthcare institutions perceived by seniors and students. *Nursing Ethics, 26*, 443–459.

Edebalk, P. (2010). Ways of funding and organising elderly care in Sweden. In T. Bengtsson içinde (Ed.), *Population ageing-a threat to the welfare state? Demographic research monographs* (pp. 65–80). Springer.

Esping-Andersen, G. (1991). *The three worlds of welfare capitalism*. Princeton University Press.

European Centre Vienna. (2013). *Active ageing index 2012 concept, methodology and final results*. UNECE.

EUROSTAT. (2023a, 12 09). *Pensions (PPS)*. https://ec.europa.eu/eurostat/databrowser/view/spr_exp_pens/default/table?lang=enadresindenalındı

EUROSTAT. (2023b, 12 19). *Pensions beneficiaries*. https://ec.europa.eu/eurostat/databrowser/view/spr_pns_ben/default/table?lang=enadresindenalındı

EUROSTAT. (2023c, 12 22). *Net social benefits by old age*. https://ec.europa.eu/eurostat/databrowser/view/tps00083/default/table?lang=enadresindenalındı

EUROSTAT. (2024a, 01 04). *Social benefits by old age*. https://ec.europa.eu/eurostat/databrowser/view/tps00106/default/table?lang=enadresindenalındı

EUROSTAT. (2024b, 01 04). *Social Protection Receipts by General Government Contributions*: https://ec.europa.eu/eurostat/databrowser/view/tps00108/default/table?lang=enadresindenalındı

EUROSTAT. (2024c, 01 04). *Social protection receipts by protected person*. https://ec.europa.eu/eurostat/databrowser/view/tps00108/default/table?lang=enadresindenalındı

Fallon, C., & Karlawish, J. (2019). Is the WHO definition of health aging well? Frameworks for "health" after three score and ten. *American Journal of Public Health, 109*, 1104–1106.

Fried, L., & Rowe, J. (2020). Health in aging past, present, and future. *The New England Journal of Medicine, 383*, 1293–1296.

Garin, N., Beatriz, O., Miret, M., Ayuso-Mateos, J., Power, M., Bucciarelli, P., & Haro, J. (2014). Built environment and elderly population health: A comprehensive literature review. *Clinical Practice and Epidemiology in Mental Health, 10*, 103–115.

Goncalves, J., Gomes, M., Fonseca, M., Teodoro, T., Barros, P., & Botelho, M. (2017). Selfie aging index: An index for the self-assessment of healthy and active aging. *Frontiers in Medicine, 4*, 236.

Hallegatte, S., & Rozenberg, J. (2017). Climate change through a poverty lens. *Nature Climate Change, 7*, 250–256.

Han, J., Kamber, M., & Pei, J. (2012). *Data mining: Concepts and techniques*. Morgan Kaufman.

Juszczak, P., Tax, D., & Duin, R. (2002). Feature scaling in support vector data description. In *8th Annual Conf. of the Advanced School for Computing and Imaging* (pp. 95–102). Lochem.

Kabisch, N., van den Bosch, M., & Lafortezza, R. (2017). The health benefits of nature-based solutions to urbanization challenges for children and the elderly-A systematic review. *Environmental Research, 159*, 362–373.

Kalkan, M. (2020). Almanya'da Sosyal Politika-Sosyal Devlet. *Düşünce ve Toplum Sosyal Bilimler Dergisi*, 167–170.

Keating, N. (2022). A research framework for the United Nations Decade of Healthy Ageing (2021–2030). *European Journal of Ageing, 19*, 775–787.

Kocabaş, F., & Kol, E. (2020). Almanya ve Türkiye'de Karşılaştırmalı Olarak Bakım Hizmetleri: Türkiye'de Bakım Sigortası Kurulmasına Yönelik Bir Öneri. *Anadolu Üniversitesi Sosyal Bilimler Dergisi, 20*, 283–310.

Lara, J., Godfrey, A., Evans, E., Heaven, B., Brown, L., Barron, E., et al. (2013). Towards measurement of the Healthy Ageing Phenotype in lifestyle-based intervention studies. *Maturitas, 76*, 189–199.

Lara, J., Cooper, R., Nissan, J., Ginty, A., Khaw, K., Deary, I., et al. (2015). A proposed panel of biomarkers of healthy ageing. *BMC Medicine, 13*, 222.

Lee, D., Aula, I., & Masoodian, M. (2023). Perspectives on creative well-being of older adults. *Journal of Aging Studies, 66*, 1–8.

Leibfried, S. (1993). *Towards a European welfare state*. Routledge Press.

Livingston, V., Jackson-Nevels, B., & Reddy, V. (2022). Social, cultural, and economic determinants of well-being. *Encyclopedia, 2*, 1183–1199.

Malderen, L., Mets, T., Vriendt, P., & Gorus, E. (2013). The active ageing–Concept translated to the residential long-term care. *Quality of Life Research, 22*, 929–937.

McCabe, E., Larson, M., Lunetta, K., Newman, A., Cheng, S., & Murabito, J. (2016). Association of an index of healthy aging with incident cardiovascular disease and mortality in a community-based sample of older adults. *The Journals of Gerontology: Series A, 71*, 1695–1701.

Mendes, F. (2013). Active ageing: A right or a duty? *Health Sociology Review, 22*, 174–185.

Michel, J., & Sadana, R. (2017). "Healthy aging" concepts and measures. *Journal of the American Medical Directors Association, 18*, 460–464.

Molina-Luque, F., Stoncikaite, I., Torres-Gonzalez, T., & Sanvicen-Torne, P. (2022). Profiguration, active ageing, and creativity: keys for quality of life and overcoming ageism. *International Journal of Environmental Research and Public Health, 19*, 1564.

Mount, S., Lara, J., Schols, A., & Mathers, J. (2016). Towards a multidimensional healthy ageing phenotype. *Current Opinion in Clinical Nutrition and Metabolic Care, 19*, 418–426.

Nelson, T. (2017). *Ageism. Stereotyping and prejudice against older persons*. MIT Press.

Newman, A., Boudreau, R., Naydeck, B., Fried, L., & Harris, T. (2008). *A physiologic index of comorbidity: Relationship to mortality and disability* (Vol. 63, pp. 603–609). Series A.

O'Caoimh, R., Cornally, N., Weathers, E., O'Sullivan, R., Fitzgerald, C., Orfila, F., et al. (2015). Risk prediction in the community: A systematic review of case-finding instruments that predict adverse healthcare outcomes in community-dwelling older adults. *Maturitas, 82*, 3–21.

Öçal, M. (2022). *Üniversite Öğrencilerine Yönelik Sosyal Politika Uygulamaları ve Öğrencilerin Yaşam Koşullarına Etkisi* (Doctoral Thesis). Pamukkale Unıversty.

Öçal, M., & Kutlu, Ö. (2023). A study on welfare and living conditions of disadvantaged groups: The case of Burdur Province. *Journal of Management and Economics Research*, 21(3), 410–425.

Öz, F. (2002). Yaşamın Son Evresi: Yaşlılık Psikososyal Açıdan Gözden Geçirme. *Kriz Dergisi*, 17–28.

Pak, K., Furunes, T., & Lange, A. (2022). Discrimination and employability in healthcare work: A double-edged sword for older workers? *Sustainability, 14*, 5385.

Panayiotou, G., & Karekla, M. (2013). Perceived social support helps, but does not buffer the negative impact of anxiety disorders on quality of life and perceived stress. *Social Psychiatry and Psychiatric Epidemiology, 48*, 283–294.

Rippon, I., Kneale, D., Oliveira, C., Demakakos, P., & Steptoe, A. (2013). Perceived age discrimination in older adults. *Age and Ageing, 43*, 379–386.

Rudnicka, E., Napierala, P., Podfigurna, A., Meczekalski, B., Smolarczyk, R., & Grymowicz, M. (2020). The World Health Organization (WHO) approach to healthy ageing. *Maturitas, 139*, 6–11.

Rugel, E., Chow, C., Corsi, D., Hystad, P., Rangarajan, S., Yusuf, S., & Lear, S. (2022). Developing indicators of age-friendly neighbourhood environments for urban and rural communities across 20 low-, middle-, and high-income countries. *BMC Public Health, 22*, 1–16.

Sadana, R., & Thiyagarajan, J. (2019). Healthy Ageing – What is it, can we measure it & use it. In *Expert Group Meeting on Measuring Population Ageing: Bridging Research and Policy*. WHO.

Sundström, G., & Johansson, L. (2005). The changing balance of government and family in care for the elderly in Sweden and other European Countries. *Australasian Journal on Ageing, 24*, 5–11.

Tamkoç, B. (2020). Esping-Andersen'in Refah Rejimleri Sınıflandırmasına Göre Farklı Refah Rejimlerinde Alzheimerlı Bireylere Yönelik Hizmetlerin İncelenmesi. *Türkiye Sosyal Hizmet Araştırmaları Dergisi*, 1–12.

Taşçı, F. (2010). Yaşlılara Yönelik Sosyal Politikalar: İsveç, Almanya, İngiltere ve İtalya Örnekleri. *Çalışma ve Toplum*, 175–202.

Timonen, V. (2008). *Ageing societies: A comparative introduction*. McGrawHill.

Titmuss, R. (1968). *Commitment to welfare*. Pantheon Books.

Toprak, D. (2015). Uygulamada Ortaya Çıkan Farklı Refah Devleti Modelleri Üzerine Bir İnceleme. *Süleyman Demirel Üniversitesi Sosyal Bilimler Enstitüsü Dergisi*, 151–175.

Tuckett, A., Banchoff, A., Winter, S., & King, A. (2018). The built environment and older adults: A literature review and an applied approach to engaging older adults in built environment improvements for health. *International Journal of Older People Nursing, 13*, 1–9.

United Nations. (2022). *World population prospects 2022*. https://www.un.org/development/desa/pd/sites/www.un.org.development.desa.pd/files/wpp2022_summary_of_results.pdfadresindenalındı

Van den Broucke, S., & Renwart, A. (2014). Health literacy mediates the relationship between education level and health behaviour: Stephan Van Den Broucke. *European Journal of Public Health, 24*, 202.

Vaudin, A., Moshfegh, A., & Sahyoun, N. (2022). Measuring food insecurity in older adults using both physical and economic food access, NHANES 2013–18. *The Journal of Nutrition Community and International Nutrition, 152*(1953–1962), 152.

WHO. (2024a). *Health Life Expectancy (HALE)*. https://www.who.int/data/gho/data/indicators/indicator-details/GHO/gho-ghe-hale-healthy-life-expectancy-at-age-60adresindenalındı

WHO. (2024b). *Life expectancy at birth*. https://www.who.int/data/gho/data/indicators/indicator-details/GHO/life-expectancy-at-birth-(years)adresindenalındı

World Health Organization. (2002). *Active ageing: A policy framework*. https://apps.who.int/iris/bitstream/handle/10665/67215/WHO_NMH_NPH_02.8.pdf? sequence=1&isAllowed=yadresindenalındı

World Health Organization. (2015). *World report on ageing and health*. https://apps.who.int/iris/bitstream/handle/10665/186463/9789240694811_eng.pdf;jsessionid=8946BF60EA4BAD389F1AD638460990C6?sequence=1adresindenalındı

World Health Organization. (2020). *Decade of healthy ageing 2020–2030*. https://www.who.int/docs/default-source/decade-of-healthy-ageing/final-decadeproposal/decade-proposal-final-apr2020-en.pdf?sfvrsn=b4b75ebc_5adresindenalındı
Wu, C., Smit, E., Sanders, J., Newman, A., & Odden, M. (2017). A modified healthy aging index and its association with mortality: The national health and nutrition examination survey, 1999–2002. *The Journals of Gerontology: Series A, 72*, 1437–1444.
Yıldırım, F. (2014). *Gri İlişkisel Analiz*. Dora Publishing.

Chapter 11
GIS Objective Measures of Walkability Are Not Always Superior to Psychometric Measures

Nestor Asiamah and Hafiz T. A. Khan

Acronyms and Abbreviations

DTA Disengagement Theory of Ageing
GIS Geographic Information Systems
SST Socioemotional Selectivity Theory

11.1 Introduction

Since the development of the first walkability measure (Saelens et al., 2003) around two decades ago, academic debate on the subject has gained momentum, with many studies on walkability published in the *Journal of Transport Geography* (Jeffrey

N. Asiamah (✉)
School of Health and Social Care, Colchester, Essex, UK

International Public Health Management Programme, University of Europe for Applied Sciences, Iserlohn, Germany

Department of Health Management, Berlin School of Business and Innovation, Berlin, Germany

Department of Gerontology and Geriatrics, Africa Centre for Epidemiology, Accra North, Accra, Ghana
e-mail: n.asiamah@essex.ac.uk

H. T. A. Khan
Public Health Group, College of Nursing, Midwifery, and Healthcare, University of West London, Brentford, UK

Oxford Institute of Population Ageing, University of Oxford, Oxford, UK
e-mail: hafiz.khan@uwl.ac.uk; hafiz.khan@ageing.ox.ac.uk

N. Asiamah et al. (eds.), *Sustainable Ageing*,
https://doi.org/10.1007/978-3-031-69475-2_11

et al., 2019; Otsuka et al., 2021). There is a growing body of empirical evidence on the positive influence of walkability on active transportation, which includes walking, bicycling, and skating (Pontin et al., 2022; Williams et al., 2018), as well as on social and physical activities (Asiamah et al., 2021a, b; Grasser et al., 2016; Pontin et al., 2022). These studies reflect the worth of walkability and investments in it.

Walkability refers to street connectivity; mixed land use, that is, commercial, residential, or domestic; and a high residential density (Saelens et al., 2003; Telega & Telega, 2021). Studies (Gan et al., 2020; Wahl & Gerstorf, 2018) have provided a more elaborate framing of walkability that encapsulates psychosocial factors including neighbourhood safety, cohesion, a sense of inclusiveness and belonging, and other architectural attributes that encourage walking. In this paper, a psychosocial factor is defined as a socio-environmental condition that influences thoughts, emotions, and behaviour. Negative psychosocial factors such as violence, extreme temperatures, ageism, outbreak of infectious diseases, racism, and abuse may cause fear and panic, rendering even the most walkable neighbourhoods less attractive for active transportation. Positive psychosocial factors, however, like social cohesion, trust, reciprocity, and a sense of attachment, can engender an atmosphere of safety and inclusiveness, which in turn will encourage active transportation. In recent literature, walkability has been shown to embody psychosocial factors and architectural features that interplay to encourage neighbourhood-based active transportation, social participation, and other health behaviours. These factors have been incorporated into psychometric measures (Gan et al., 2020; Oyeyemi et al., 2016; Saelens et al., 2003; Sallis et al., 2010), including the more recent OpenX tool (Gan et al., 2020).

Like all other psychometric measures, walkability scales are vulnerable to response bias and can result in biased data (Westland, 2022). For this reason, studies utilising them are expected to take measures, such as steps against common methods bias, to minimise response bias and acknowledge this weakness as a limitation. On the other hand, walkability measured with the geographical information system (GIS) is considered objective (Lam et al., 2022; Telega & Telega, 2021), because it is independent of human psychology and the threat of response bias. However, the future of walkability research may undermine human psychology, which plays a central role in identifying and understanding interventions for ageing-in-place and active transportation. Ageing-in-place refers to the maintenance of optimal health and a sense of attachment to one's home or neighbourhood (Pani-Harreman et al., 2020).

The Decade of Healthy Ageing 2021–2030 is a flagship campaign seeking to support older adults and their communities (Keating, 2022; Rudnicka et al., 2020). It recognises quality data as a resource for fostering healthy ageing, which is the maintenance of the functional ability necessary for well-being in later life (Menassa et al., 2023; Rudnicka et al., 2020). The campaign advocates widening the network of age-friendly cities and communities to enhance access to walkable neighbourhoods. It also emphasises the collection and application of quality data to make effective decisions regarding ageing in a healthy manner. Stakeholders need data on people's feelings and thoughts about initiatives and interventions. For instance, there is a need to understand people's thoughts and feelings about interventions aimed at improving walkability and age-friendliness of neighbourhoods. These thoughts and feelings cannot be fully captured with GIS measures, so psychometric measures are needed to generate data that will provide insights into the opinions and feelings of target groups, such as older adults.

This chapter aims to guide students, peer reviewers, editors, researchers, and publishers to reassess the worth of psychometric measures of walkability. Ideally, such a reassessment would bring these stakeholders to an understanding of the value of a balance between subjective and GIS-based measures. The goal is not to question the significance of GIS-based measurement or to undermine the limitations of subjective measures but to provide a plausible theoretical basis for re-evaluating subjective measures and pre-empting widespread discrimination and editorial bias against them. The unique significance of subjective measures is presented in this chapter, in the context of ageing-in-place, through the lens of psychology. A theoretical premise is provided within which these measures cannot be avoided, which is then followed by a discussion of some of the implications for research and the Decade of Healthy Ageing 2021–2030.

This chapter comprises five sections. The introductory section has provided a background for discussing the aim and rationale of the chapter. The second section provides a theoretical foundation of the argument and demonstrates the role of human psychology in active transportation. The unique advantages of psychometric measures over GIS measures are discussed in the third section, setting the basis for analysing implications for research. The Decade of Healthy Ageing 2021–2030 is covered in the fourth section, with concluding remarks presented in the fifth section.

11.2 Psychology Plays a Role in Active Transportation for Ageing: A Theoretical Framework

Recent projections by the United Nations and World Health Organization (Professions, 2021; Rudnicka et al., 2020) suggest that, in the future, most residents of neighbourhoods may be aged 65 years or older. Ageing is characterised by a gradual decline in physical functional and cognitive ability (Asiamah et al., 2021a, b; Rudnicka et al., 2020), so many residents in the future may well live with disability or frailty. This fact upholds calls for designing neighbourhoods to meet the evolving needs of older adults. Meeting these needs requires enriching neighbourhoods with psychosocial factors such as safety, social cohesion, and a sense of belonging (Gan et al., 2020; Wahl & Gerstorf, 2018).

There is a consensus among bio-ecological models, including the COntext Dynamics in Ageing framework (Wahl & Gerstorf, 2018), that psychosocial conditions are an important facet of walkability. Unfortunately, these factors are being obliterated by climate change events such as extreme temperatures (Yang et al.,

2021), the outbreak of infectious diseases (Honey-rosés et al., 2021), and violence or war (Luckham & Luckham, 2018). Abuse of older adults may increase over time as the size of the human population increases (Asiamah et al., 2021b). These developments threaten the walkability of every neighbourhood, and even the most walkable neighbourhoods are unlikely to encourage active transportation and social participation if they become a hotbed of war or violence, as well as ageist stereotypes. As such, it is necessary for measures of walkability to incorporate psychosocial factors in the interest of older adults and other segments of the population more susceptible to these events.

The socioemotional selectivity theory (SST) contends that older adults prioritise activities and social networks that meet their current physical, emotional, and psychological needs in later life (Cleveland & Agbeke, 2019; Löckenhoff & Carstensen, 2004). It adds that a change in life goals in the ageing process impels older adults to create new meanings of life, which causes instability in their priorities, perceptions, and lived experiences in their neighbourhoods. An adaptation of the service quality model (Dekker et al., 2011; Local et al., 1996) indicates that older adults are among the end-users of neighbourhood attributes implicit in walkability like services, parks, and streets, so the best way to meet and improve their satisfaction is to improve neighbourhoods in harmony with their current lived experiences, opinions, and choices.

The disengagement theory of ageing (DTA) (Asiamah, 2017; Nilsson et al., 2015) also recognises that ageing accompanies a change in life choices due to changes in life goals and declines in physical, emotional, and psychological well-being over the life course. The DTA posits that this change in choices alters behaviours such as social participation and physical activities, including active transportation. Recent advances in environmental gerontology (Bempong & Asiamah, 2022; D'Haese et al., 2016; Wahl & Gerstorf, 2018, 2020) suggest that the preference of older adults for active types of transportation, be it walking, bicycling, or skating, over travelling by car will depend on the availability of psychosocial environmental factors such as safety, cohesion, inclusiveness, and a sense of belonging. It will also depend on whether their changing goals, as well as physical, emotional, and psychological well-being, are supported by these factors.

Drawing on the SST and DTA, older adults' transportation choices and health behaviours over the life course are based on their current physical, emotional, and psychological well-being and how this status shapes their evolving perceptions about their neighbourhood. If older adults grow frail over time in a neighbourhood where violence has grown from bad to worse, for example, they are likely to choose an alternative and a safer form of transportation, such as travelling by a public bus rather than walking. Thoughts and feelings about context emanate from evolving personal situations and current experiences and are, therefore, referred to in this paper as *the psychology of transportation choices*. It is, thus, understandable why users of GIS-based measures (Grasser et al., 2016; Jeffrey et al., 2019) have acknowledged a need for future research to measure this psychology.

11.3 Why GIS Objective Measures Are Not Always Better than Psychometric Measures

The main limitation of GIS objective measures of walkability is its inability to capture either the psychology described in the previous section or the clues for age-friendly community design enshrouded in this psychology. Some researchers (Grasser et al., 2016; Jeffrey et al., 2019; Otsuka et al., 2021; Williams et al., 2018) utilising this objective measure have acknowledged this shortcoming as a limitation that decision-makers should consider and have combined GIS measures with subjective measures (Otsuka et al., 2021). GIS objective measures typically capture street connectivity, residential density, mixed land use, and the spatial distribution and location of walkability attributes such as services, traffic lights, pavements, and parks. A recent study (Telega & Telega, 2021) reveals that the crime rate in an area is the only psychosocial factor of walkability that is measured, with only a few GIS techniques, meaning that data from an assessment of this nature may not reflect the current situation and experiences of residents. Core psychosocial conditions such as the absence of racism, neighbourhood social cohesion, and a sense of attachment provided by the neighbourhood, which is an important part of walkability (Gan et al., 2020; Morris et al., 2020), are not measured with any GIS-based tool. Yet, these factors could change and affect people's thoughts and experiences of walkability over time.

If GIS objective measures replaced psychometric scales, then this would undermine the experiences, opinions, and feelings of residents, who ideally should be able to say what walkability in their neighbourhood would look like. In this situation, psychometric measures would be regarded as an inferior option, thereby undermining the significant effort made by psychometricians (Oyeyemi et al., 2016; Saelens et al., 2003; Sallis et al., 2010) to construct subjective measures of walkability. Psychometric tools generally measure the traditional domains of walkability, such as street connectivity, mixed land use, and high residential density (Oyeyemi et al., 2016; Saelens et al., 2003; Sallis et al., 2010), as well as psychosocial factors (Gan et al., 2020; Oyeyemi et al., 2016). This gives them an advantage over the GIS-based method, particularly where human psychology is needed as part of actionable empirical evidence.

Recent studies have shown how the psychosocial factors already mentioned have been affected by the coronavirus disease 2019 pandemic (Honey-rosés et al., 2021), war and violence (Luckham & Luckham, 2018), and unforgiving climate change events (Yang et al., 2021). Fears about these issues may compel individuals to flee their neighbourhoods or abandon community centres where services can be accessed (Honey-rosés et al., 2021; Luckham & Luckham, 2018; Yang et al., 2021). Violence may also compel residents to give up active transportation for travelling in public buses and cars since active transportation, such as walking, makes them more vulnerable to robbery and social unrest. As the SST suggests, these changes in behaviour among older people are a swift response to psychosocial environmental conditions that are detrimental to their physical, emotional, and psychological well-being.

Arguably, humans cannot completely eradicate climate change, infectious diseases, and violence in the short-term, so preparation to measure changes in transportation and other behaviours driven by these adverse events is imperative. When it comes to transportation choices and other behaviours of older people, GIS objective measures cannot always convey an understanding of changes and pressing concerns. This being so, the psychology of transportation and behavioural choices must be measured with subjective scales to meet the ever-changing needs of the ageing population. From this perspective, psychometric measures are ideal as they can assess psychosocial factors affecting transportation and health behaviour and how they change within human ecosystems.

11.4 Implications for Research and the Decade of Healthy Ageing 2021–2030

Groups that are targeted by the Decade of Healthy Ageing 2021–2030, such as older adults, are important stakeholders whose views and feelings must be considered in evaluating the impact and effectiveness of campaign-related activities. Widening the network of age-friendly cities and communities to increase access to walkable neighbourhoods is laudable. Yet, stakeholders must ensure that people living in these communities have positive active travel experiences, like walking and bicycling, that encourage them to engage in active transportation over their life course. It can, therefore, be inferred that data needed for understanding and improving these experiences would ultimately come from research utilising psychometric tools. For this reason, those responsible for generating data and evidence to facilitate healthy ageing interventions, be they students, researchers, or journal editors, should not undermine psychometric measures of walkability and other variables. Failure to accurately use psychometric scales and data generated by them would mean that beneficiaries of healthy ageing interventions are disregarded and not allowed to influence the design of their neighbourhoods. Although qualitative studies can be utilised to understand experiences and opinions, they must be complemented with quantitative studies employing larger representative samples. Quantitative studies utilising cross-sectional designs and subjective measures, for instance, can provide generalisable evidence relating to opinions and experiences.

Researchers and publishers should not lose sight of the potential of psychometric measures to measure feelings and thoughts, which ultimately convey unique lessons for improving neighbourhood design and services to meet the needs of residents. Researchers, nevertheless, must acknowledge the limitations of their subjective measures even in contexts where the use of these tools mitigates the abovementioned weaknesses of GIS-based measures. Journals and editors should expect authors to apply appropriate study design techniques to avoid or minimise the weaknesses of the subjective measures. Examples are techniques against common methods bias (Bempong & Asiamah, 2022; Jakobsen & Jensen, 2015), a robust assessment of the properties of psychometric scales such as internal consistency and validity, and coding and scoring of the measures based on established standards (Sullivan & Artino, 2013). These techniques, however, do not eliminate the susceptibility of subjective measures to response and recall biases, which can be high among older adults with cognitive limitations.

Likewise, researchers utilising GIS-based measures should acknowledge the limitations of their measures and admit that these measures do not capture human psychology, which is necessary for understanding feelings and experiences that determine transportation choices. In the context of ageing, an acknowledgement of this limitation is crucial since these choices are driven by the lived experiences of older adults and feelings about their well-being. In many contexts, feelings and thoughts must be captured through subjective measures to identify new ways to design neighbourhoods to maximise residents' satisfaction. Editors and reviewers should assess the merit of manuscripts by considering the study context and evaluating the role of human psychology in the ideal evidence. Thus, the mere use of GIS measures should not determine or override the merit of manuscripts.

Since the two measures are unique, as discussed earlier, they should not be viewed as competing methods. It is possible to use both measures in situations where the psychology of healthy transportation choices would complement the objective measurement of walkability. Ultimately, the simultaneous use of both measures, as performed by some researchers (Otsuka et al., 2021), should be accompanied by a sensitivity analysis assessing how the results of the two techniques differ and change across different neighbourhoods, such as between high and low socioeconomic areas. This analysis could also provide an understanding of how the two methods correlate or overlap.

Finally, researchers ought to distinguish GIS-based measures from subjective measures by referring to the latter as 'perceived walkability', which mirrors the psychology captured by subjective measures. A clear distinction between the two measures is necessary for applying existing evidence for the right purposes and the replication of research. Decision-makers are likely to be confused by the literature if researchers continue to insinuate that both methods measure the same thing.

11.5 Conclusion

GIS objective measures produce more accurate data, but they do not measure psychosocial factors that are now recognised as a key part of walkability. High walkability measured with GIS is independent of the thoughts of residents and may, therefore, produce no clues for interventions that are harmonious with the expectations and needs of end-users. Psychometric tools measure psychosocial factors and the primary domains of walkability, which means they can overcome the shortcomings of GIS measures. GIS walkability measures should not replace subjective measures, and their existence should not compel students, researchers, editors, and peer reviewers to discriminate against psychometric measures. The use of psychometric measures to provide data-rich insights into the experiences and thoughts of groups targeted by the Decade of Healthy Ageing 2021–2030 is essential. These experiences will reveal shortcomings associated with campaign-related activities and will better inform ways to design communities and services that meet the expectations of target groups.

Review Questions

1. What are the unique strengths of GIS measures of walkability?
2. What is a psychometric measure of walkability?
3. Enumerate three reasons why psychometric measures of walkability are not always inferior to their counterpart GIS measures.
4. How would the use of psychometric measures of walkability facilitate the realisation of the Decade of Healthy Ageing 2020–2023 campaign?
5. Why is it necessary for students to acknowledge the limitations of psychometric and GIS measures when using them?

References

Asiamah, N. (2017). Social engagement and physical activity: Commentary on why the activity and disengagement theories of ageing may both be valid. *Cogent Medicine, 4*(1), 1289664. https://doi.org/10.1080/2331205x.2017.1289664

Asiamah, N., Conduah, A. K., & Eduafo, R. (2021a). Social network moderators of the association between Ghanaian older adults' neighbourhood walkability and social activity. *Health Promotion International*, 1–11. https://doi.org/10.1093/heapro/daaa156

Asiamah, N., Kouveliotis, K., Eduafo, R., & Borkey, R. (2021b). Psychometric properties of a new scale measuring neglect and abuse of older adults in the community: Implications for social activity. *International Quarterly of Community Health Education, 41*(2), 163–172. https://doi.org/10.1177/0272684X20915384

Bempong, A. E., & Asiamah, N. (2022). Neighbourhood walkability as a moderator of the associations between older Ghanaians' social activity, and the frequency of walking for transportation: A cross-sectional study with sensitivity analyses. *Archives of Gerontology and Geriatrics, 100*(January), 104660. https://doi.org/10.1016/j.archger.2022.104660

Cleveland, J. N., & Agbeke, D. V. (2019). *Socioemotional selectivity theory lifespan perspectives on job performance, performance appraisal / management and creative performance*. 2009.

D'Haese, S., Gheysen, F., De Bourdeaudhuij, I., Deforche, B., Van Dyck, D., & Cardon, G. (2016). The moderating effect of psychosocial factors in the relation between neighborhood walkability and children's physical activity. *International Journal of Behavioral Nutrition and Physical Activity, 13*(1), 1–16. https://doi.org/10.1186/s12966-016-0452-0

Dekker, K., De Vos, S., Musterd, S., & Van Kempen, R. (2011). Residential satisfaction in Housing Estates in European cities: A multi-level research approach. *Housing Studies, 26*(04), 479–499. https://doi.org/10.1080/02673037.2011.559751

Gan, D. R. Y., Fung, J. C., & Cho, I. S. (2020). Neighborhood experiences of people over age 50: Factor structure and validity of a scale. *Gerontologist, 60*(8), E559–E571. https://doi.org/10.1093/geront/gnz111

Grasser, G., Van Dyck, D., Titze, S., & Stronegger, W. J. (2016). A European perspective on GIS-based walkability and active modes of transport. *European Journal of Public Health, 27*(1), 145–151. https://doi.org/10.1093/eurpub/ckw118

Honey-rosés, J., Anguelovski, I., Chireh, V. K., Daher, C., Van Den Bosch, C. K., Litt, J. S., Mawani, V., Michael, K., Orellana, A., Oscilowicz, E., Sánchez, U., Senbel, M., Tan, X., Villagomez, E., Zapata, O., Nieuwenhuijsen, M. J., Anguelovski, I., Chireh, V. K., Daher, C., et al. (2021). The impact of COVID-19 on public space: An early review of the emerging questions—design, perceptions and inequities. *Cities & Health, 5*(1), 263–279. https://doi.org/10.1080/23748834.2020.1780074

Jakobsen, M., & Jensen, R. (2015). Common method bias in public management studies. *International Public Management Journal, 18*(1), 3–30. https://doi.org/10.1080/10967494.2014.997906

Jeffrey, D., Boulangé, C., Giles-Corti, B., Washington, S., & Gunn, L. (2019, April). Using walkability measures to identify train stations with the potential to become transit oriented developments located in walkable neighbourhoods. *Journal of Transport Geography, 76*, 221–231. https://doi.org/10.1016/j.jtrangeo.2019.03.009

Keating, N. (2022). A research framework for the United Nations decade of healthy ageing (2021–2030). *European Journal of Ageing, 19*(3), 775–787. https://doi.org/10.1007/s10433-021-00679-7

Lam, T. M., Wang, Z., Vaartjes, I., Karssenberg, D., Ettema, D., Helbich, M., Timmermans, E. J., Frank, L. D., Den Braver, N. R., Wagtendonk, A. J., Beulens, J. W. J., & Lakerveld, J. (2022). Development of an objectively measured walkability index for The Netherlands. *International Journal of Behavioral Nutrition and Physical Activity, 19*, 1–16. https://doi.org/10.1186/s12966-022-01270-8

Local, S., Management, A., Quality, S., & Centre, M. (1996). *Adapting the SERVQUAL scale and approach to meet the needs of local authority services*. 1995.

Löckenhoff, C. E., & Carstensen, L. L. (2004). Socioemotionol selectivity theory, aging, and health: The increasingly delicate balance between regulating emotions and making tough choices. *Journal of Personality, 72*(6), 1395–1424. https://doi.org/10.1111/j.1467-6494.2004.00301.x

Luckham, R., & Luckham, R. (2018). Building inclusive peace and security in times of unequal development and rising violence development and rising violence. *Peacebuilding, 7259*, 1–24. https://doi.org/10.1080/21647259.2018.1449185

Menassa, M., Stronks, K., Khatmi, F., Roa Díaz, Z. M., Espinola, O. P., Gamba, M., Itodo, O. A., Buttia, C., Wehrli, F., Minder, B., Velarde, M. R., & Franco, O. H. (2023). Concepts and definitions of healthy ageing: A systematic review and synthesis of theoretical models. *EClinicalMedicine, 56*, 101821. https://doi.org/10.1016/j.eclinm.2022.101821

Morris, K. A., Arundell, L., Cleland, V., & Teychenne, M. (2020). Social ecological factors associated with physical activity and screen time amongst mothers from disadvantaged neighbourhoods over three years. *International Journal of Behavioral Nutrition and Physical Activity, 17*(1), 110. https://doi.org/10.1186/S12966-020-01015-5

Nilsson, H., Bülow, P. H., & Kazemi, A. (2015). Theoretical contributions mindful sustainable aging: advancing a comprehensive approach to the challenges and opportunities of old age. *Europe's Journal of Psychology, 11*, 494. https://doi.org/10.5964/ejop.v11i3.949

Otsuka, N., Wittowsky, D., Damerau, M., & Gerten, C. (2021, July). Walkability assessment for urban areas around railway stations along the Rhine-Alpine Corridor. *Journal of Transport Geography, 93*, 103081. https://doi.org/10.1016/j.jtrangeo.2021.103081

Oyeyemi, A. L., Kasoma, S. S., Onywera, V. O., Assah, F., Adedoyin, R. A., Conway, T. L., Moss, S. J., Ocansey, R., Kolbe-Alexander, T. L., Akinroye, K. K., Prista, A., Larouche, R., Gavand, K. A., Cain, K. L., Lambert, E. V., Aryeetey, R., Bartels, C., Tremblay, M. S., & Sallis, J. F. (2016). NEWS for Africa: Adaptation and reliability of a built environment questionnaire for physical activity in seven African countries. *International Journal of Behavioral Nutrition and Physical Activity, 13*(1), 1–12. https://doi.org/10.1186/s12966-016-0357-y

Pani-Harreman, K. E., Bours, G. J. J. W., Zander, I., Kempen, G. I. J. M., & Van Duren, J. M. A. (2020). Definitions, key themes and aspects of "ageing-in-place": A scoping review. *Ageing and Society, 1–34*, 2026. https://doi.org/10.1017/S0144686X20000094

Pontin, F. L., Jenneson, V. L., Morris, M. A., Clarke, G. P., & Lomax, N. M. (2022). Objectively measuring the association between the built environment and physical activity: A systematic review and reporting framework. *International Journal of Behavioral Nutrition and Physical Activity*, 1–22. https://doi.org/10.1186/s12966-022-01352-7

Professions, C. (2021). *Socially active Neighbourhoods for older adults: A consolidation of evidence from psychometric tests and cross-sectional studies.*

Rudnicka, E., Napierała, P., Podfigurna, A., Męczekalski, B., Smolarczyk, R., & Grymowicz, M. (2020, February). The World Health Organization (WHO) approach to healthy ageing. *Maturitas, 139*, 6–11. https://doi.org/10.1016/j.maturitas.2020.05.018

Saelens, B. E., Sallis, J. F., Black, J. B., & Chen, D. (2003). Comité Européen des Entreprises Vins (CEEV) (2016b) Internal market and food safety. Comité Vins, Brussels. http://ceev.eu/policy-dossiers/internal-market-food-safety. Accessed 02 Nov 2016. *American Journal of Public Health, 93*(9), 1552–1558. http://ceev.eu/policy-dossiers/internal-market-food-safety

Sallis, J. F., Kerr, J., Carlson, J. A., Norman, G. J., Saelens, B. E., Durant, N., & Ainsworth, B. E. (2010). Evaluating a brief self-report measure of neighborhood environments for physical activity research and surveillance: Physical Activity Neighborhood Environment Scale (PANES). *Journal of Physical Activity and Health, 7*(4), 533–540. https://doi.org/10.1123/jpah.7.4.533

Sullivan, G. M., & Artino, A. R. (2013). Analyzing and interpreting data from Likert-type scales. *Journal of Graduate Medical Education, 5*(4), 541–542. https://doi.org/10.4300/jgme-5-4-18

Telega, A., & Telega, I. (2021). Measuring walkability with GIS — Methods overview and new approach proposal. *Sustainability, 13*(4), 1883.

Wahl, H. W., & Gerstorf, D. (2018, August). A conceptual framework for studying COntext Dynamics in Aging (CODA). *Developmental Review, 50*, 155–176. https://doi.org/10.1016/j.dr.2018.09.003

Wahl, H. W., & Gerstorf, D. (2020). Person-environment resources for aging well: Environmental docility and life space as conceptual pillars for future contextual gerontology. *Gerontologist, 60*(3), 368–375. https://doi.org/10.1093/geront/gnaa006

Westland, J. C. (2022). Information loss and bias in likert survey responses. *PLoS One, 17*(7), e0271949. https://doi.org/10.1371/journal.pone.0271949

Williams, G. C., Borghese, M. M., & Janssen, I. (2018, December). Neighborhood walkability and objectively measured active transportation among 10–13 year olds. *Journal of Transport and Health, 8*, 202–209. https://doi.org/10.1016/j.jth.2017.12.006

Yang, J., Zhou, M., Ren, Z., Li, M., Wang, B., Liu, D. L., Ou, C., Yin, P., Sun, J., Tong, S., Wang, H., Zhang, C., Wang, J., Guo, Y., & Liu, Q. (2021). Projecting heat-related excess mortality under climate change scenarios in China. *Nature Communications*, 1–11. https://doi.org/10.1038/s41467-021-21305-1

Chapter 12
The Role of PROMs in Mitigating Infectious Disease Crises: A Healthy Ageing Perspective

Kasturi Shukla and Asiya Attar

Acronyms and Abbreviations

AAFP	American Academy of Family Physicians
AARP	American Association of Retired Persons
AFCCs	Age-Friendly Cities and Communities
CDC	Centre for Disease Control and Prevention
CHI	Community Health Initiatives
GSAP	Global Strategy and Action Plan
ICOPE	Integrated Care for Older People
PHAB	Public Health Accreditation Board
PROMs	Patient-Reported Outcome Measures
QoL	Quality of Life
SDGs	Sustainable Development Goals
UN	United Nations
WHO	World Health Organization

12.1 Introduction

The value and productivity of a long-living individual are decided not just by the length of life but also by the health status of the living individual. Combined with the declined fertility rates, the reduced incidence of infectious diseases has resulted in higher life expectancy worldwide (World Health Organization, 2015a). According

K. Shukla (✉) · A. Attar
Symbiosis Institute of Health Sciences, Symbiosis International (Deemed University), Pune, India
e-mail: drkasturi@sihs.edu.in; asiya.attar@gmail.com

N. Asiamah et al. (eds.), *Sustainable Ageing*,
https://doi.org/10.1007/978-3-031-69475-2_12

to the World Report on Ageing and Health, the elderly and the ageing are being given importance in the global agenda to ensure that no one is left behind. WHO World Report on Ageing and Health thoroughly reviews the body of knowledge currently existing about how ageing and health interact (World Health Organization, 2015b).

Based on the findings of the 2015 report, the World Health Assembly requested the WHO to create a thorough plan called the Global Strategy and Action Plan (WHO GSAP 2016–2020) on Ageing and Health (World Health Organization, 2016). Consequently, 'The Decade of Healthy Ageing 2021–2030' programme was initiated under the WHO-GSAP and is in alignment with the United Nations Madrid International Plan of Action on Ageing 2002. Therefore, coinciding with the Sustainable Development Goals (SDGs) and the United Nations Agenda 2030 on Sustainable Development (Keating, 2022). The Decade of Healthy Ageing calls for 'concerted, catalytic, and collaborative action to improve the lives of older people, their families, and the communities in which they live', with shared accountability (World Health Organization, 2020a). Keeping older people at the centre, this plan brings together governments, civil society, international agencies, professionals, academia, the media, and the business sector to better the lives of older people, their families, and their communities.

The United Nations (UN) endorsed the Decade of Healthy Ageing in December 2020. It aims to enhance the lives of older individuals, their families, and communities. The UN agencies, along with WHO, have developed a Healthy Ageing Framework that concentrates on older people in various environments and describes both desired processes and outcomes. Several strategies have been introduced to achieve this goal. WHO has suggested implementing Integrated Care for Older People (ICOPE) as a key measure for the Decade of Healthy Ageing. To put this into practice, WHO formulated four plans of action based on an equity perspective to maximise the health outcomes for all older adults. Out of the four plans of action, the third plan of action is to 'deliver person-centred, integrated care and primary health services with higher responsiveness to older people' (World Health Organization, 2020a). This action aims to provide older people with non-discriminatory access to basic health care for older persons without causing financial hardship (Keating, 2022). Given the ongoing difficulties in combating the infectious disease crises, it is crucial to strengthen public health promotion and address the specific health needs of the ageing population (Assar et al., 2016). With its importance on person-centred care and coordination, ICOPE and the third action area represent a continuum of care that will assist in reorienting social and health services during infectious disease crises.

Healthcare professionals need to be enabled to better identify the challenges that older patients encounter while fighting against infectious diseases. One of the recent solutions is to integrate Patient-Reported Outcome Measures (PROMs) into standard clinical practice. This is a major development in the current healthcare discourse, as utilising PROMs in the process of mitigating infectious diseases can provide clear documentation of the patients' perspective regarding relief from symptoms, the effectiveness of treatment, and the general improvement of their well-being. There are numerous pieces of evidence that these patient-centred approaches have been significant in mitigating the healthcare requirements of older individuals and promoting healthy and sustainable ageing. However, PROMs are not an integral component of international guidelines like ICOPE and various WHO and UN guidelines that are focused on ageing. Therefore, this chapter emphasises the impact of infectious diseases on ageing populations. Furthermore, the authors have also explored the application of PROMs to supplement the achievement of goals set as a part of the Decade of Healthy Ageing for the ageing populations suffering from infectious diseases.

The chapter explores the possibility of adding more value to the older patients' voices to acknowledge their unique viewpoints and the complicated issues and subtle difficulties that they encounter when trying to manage infectious diseases. Additionally, the individualised, patient-centred care strategies catered to the unique requirements and preferences of older adults, might diverge greatly from those of younger demographics. Hence, policymakers, academics, and practitioners in the healthcare industry can better understand the complex nature of these infections and create focused interventions that support healthy and sustainable ageing. In addition to improving the standard of care for older patients with infectious diseases, this move towards patient-centred care aims to foster a culture of dignity, respect, and empowerment, all of which are critical for encouraging healthy and sustainable ageing.

While PROMs are increasingly recognised as valuable tools in many healthcare domains, their application in the specific context of infectious diseases and ageing brings a distinct perspective to the literature, which is the aim of this chapter. Overall, this chapter shall contribute by focusing on the importance of individualised treatment for older adults during infectious disease crisis and documenting PROMs as an essential resource for addressing challenges encountered by this cohort. Additionally, the authors have attempted to present strategies to enable proactive healthcare for older individuals and the application of PROMs to combat the infectious disease crisis.

To elaborate on the points mentioned above and address the knowledge gaps, the chapter has been organised into eight sections. The first section, the introduction, provides a background to the chapter, whereas the second section sets the overview and provides data on infectious diseases and ageing. The basis and comprehension of the related concepts of sustainable ageing are clarified by providing the various definitions in the third section. In the fourth section, the 'co-design strategy' and the stakeholders' approach, along with an overview of the global initiatives, have been stated. The significance of PROMs in sustainable ageing is explained in the fifth section, whereas the global response towards the Decade of Healthy Ageing is explained in the sixth section. The authors then propose a multilevel programme framework to attain sustainable ageing in the seventh section. The eighth section presents the concluding remarks.

12.2 An Overview on Infectious Diseases and Ageing

According to the Centres for Disease Control and Prevention, infections are the main cause of mortality and morbidity for individuals above 65 years of age (CDC, 2022; Jing et al., 2023; Serenity care, 2022). In fact, one-third of all deaths in adults 65 years of age and older are caused by infectious diseases (American Academy of Family Physicians, 2022). Pneumonia, skin infections, and urinary tract infections are the top three infectious diseases among the elderly (Duvall, 2020). It is more difficult to diagnose common diseases such as pneumonia, urinary tract infections, and skin infections in adults over 65 years of age. This can result in chronic illness, continuous discomfort, and an increased risk of hospitalisation (Kline & Bowdish, 2016; Serenity Care, 2022). It is an accepted fact that unpredictability, transmissibility, and preventability, which distinguish infectious diseases from other ailments, are also dangerous for public health and significantly impact older adults (Jing et al., 2023).

There is a serious risk to nations from infectious or communicable diseases. Older adults have lowered resistance thresholds. The presence of underlying medical disorders and/or frailty makes them more susceptible to infectious diseases (United Nations, 2020). Systems must adapt and change to meet the demands of the ageing population with a growing number of complex health problems, particularly in the face of the ongoing threat of infectious diseases (United Nations, Economic and Social Commission for Asia and the Pacific, 2021). The interaction of infectious diseases and ageing needs new approaches to identification, monitoring, and resilience, emphasising the importance of holistic care (Conroy & van Oppen, 2023). Due to the variations in the way infections affect people of different ages, older patients may not exhibit the symptoms commonly seen in younger patients. Consequently, diagnosing infections in older adults can be challenging at times. Therefore, during such crises and emergencies, older people with infectious diseases are particularly vulnerable (HelpAge International, 2020). These scenarios have led to the evolution of frameworks, one of which is sustainable ageing, which is discussed in further sections.

12.3 Gaining Insight into Sustainable Ageing

The growing paradigm of ageing has led to terms such as 'successful', 'active', and 'healthy' ageing, which shapes the political debate and influences the academic discourse on the positive elements of ageing (Yazdanpanahi & Hussein, 2021). The hallmark of healthy, successful, and active ageing is preserving well-being and functional capacity. Maintaining one's well-being in old age can be difficult, and global crises (i.e. infectious disease, war and violence, climate change, and extreme industrialisation) can make ageing interventions less effective (Asiamah, 2023).

Sustainable ageing needs to be adopted as a new approach to enable older individuals to age well with little or no impact on the global crises. Sustainable ageing is defined as the 'maintenance of a high physical functional ability and engagement with life at an individual level, for well-being with little or no impact of the global crises in later life' (Asiamah, 2023). According to this definition, even when a person lives in a community that is experiencing a crisis, sustainable ageing leads to strong functional ability, life involvement, and health in later life (Asiamah, 2023). 'No or limited impact of the crises' conveys two different meanings. First, older people have the opportunity to avert crises through their own actions or through proactive measures by responsible authorities. Second, by taking comparable actions, the crises effects can be reduced (Asiamah, 2023). Promoting healthy ageing is vital for sustainable ageing, enabling meaningful social and economic contributions across individuals' lifespans (Yazdanpanahi & Hussein, 2021).

To guarantee that every person makes significant social and economic contributions throughout their life, healthy ageing is promoted as a crucial element of sustainable ageing (Sadana & Michel, 2019; Yazdanpanahi & Hussein, 2021). Over the last 40 years, numerous attempts have been made to define healthy ageing and its counterparts. This reflects changing attitudes and a growing public interest in the well-being and health of older people (Browning et al., 2017). The major concern associated with global crises is their potential to worsen the environment in which people age, jeopardise the ability of older adults to lead normal lives, and undermine public health spending and collaboration (Asiamah, 2022; Li et al., 2018; Quinn et al., 2022).

The definitions of healthy and sustainable ageing are more than just semantic quirks. They signify a conceptual framework that supports the overall objectives of encouraging senior citizens' security, involvement, and well-being. When the focus is on holistic well-being, which encompasses the social, psychological, and physical aspects of older adults' health, the integration of these objectives becomes even more evident.

The growing number of older persons should be embraced as a success for improving human health rather than viewed as a challenge to a productive society (Irving, 2014). Healthy ageing is embracing positive viewpoints that lead to an increase in longevity (Aula & Masoodian, 2023). With an increasing number of older people, beliefs and conventions around ageing are changing (Higgs & Gilleard, 2017). In the past few decades, there has been a conscious effort to refocus discussions surrounding old age. There has been a shift in the perception of ageing populations from a more negative perspective, like perceived economic burden, to a more positive perspective, like being valuable economic and social assets (Foster & Walker, 2015). Thus, sustainable ageing also has implications for the caretakers of older individuals, who are the critical stakeholders in their overall healthcare. Sustainable ageing cannot be approached unless all stakeholders are considered, which is discussed further.

12.4 Stakeholder Approach for Sustainable Ageing and Global Initiatives

A 'co-design strategy', which is defined as a multidisciplinary endeavour to support individuals and populations in ageing well, can optimise sustainable ageing (Asiamah, 2023). This principle emphasises the participation of all stakeholders (such as individuals, governments, opinion leaders, and civil society organisations) in healthy ageing projects (Asiamah, 2023). The need for governments and other key stakeholders (such as the WHO) to educate all stakeholders about their individual responsibilities is an essential part of the co-design method. In situations where there are multiple crises and people are needed to create and implement policies, this effort would create enough synergy to continue campaigns for healthy ageing. The sustainability of the co-design strategy is essential, as the global crises may have long-term effects on society (Asiamah et al., 2021). Hence, the next few subsections talk about the various national and international bodies that are critical stakeholders in developing effective programmes for sustainable and healthy ageing.

12.4.1 Decade of Healthy Ageing by WHO

The Decade of Healthy Ageing (2016–2020), an initiative by the WHO, its member states, and the SDGs stakeholders, overlapped with the purpose of active ageing and physical activity promotion campaigns (Rudnicka et al., 2020; World Health Organization, 2021a). The initiative was renewed since diversity and inequity were not eradicated by the end of 2020 (Asiamah, 2023). The updated version of the aforementioned plan, known as the Decade of Healthy Ageing (2021–2030), came with ten goals, one of which was to match health systems to the needs of the older population (Rudnicka et al., 2020; Schick-Makaroff, 2021) While this is a promising approach towards healthy ageing, increasing global crises like infectious disease crises may slow it down (Asiamah, 2023). In such situations, self-reported patient outcome measures can contribute to maintaining the Quality of Life (QoL) among ageing populations. However, this will be dealt with in detail in the later sections.

12.4.2 WHO—Global Strategy Action Plan

WHO has listed its key goals, which include enhancing global data collection, implementation of policies, and doing research on healthy ageing to satisfy the needs of older adults. These key goals ensure that professionals trained in long-term care are instigating a global campaign by expanding the network for age-friendly cities and communities (Rudnicka et al., 2020). The Decade of Healthy Ageing and WHO-GSAP are providing a rather strong base for this action. The successful implementation of these programmes and strategies may be hampered in a crisis situation. There are two goals in the strategy (2016–2020):

1. A five-year plan based on evidence to maximise each person's functional capacity.
2. Develop collaborations and evidence by 2020 to enable a Decade of Healthy Ageing, which runs from 2020 to 2030 (World Health Organization, 2016). The strategy aims to address five strategic objectives:

    (a) Promoting healthy ageing in all countries.
    (b) Creating age-friendly environments.
    (c) Aligning health systems with older populations needs.
    (d) Creating sustainable and equitable long-term care systems (home, communities, and institutions).
    (e) Enhancing measurement, evaluation, and research on healthy ageing.

The last strategic objective, which is improving measurement evaluation, can be better achieved through self-reported patient assessments such as PROMs. The PROMs can be used for a deeper understanding of the individual experiences, health-related behaviours, and outcomes of the older population. On a national level, countries worldwide are formulating responses to the Decade Action Plan. They are committed to the strategy and identify key areas where policy decisions can be supported by knowledge development to achieve the objectives of the Decade of Healthy Ageing (Keating, 2022). The initiatives by different countries are elaborated in Sect. 12.6. The UN Decade Plan is based on global research. However, the data for understanding the environment, life cycles, and well-being will be based on specific countries and regions. This is further supported by WHO's ten priorities for achieving the Decade of Healthy Ageing objectives (2021–2030). The fifth priority, 'Aligning health systems to the needs of older people' introduces the ICOPE strategy, which provides standards for systems, services, and primary care providers (World Health Organization, 2019a, b).

12.4.3 *Integrated Care for Older People (ICOPE)*

The WHO-ICOPE guidelines for community-level interventions were issued in October 2017. The ICOPE guidelines provide advice on preventing, slowing, or reversing the decline in physical and mental abilities in older people (World Health Organization, 2019a). These guidelines provide healthcare providers with 13 evidence-based suggestions to support the development and implementation of person-centred ICOPE in the community. These suggestions demand countries prioritise older individuals' needs and choices while also coordinating care. The ICOPE guidelines will enable countries to improve the health and well-being of their older populations while moving closer to achieving universal health care for people of all ages (Integrated Care for Older People, 2017).

Sustainable ageing emerges as a central theme within the ICOPE initiative in the context of infectious disease crises. ICOPE stands out as an important component, calling for a comprehensive approach to the well-being of the elderly. In order to promote active and healthy ageing, it is necessary to acknowledge and address the social, psychological, and physical aspects of health. The ICOPE strategy embodies the optimisation of intrinsic capacity and functional ability as the basis of healthy ageing (Integrated Care for Older People, 2017). For this reason, the WHO Decade of Healthy Ageing (2021–2030) provides a framework to carefully address the many needs of older people within the global health objectives, especially those that align with the SDGs (United Nations, 2015; World Health Organization, 2019b).

ICOPE recognises the particular difficulties posed by infectious diseases in older populations. It is, therefore, in line with SDG 3 (Good Health and Well-Being) and helps attain universal health coverage. The chapter acknowledges the importance of health on the overall sustainability of communities and links with SDGs 11 (sustainable cities and communities) and 12 (responsible consumption and production) by viewing infectious disease crises through a sustainable ageing lens. ICOPE emphasises the importance of using landmark campaigns to improve care in the community. The importance of person-centred care and community-based interventions for older people is recognised through this strategic approach.

ICOPE prioritises better community care by encouraging inclusivity and older people's access to high-quality healthcare services. Hence, it is in line with SDGs 10 (reduced inequalities) and 16 (peace, justice, and strong institutions). The implementation of ICOPE requires a rigorous monitoring and evaluation plan and continuous sensitisation of older people about the risks to their physical and mental health and to infectious diseases crises. It is critical to correctly examine the health and needs of older adults while dealing with infectious disease crises. In order to encourage sustainable ageing, it is imperative to incorporate a self-reported measure to gather information directly from older individuals. PROMs are a widely used metric that would be quite applicable in this case.

12.5 Patient-Reported Outcome Measures (PROMs) as a Tool for Sustainable Ageing

12.5.1 Definition and Framework of PROMs

Patient-reported outcome measures (PROMs) entail asking patients directly about their symptoms, functional abilities, and overall health (Conroy & van Oppen, 2023). PROMs can be used to evaluate a broad range of health-related concepts, in particular for measuring performance and QoL (Cella et al., 2015). PROMs are tools that help determine whether patient goals have been reached and can help initiate a beneficial dialogue with them about their priorities (Horn et al., 2021). With the interactions between patients and clinicians, PROMs can assist in obtaining opinions on health at the Micro Level (Schick-Makaroff et al., 2021). PROMs go a long way in evaluating the impact on health-related behaviours and concerns. PROMs that identify social and emotional needs can play an important role in collecting important data that helps with the creation of personalised treatment plans (Campbell et al., 2021).

A carefully constructed and validated PROM can be used in various contexts (different nations and care settings), populations (older patients), and goals (decision-making with individual patients) (Printza & Triaridis, 2022). Depending on the objectives of the application of PROMs, different kinds of instruments (measures that are generic or disease-specific) and methods of administration (self-reporting, interviews, telephone administration, or online kiosk applications) can be utilised (Silveira et al., 2018). PROMs are applied at an individual or clinical level. To understand its role in crisis situations, the further subsections will explore the application of PROMs to supplement the achievement of goals set as a part of the WHO GSAP, Decade of Healthy Ageing, and ICOPE.

12.5.2 Integration with WHO GSAP

A comprehensive approach to health and person-centred care is prioritised in sustainable ageing, which acknowledges the diverse needs of the senior population (World Health Organization, 2016). PROMs enable older people to self-report their health and give a comprehensive picture of their circumstances by emphasising the specific experiences from their perspectives (Newlands et al., 2023). This aligns with WHO principles to promote healthy ageing. Accordingly, PROMs are crucial in enabling older persons to directly describe their functional skills, general health, and symptoms, thereby facilitating a tailored treatment strategy.

12.5.3 Integration with Decade of Healthy Ageing

Countries must provide person-centred, integrated care, and comprehensive primary health services in order to achieve universal health coverage for more people by 2030 (WHO, 2020b). PROMs frequently centre on the effects of symptoms, such as how much pain interferes with daily functioning. These are essentially functional status metrics that align with the definition of healthy ageing (Cella et al., 2015). PROMs provide data on the efficacy of healthcare policies and interventions, thereby supporting evidence-based decision-making that is consistent with the third action plan of the Decade of Healthy Ageing (Campbell et al., 2021).

12.5.4 Integration with ICOPE

The changing requirements of healthcare provision for older adults can be adjusted flexibly through PROM-enabled monitoring. This reinforces the adaptable nature of sustainable ageing. Hence, older populations could experience improved health outcomes and an overall improvement in QoL (Rikkert et al., 2018). PROMs and ICOPE are comparable, wherein both offer an all-encompassing strategy for the well-being of the elderly. Thus, the incorporation of PROMs into the ICOPE can signify an important advancement in the evaluation and management of older individuals' health.

It highlights the need for a person-centred approach and encourages older people to actively report their health status (World Health Organization, 2019a). The use of PROMs in programmes such as ICOPE shall promote resilience by ensuring targeted treatments that improve overall health and well-being. These outcomes also place a high value on QoL to enhance their well-being. Prioritising outcomes will have the potential to improve systems and services that matter most to patients, particularly in times of infectious disease crisis (Conroy & van Oppen, 2023).

Inclusiveness is highly prioritised by ICOPE, which ensures older people have access to excellent healthcare to meet their urgent needs by minimising inequalities. Thus, the increased susceptibility of older people to infections emphasises the critical need for effective health strategies. It also underlines the indispensable function of PROMs in situations involving infectious diseases. One way to address this is by integrating PROMs in flagship campaigns, but prior to that, a global response to healthy ageing needs to be explored.

12.6 Global Response Towards Healthy and Sustainable Ageing

Stereotypes (how we think), prejudice (how we feel), and discrimination (how we act) against people or oneself because of one's age are together referred to as ageism (World Health Organization, 2021b). One of the main concerns about the growing global population and its share of older people is whether or not they would have better health, a higher QoL, social inclusion, and stable income. Negative perceptions and presumptions about the older population have the power to shape social norms, individual behaviour, and societal values. Therefore, it is necessary to enact laws against age-based discrimination, both directly and indirectly (Burnes et al., 2019; Officer & de la Fuente-Núñez, 2018).

Understanding sustainable ageing requires a shift from conventional healthcare methods and an integrated approach that recognises the mutual dependency of these elements. The holistic viewpoint was made possible by the Decade of Healthy Ageing and the WHO guidelines. This emphasises the value of complete health promotion that extends beyond the absence of disease.

The Decade of Healthy Ageing is not a mandate. Rather, it is a strategic framework that facilitates a wide range of national ageing policies. To achieve the SDGs, policy measures to manage the ageing population are essential (United Nations 2019; United Nations 2021). When crises of infectious diseases occur, these regulations become more significant. Of the 14 measures listed in the UN's Twelfth Inquiry, the three most common ageing policies have been implemented by governments in the last 5 years. This includes the promotion of personal savings (65%), expansion of lifelong learning (66%), and promotion of active and healthy ageing (76%) (UN Population Division, 2019). These actions reflect a global commitment to age-friendly communities and support the initiatives that improve the overall health of older people. These activities are encouraged across the developed continents such as Europe, North America, and Oceania. Consequently, the development of long-term and institutional care programmes was a widespread response to the ageing population in Northern Africa and Western Asia (United Nations, 2015; United Nations, 2019).

In developing countries like India, many activities are being undertaken throughout the year, aimed at mainstreaming issues related to the older population and deliberating upon the ways to ensure better and more effective health delivery of services (Lamb & Goswami, 2024). Indonesia emphasises the relevance of all action items in its National Strategic Plan on Ageing (Ministry of Justice and Human Rights, Republic of Indonesia, 2021). Chile supports decade action items and sees its national plan as an opportunity to develop social healthcare and rights policies (Gobierno de Chile, 2021). African countries have adopted unique approaches to defining regional objectives in response to the Decade Action Plan. The African Union is considering the adoption of a draft set of priorities developed by regional academics and civil society organisations.

When it comes to the implementation of ICOPE, several nations have embraced its guidelines. In March 2023, with the cooperation of WHO, the ICOPE strategy and action plan 2022–2026 were brought into force in Mauritius. The important aspects of implementing and scaling up the ICOPE technique were to ensure ICOPE's long-term viability and a rigorous training strategy (WHO, 2020a). The training manual for ICOPE trainers, initially created and published by the WHO Southeast Asia Regional Office, underwent adoption for use in Sri Lanka (WHO, 2020b).

Although developed nations have made headway in implementing these guidelines, a global approach is needed to take into account the cultural differences and national capacities of other countries (Rudnicka et al., 2020). This approach will allow different countries having varying priorities to develop their own unique strategies. Although there is an optional adoption of recommendations, there is a lack of clearly defined evaluation criteria, resulting in uneven submissions of descriptive, fragmented, and self-defined material. This results in a lack of research regarding the relationship between outcomes and policy impact (Rudnicka et al., 2020).

Various disease-specific PROMs are recognised and used worldwide for infectious diseases. The most often utilised PROM tools in cases of pneumonia are the 36-item Short Form Survey (SF-36), the CAP-symptom questionnaire (CAP-Sym), and the CAP burden of illness questionnaire (CAP-BIQ) (Lloyd et al., 2019). Numerous PROMs have been created and proven in dermatology for a variety of skin infections and conditions. Since PROMs capture the voice of the patient regarding the effects of their skin infections (and its treatments), they may serve as an important indicator during infectious disease crises (Snyder et al., 2023). Isotretinoin, for instance, can be used to treat skin infections since it clinically and substantially improves HRQL as determined by Skindex-16 (Secrest et al., 2020).

The most commonly used PROMs for urinary tract infections are the Urinary Tract Infection-Symptom and Impairment Questionnaire (UTI-SIQ-8), the Urinary Tract Infection Symptom Assessment Questionnaire (UTISA), and the International Consultation on Incontinence Questionnaire for Female Lower Urinary Tract Symptoms (ICIQ-FLUTS) (Piontek et al., 2023).

12.6.1 Prioritisation

The size of the world population has increased by more than three times since the middle of the twentieth century. Furthermore, the global population's age distribution is progressively moving older (United Nations, 2019). The United Nations Population Division projects that over the next three decades, the number of people 65 and older will double, reaching 1.6 billion by 2050. Nearly every country in the world is experiencing a higher proportion of an ageing population, albeit at varying rates and degrees. The percentage of older people and the median age of the population are expected to rise in all nations, but the extent and effects of ageing will differ greatly. In many developing nations, for instance, the population is still comparatively young but is ageing quicker than in developed countries (United Nations, 2019; United Nations 2021)Ageing populations around the world are placing increased demands on people's well-being and access to healthcare, among other demands on individuals, families, communities, and society. Consequently, from a sustainability viewpoint, the ageing population should be considered more rigorously in policymaking (Grazuleviciute-Vileniske et al., 2020). In order to achieve this, sustainable ageing should be advanced through community campaigns.

12.6.2 Advancing Sustainable Ageing Through Community Care Campaigns

Healthy ageing campaigns are perhaps the best way to tackle the ageing population. However, it is unclear whether global crises can jeopardise the efforts of the advocates or the ageing process itself (Asiamah, 2023). Sustainable ageing is greatly aided by community-level interventions. Community awareness and engagement campaigns are essential to support older people and encourage their active participation in many aspects of life. These initiatives are of great importance as they can create an age-friendly environment, which is in line with the World Health Organization's Decade of Healthy Ageing (World Health Organization, 2020b, c). These communities help older people come out of poor health.

The longer the people live in poor health, the greater the demand for health and social services. Although life expectancy has increased, years spent in good health have not increased. Therefore, it is critical to support ageing individuals in a healthy way (Health Action Research Group, 2021). Thus, a number of programmes and frameworks have been formed to promote sustainable ageing.

The John A. Hartford Foundation's Age-Friendly Public Health Systems 6 Cs Framework, the WHO Age-Friendly Cities Framework (World Health Organization, 2015a, b, c), and the American Association of Retired Persons (AARP, 2014) 8 Domains of Liveability offer a structured system for cultivating a culture of healthy ageing across the lifespan, especially within public health and Community Health Initiatives (CHI). These frameworks emphasise the dynamic interplay of multiple factors and provide a basis for improving opportunities for healthy ageing through public health practices, policies, and research.

A number of additional tools and frameworks (e.g., Age-Friendly Framework (AARP, 2014), age-friendly public health system (AFPHS) framework (TFAH, 2024), and Healthy People 2030 (NASEM, 2019)) have been developed to promote and research healthy ageing. They focus on ways to address social determinants of health and promote health equity. With the aim of improving the health and overall well-being of older populations, Healthy People 2030 provides a range of objectives and evidence-based materials that should serve as a guideline for health policy and practise focused on older people. With health equity as the basis, the Public Health Accreditation Board (PHAB) provides a framework that assists local health departments to enhance and bring about advancements in public health practice through performance improvement (Public Health Accreditation Board, 2021). Approaches like these will tackle the social issues surrounding health and promote health equity by reducing the risk in crisis situations.

12.6.3 Mitigating Infectious Disease Crises

The proactive way of mitigating infectious disease crises offers a way to reduce the impact of such outbreaks. As individuals get older, health problems become chronic, and many illnesses and disorders frequently coexist. However, treating acute illnesses is the main emphasis of most health services (De Carvalho et al., 2017). The accurate assessment of the functional, psychological, and medical abilities of an older individual requires relevant tools and trained professionals. These tools are necessary to organise an integrated plan for treatment and long-term care (Stoop et al., 2019).

Infections like pneumonia, urinary tract disease, and skin infections have been linked with a high mortality rate and have a significant negative impact on patient's

QoL and functionality (Rowe & Juthani-Mehta, 2013). Early symptom detection is especially important in the context of these most common infectious disorders (Cilloniz et al., 2023). In the middle of an infectious disease crisis, PROMs not only help to standardise patient outcome monitoring, but they also improve the patient-clinician connection. They encourage active patient participation, improve the emphasis of consultations, and, ultimately, contribute to the overall goal of sustainable ageing throughout the Decade of Healthy Ageing. PROMs could provide a unique perspective by measuring patients' assessments of their health. They could help with early symptom detection and contribute to remote monitoring, allowing healthcare providers to monitor changes in health status and intervene proactively. Hence, there is a requirement for a framework that provides a basis for the use of PROMs to attain sustainable ageing. In the next section, the authors have proposed a multilevel framework for the same.

12.7 Multi-level Programme Framework Proposed for Sustainable Ageing

Approaches for sustainable ageing should prevent global crises or lessen their detrimental effects on collaborative initiatives and the ageing process. One of these methods is a co-design approach that combats the crises through interdisciplinary cooperation (Asiamah, 2023). With the help of this strategy, we have assembled a framework that assists in monitoring the outcomes of sustainable ageing.

Long-term solutions for sustainable ageing are even more important given the rise in infectious diseases and the challenges that an ageing population poses to the current healthcare system. In line with this notion, a multidisciplinary strategy that operates at the Mmacro, Meso, and Micro Levels ought to include PROMs (Rudnicka et al., 2020). Promising approaches to ageing include the Decade of Healthy Ageing, but they are being implemented at a time when crises are getting worse (Asiamah, 2023). The authors propose a framework that incorporates the needs and constructs required to achieve sustainable ageing (Fig. 12.1). It is consistent with the ICOPE programme's guiding principles (World Health Organization, 2019a) and also offers a model for addressing the multifaceted issues brought in by infectious disease crises.

People should continue to participate in the larger economy and society well into old age, as this is essential to long-term financial independence (Asiamah, 2023). The old-age dependency ratio—the number of older persons per 100 people of working age between the ages of 20 and 64—is expected to decrease (Muszyńska & Rau, 2012). Reducing the old-age dependency ratio, as much as possible, helps to promote economic development and reduces the financial burden on younger generations. Given this perspective, the proposed model emphasises the need for both financial investment and legislative initiatives at the Macro Level. Legal frameworks that promote adaptability and responsiveness provide the regulatory foundation needed to manage the complexity of healthcare in emergencies. Obtaining

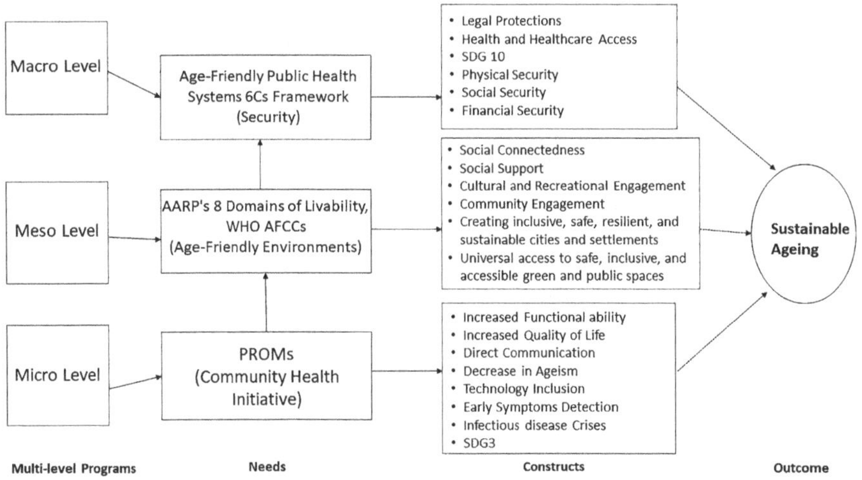

Fig. 12.1 Authors' multi-level framework for attaining sustainable ageing

enough funds at the same time becomes crucial for the efficient implementation of plans, resource allocation, and the development of strong healthcare systems that are tailored to the needs of the older population. This further aligns with the SDG 10 that urges the reduction of income inequalities as well as those that exist within a nation according to factors like age, sex, handicap, colour, ethnicity, origin, religion, or economic or other status (United Nation, 2015).

Additionally, the Age-Friendly Public Health Systems 6 Cs Framework from the campaigns can be seamlessly integrated at the Macro Level. The 6Cs are: Creating—explore socioeconomic elements of health, Connecting—bringing together and integrating stakeholders, Coordinating—identify the gaps in the community offerings to overcome the obstacles to their effectiveness, Collecting—relevant data can call attention to the needs of ageing adults, Communicating—to educate, enlighten, and empower the older people, and Complementing—Taking older persons' needs into consideration by integrating public health with the larger healthcare system promote healthy ageing at its core (TFAH, 2024).

A goal in the WHO's GSAP 2016 emphasises the creation of inclusive, safe, resilient and sustainable cities, and human settlements. The cities would ensure universal access to safe, inclusive and accessible green, and public spaces, especially for older people (Rugel et al., 2022). The WHO Global Network of Age-Friendly Cities and Communities (AFCCs), formed in 2010 and now spanning over 1000 cities and communities, exemplifies effective actions implemented at various levels (Van Hoof et al., 2018; Marston & Van Hoof, 2019). AARP's 8 Domains of Liveability and Age-Friendly Environment Design is critical in reducing the Meso Level effects of infectious disease crises on the aged population. ICOPE guidelines encourage social inclusion and community involvement. In times of infectious disease outbreaks, an age-friendly environment encompasses not only the physical infrastructure but also the social support networks that play a critical role in the overall well-being of older people. Investing in age-friendly infrastructure, access to basic services, and the creation of supportive social structures can significantly improve the sustainability of ageing populations during health crises.

Ageism not only has an extremely negative impact on our health, longevity, and overall well-being but can also weaken intergenerational bonds, alter our self-perception, and limit our ability to benefit from the contributions of the older population (World Health Organization, 2021b). The elimination of ageism is one of the ten goals in the Decade of Healthy Ageing (2021–2030) strategy. When dealing with ageism, the use of PROMs becomes crucial. These measures provide a personalised view of the challenges faced by senior citizens and their families. Integrated care models at the Micro Level ensure that healthcare interventions are effective. Additionally, it also complements the ICOPE programme by promoting a patient-centred approach and taking into account the specific needs and preferences of the older population. The effective use of resources in the security level of the needs column of the framework ensures the long-term viability of healthcare systems. An age-friendly environment is intrinsically tied to the promotion of healthcare practices that lessen their environmental impact, such as telemedicine solutions. It is the responsibility of residents to keep their neighbourhoods age-friendly. These appeals stress the importance of the involvement of the residents in adopting environmentally friendly practices (Danquah et al., 2022; Dugan et al 2022; Rodrigues & Franco, 2021).

Views of older individuals must be heard during infectious disease crises. In such instances, PROMs can help to advance social justice, inclusivity, and community resilience while also acknowledging the interconnection of all people. By following the ICOPE initiative's objectives, this theory seeks to overcome the intricate problems caused by infectious diseases. Integrating PROMs during infectious disease crises offers a flexible and all-encompassing approach to sustainable ageing. Addressing the Macro, Meso, and Micro Levels not only protects older adults during health crises but also increases the resilience and adaptability of healthcare systems.

12.8 Conclusion

The global population is getting older, which emphasises the need to change healthcare to an integrated, person-centred approach that puts older people's needs first. The issues of infectious diseases, ageing, and health discussed here bring to light some important concepts that are necessary for an increasingly sustainable and healthy future for older people. The WHO's key components for active and healthy ageing emphasise the need for a comprehensive approach that includes social, psychological, and physical well-being. Notable frameworks with ambitious goals for improving global health are the Decade of Healthy Ageing and the World Health Organization's Global Strategy and Action Plan on Ageing and Health. The innovative potential of PROMs in assessing health outcomes for the older population could be an important topic of discussion. As PROMs focus on individual experiences and reported symptoms, they are particularly helpful for person-centred, personalised therapy in infectious disease outbreaks. As we address the issues posed by an ageing global population, there is an evident need for action. Coordinated initiatives and improved community care are necessary for sustainable ageing, with flagship campaigns serving as catalysts for change. These initiatives should raise awareness and promote community engagement as well as active engagement in the civic, cultural, and economic arenas. When we embrace all of these concepts, we can work towards a time when ageing is not only a normal process but also a fulfilling and enriching experience for people and communities. This is the moment for unwavering commitment and collaboration to create a more resilient, diverse, and health-conscious environment for our ageing population.

Review Questions

1. How does the Decade of Healthy Ageing complement the objectives of the WHO's Global Strategy and Action Plan on Ageing and Health?
2. What are the key components of the ICOPE approach, and how does it relate to the Decade of Healthy Ageing's overarching objectives?
3. What strategies and policy measures are suggested to address the issues brought about by the world's ageing population?
4. Explain how the inclusion of PROMs can support better decision-making and person-centred care in ageing populations.
5. Examine the necessity of integrating PROMs into the WHO GSAP, Decade of Healthy Ageing, and ICOPE plan for senior citizens during infectious disease crises.

References

American Association of Retired Persons. (2014). *Introduction to the 8 domains of liveability*. Available at: https://www.aarp.org/livable-communities/info-2014/age-friendly-world-tour.html

American Academy of Family Physicians. (2022). Available at: https://www.aafp.org/home.html.

Asiamah, N. (2022). Walkable urban neighbourhoods: The adverse effects of industrialization and climate change in developing countries. In *Sustainable urbanism in developing countries* (pp. 247–262). Available at: https://www.taylorfrancis.com/chapters/edit/10.1201/9781003131922-16/walkable-urban-neighborhoods-nestor-asiamah

Asiamah, N. (2023). 'Sustainable ageing' in a world of crises. In *Sustainable Neighbourhoods for ageing in place: An interdisciplinary voice against global crises* (pp. 217–236). Available at: https://link.springer.com/chapter/10.1007/978-3-031-41594-4_12

Asiamah, N., Opuni, F. F., Mends-Brew, E., Mensah, S. W., Mensah, H. K., & Quansah, F. (2021). Short-term changes in behaviours resulting from COVID-19-related social isolation and their influences on mental health in Ghana. *Community Mental Health Journal, 57*(1), 79–92.

Assar, S., Mirzaei, T., Ravari, A., Vakilian, A. R., Rezahosseini, O., Hosseini, F., & Assar, S. (2016). A study of the status of the elderly; Bacterial infections, their causes, prevention, and control methods. *Journal of Occupational Health and Epidemiology, 5*(3), 182–193.

Aula, I., & Masoodian, M. (2023). *Creativity and healthy ageing: Future research directions*. Available at: https://link.springer.com/article/10.1007/s12062-023-09431-8

Browning, C. J., Thomas, S. A., Kendig, H., & Ory, M. G. (2017). Healthy aging. In N. A. Pachana (Ed.), *Encyclopaedia of geropsychology*. Springer. Available at: https://link.springer.com/referenceworkentry/10.1007/978-981-287-082-7_323

Burnes, D., Sheppard, C., Henderson, C. R., Jr., Wassel, M., Cope, R., Barber, C., & Pillemer, K. (2019). Interventions to reduce ageism against older adults: A systematic review and meta-analysis. *American Journal of Public Health, 109*(8), e1–e9.

Campbell, R., Ju, A., King, M. T., & Rutherford, C. (2021). Perceived benefits and limitations of using patient-reported outcome measures in clinical practice with individual patients: A systematic review of qualitative studies. *Quality of Life Research, 31*, 1596–1620.

Cella, D., Hahn, E. A., Jensen, S. E., Butt, Z., Nowinski, C. J., Rothrock, N., & Lohr, K. N. (2015). *Patient-reported outcomes in performance measurement*. Available at: https://books.google.co.in/books?hl=en&lr=&id=K9gREAAAQBAJ&oi=fnd&pg=PP2&dq=Cella,+D.,+Hahn,+E.+A,+Jensen,+S.+E.,+Butt,+Z.,+Nowinski,+C.+J.,+Rothrock,+N.,+%26+Lohr,+K.+N.+(2015)

Centres for Disease Control and Prevention. (2022). *Trends in health and ageing*. U.S. Department of Health and Human Services. Available at: https://www.cdc.gov/nchs/hus/index.htm

Cilloniz, C., Pericas, J. M., & Curioso, W. H. (2023). Interventions to improve outcomes in community-acquired pneumonia. *Expert Review of Anti-Infective Therapy, 21*(10), 1071–1086.

Conroy, S. P., & van Oppen, J. D. (2023). Are we measuring what matters to older people? *The Lancet Healthy Longevity, 4*(7), e354–e356.

Danquah, E., Asiamah, N., Opuni, F. F., Ocloo, E. C., & Ricky-Okine, C. K. (2022, June). Pro-environment behavioural moderators of the association between perceived walkability and social activity. *Journal of Transport and Health, 27*, 101533. Available at: https://www.sciencedirect.com/science/article/pii/S2214140522002055.

De Carvalho, I. A., Epping-Jordan, J., Pot, A. M., Kelley, E., Toro, N., Thiyagarajan, J. A., & Beard, J. R. (2017). Organizing integrated health-care services to meet older people's needs. *Bulletin of the World Health Organization, 95*(11), 756.

Dugan, E., Porell, F., Silverstein, N. M., & Lee, C. M. (2022). Healthy aging data reports: Measures of community health to identify disparities and spur age-friendly-progress. *The Gerontologist, 62*(1), e28–e38.

Duvall, A. (2020). *Top 3 most common infections seen in elderly | #3. Pneumonia in the elderly — Alee solutions*. Alee Solutions. Available at: https://www.aleesolutions.org

Foster, L., & Walker, A. (2015). Active and successful aging: A European policy perspective. *The Gerontologist, 55*(1), 83–90.

Gobierno de Chile. (2021). *Chile leads launch of Decade of Healthy Ageing 2021–2030, which seeks to improve conditions for older people*. Available at: https://www.gob.cl/en/news/chile-leads-launchdecade-healthy-ageing-2021-2030-which-seeks-improve-conditions-older-people

Grazuleviciute-Vileniske, I., Seduikyte, L., Teixeira-Gomes, A., Mendes, A., Borodinecs, A., & Buzinskaite, D. (2020). Aging, living environment, and sustainability: What should be taken into account? *Sustainability, 12*(5), 1853.

Health Action Research Group. (2021). *Implications for healthy ageing*. Health Action Campaign. Health Canada. Workshop on healthy aging. Available at: https://www.healthactionresearch.org.uk/tackling-obesity/implications-for-healthy-ageing

HelpAge International. (2020). *If not now, when? Keeping promises to older people affected by humanitarian crises*. Available at: https://www.helpage.org/what-we-do/if-notnow-when

Higgs, P., & Gilleard, C. (2017). *Rethinking old age: Theorising the fourth age*. Bloomsbury Publishing. Available at: https://books.google.co.in/books?hl=en&lr=&id=SCVHEAAAQBAJ&oi=fnd&pg=PR1&dq=Higgs,+P.,+%26+Gilleard,+C.+(2017)

Horn, M. E., Reinke, E. K., Mather, R. C., O'Donnell, J. D., & George, S. Z. (2021). Electronic health record–integrated approach for collection of patient-reported outcome measures: A retrospective evaluation. *BMC Health Services Research, 21*(1), 1–11.

Integrated Care for Older People. (2017). *Guidelines on community-level interventions to manage declines in intrinsic capacity*. World Health Organization; 5, Publication, dissemination and evaluation. Available at: https://www.who.int/publications/i/item/9789241550109

Irving, P. (2014). *The upside of aging: How long life is changing the world of health, work, innovation, policy, and purpose*. Wiley. Available at: https://books.google.co.in/books?hl=en&lr=&id=tIZPAwAAQBAJ&oi=fnd&pg=PR11&dq=Irving,+P.+(2014)

Jing, F., Li, Z., Qiao, S., Zhang, J., Olatosi, B., & Li, X. (2023). Using geospatial social media data for infectious disease studies: A systematic review. *International Journal of Digital Earth, 16*(1), 130–157.

Keating, N. (2022). A research framework for the United Nations decade of healthy ageing (2021–2030). *European Journal of Ageing, 19*(3), 775–787.

Kline, K. A., & Bowdish, D. M. (2016). Infection in an aging population. *Current Opinion in Microbiology, 29*, 63–67.

Lamb, S., & Goswami, N. (2024, March). Healthy aging, self-care, and choice in India: Class-based engagements with globally circulating ideologies. *Journal of Aging Studies, 68*, 101194.

Li, M., Li, C., & Zhang, M. (2018). Exploring the spatial spillover effects of industrialization and urbanization factors on pollutants emissions in China's Huang-Huai-Hai region. *Journal of Cleaner Production, 195*, 154–162.

Lloyd, M., Callander, E., Karahalios, A., Desmond, L., & Karunajeewa, H. (2019). Patient-reported outcome measures in community-acquired pneumonia: A systematic review of application and content validity. *BMJ Open Respiratory Research, 6*(1), e000398.

Marston, H. R., & Van Hoof, J. (2019). WHO doesn't think about technology when designing urban environments for older people? A case study approach to a proposed extension of the WHO's age-friendly cities model. *International Journal of Environmental Research and Public Health, 16*(19), 3525.

Muszyńska, M. M., & Rau, R. (2012). The old-age healthy dependency ratio in Europe. *Journal of Population Ageing, 5*(3), 151–162.

National Academies of Sciences, Engineering, and Medicine (NASEM). (2019). *Criteria for selecting the leading health indicators for healthy people 2030*. The National Academies Press. Available at: https://doi.org/10.17226/25531

Newlands, A. F., Roberts, L., Maxwell, K., Kramer, M., Price, J. L., & Finlay, K. A. (2023). Development and psychometric validation of a patient-reported outcome measure of recurrent urinary tract infection impact: The recurrent UTI impact questionnaire. *Quality of Life Research, 32*, 1745–1758.

Officer, A., & de la Fuente-Núñez, V. (2018). A global campaign to combat ageism. *Bulletin of the World Health Organization, 96*(4), 295.

Piontek, K., Donhauser, T., Kann, G., Fechtner, M., Apfelbacher, C., & Gabes, M. (2023). Patient-reported outcome measures for uncomplicated urinary tract infections in women: A systematic review. *Quality of Life Research, 32*, 2137–2153.

Printza, A., & Triaridis, S. (2022). Is the ability of the Eating Assessment Tool (EAT-10) to screen for aspiration in patients with dysphagia depending on the patients' disease? *European Archives of Oto-Rhino-Laryngology, 279*(7), 3745–3746.

Public Health Accreditation Board. (2021). *Version 2.0 work in progress, healthy aging commissioned paper and think tank summary*. Available at: https://phaboard.org/wp-content/uploads/Healthy-Aging.pdf

Quinn, V. J. M., Dhabalia, T. J., Roslycky, L. L., Wilson, V. J. M., Hansen, J. C., Hulchiy, O., et al. (2022). COVID-19 at war: The joint forces operation in Ukraine. *Disaster Medicine and Public Health Preparedness, 16*(5), 1753–1760.

Rikkert, M. G. O., van der Wees, P. J., Schoon, Y., & Westert, G. P. (2018). Using patient reported outcomes measures to promote integrated care. *International Journal of Integrated Care, 18*(2), 8.

Rodrigues, M., & Franco, M. (2021). The role of citizens and transformation of energy, water, and waste infrastructure for an intelligent, sustainable environment in cities. *Smart and Sustainable Built Environment, 12*(2), 385–406.

Rowe, T. A., & Juthani-Mehta, M. (2013). Urinary tract infection in older adults. *Aging Health, 9*(5), 10.

Rudnicka, E., Napierała, P., Podfigurna, A., Męczekalski, B., Smolarczyk, R., & Grymowicz, M. (2020, February). The World Health Organization (WHO) approach to healthy ageing. *Maturitas, 139*, 6–11.

Rugel, E. J., Chow, C. K., Corsi, D. J., Hystad, P., Rangarajan, S., Yusuf, S., & Lear, S. A. (2022). Developing indicators of age-friendly neighbourhood environments for urban and rural communities across 20 low-, middle-, and high-income countries. *BMC Public Health, 22*(1), 1–16.

Sadana, R., & Michel, J. P. (2019). *Healthy ageing: What is it and how to describe it? Prevention of chronic diseases and age-related disability* (pp. 11–24). Available at: https://link.springer.com/chapter/10.1007/978-3-319-96529-1_2

Schick-Makaroff, K., Karimi-Dehkordi, M., Cuthbertson, L., Dixon, D., Cohen, S. R., Hilliard, N., & Sawatzky, R. (2021). Using patient-and family-reported outcome and experience measures across transitions of care for frail older adults living at home: A meta-narrative synthesis. *The Gerontologist, 61*(3), e23–e38.

Secrest, A. M., Hopkins, Z. H., Frost, Z. E., Taliercio, V. L., Edwards, L. D., Biber, J. E., et al. (2020). Quality of life assessed using Skindex-16 scores among patients with acne receiving isotretinoin treatment. *JAMA Dermatology, 156*(10), 1098–1106.

Serenity Care. (2022). *The 5 most common infections in the elderly*. Serenity Home Care. Available at: https://serenitycarehealth.com

Silveira, A., Monteiro, E., & Sequeira, T. (2018). Head and neck cancer: Improving patient-reported outcome measures for clinical practice. *Current Treatment Options in Oncology, 19*, 1–10.

Snyder, A. M., Chen, S. C., Chren, M. M., Ferris, L. K., Edwards, L. D., Swerlick, R. A., et al. (2023). Patient-reported outcome measures and their clinical applications in dermatology. *American Journal of Clinical Dermatology, 24*, 499–511.

Stoop, A., Lette, M., van Gils, P. F., Nijpels, G., Baan, C. A., & De Bruin, S. R. (2019). Comprehensive geriatric assessments in integrated care programs for older people living at home: A scoping review. *Health & Social Care in the Community, 27*(5), e549–e566.

The Ministry of Justice and Human Rights the Republic of Indonesia. (2021). *Regulation of the President of the Republic of Indonesia, No. 88 year 2021 about National Strategic Plan on Ageing*. Available at: https://jdih.bappenas.go.id/peraturan/detailperaturan/2700

Trust for America's Health (TFAH). (2024). *Creating Age Friendly Public Health Systems (AFPHS)*. Available at: https://www.tfah.org/initiatives/age-friendly-public-health

United Nations. (2020). *Policy brief: The impact of COVID-19*. Available at: https://unsdg.un.org/resources/policy-brief-impact-covid-19-older-persons

United Nations. (2021). *Leaving no one behind.* Available at: https://www.un.org/fr/desa/leaving-no-one-behind

United Nations, Department of Economic and Social Affairs, Population Division. (2019). *World population prospects 2019, Volume I: Comprehensive tables*. Available at: https://population.un.org/wpp/Publications/Files/WPP2019_Volume-I_Comprehensive-Tables.pdf

United Nations, Economic and Social Commission for Asia and the Pacific. (2021). *Key elements for developing policies on ageing in Asia and the Pacific*. Available at: http://www.unescap.org/kp/2021/key-elements-ageing-policies-asia-and-pacific

United Nations General Assembly. (2015). *Transforming our world: the 2030 Agenda for Sustainable Development*. Available at: https://sdgs.un.org/2030agenda

Van Hoof, J., Kazak, J. K., Perek-Białas, J. M., & Peek, S. T. (2018). The challenges of urban ageing: Making cities age-friendly in Europe. *International Journal of Environmental Research and Public Health, 15*(11), 2473.

World Health Organization. (2015a). *World report on ageing and health*. Available at: https://apps.who.int/iris/handle/10665/186463

World Health Organization. (2015b). *WHO global strategy on people-centred and integrated health services*. WHO Press. Available at: https://interprofessional.global/wp-content/uploads/2019/11/WHO-2015-Global-strategy-on-integrated-people-centred-health-services-2016-2026.pdf

World Health Organization. (2015c). *Measuring the age-friendliness of cities: A guide to using core indicators*. Available at: https://www.who.int/publications/i/item/9789241509695

World Health Organization. (2016). *Global Strategy Action Plan. Plan of Action on ageing and health 2016–2020: Towards a World in Which All People Can Live a Long and Healthy Life*. A69/A/CONF./8. Agenda item 13.4. Available at: https://www.who.int/publications/i/item/9789241513500

World Health Organization. (2019a). *Integrated care for older people (ICOPE): Guidance for person-centred assessment and pathways in primary care*. Available at: https://www.who.int/publications/i/item/WHO-FWC-ALC-19.1

World Health Organization. (2019b). *World population ageing 2019*. Available at: https://www.un.org/en/development/desa/population/publicatio ns/pdf/ageing/WorldPopulationAgeing2019-Report.pdf

World Health Organization. (2020a). *UN decade of healthy ageing: Plan of action*. Available at: https://www.who.int/initiatives/decade-of-healthy-ageing

World Health Organization. (2020b). *WHO's work on the UN Decade of Healthy Ageing (2021–2030)*. Available at: https://www.who.int/initiatives/decade-of-healthy-ageing

World Health Organization. (2020c). *Healthy ageing and functional ability*. Available at: https://www.who.int/news-room/questions-and-answers/item/healthy-ageing-and-functional-ability

World Health Organization. (2021a). *Decade of healthy ageing: Baseline report*. Available at: https://www.who.int/publications/i/item/9789240017900

World Health Organization. (2021b). *Global Report on Ageism Global report on ageism*. World Health Organization; 2021. Licence: CC BY NC-SA 3.0 IGO. Available at: https://www.who.int/publications/i/item/9789240016866

Yazdanpanahi, M., & Hussein, S. (2021). Sustainable ageing: Supporting healthy ageing and independence amongst older Turkish migrants in the UK. *Sustainability, 13*(18), 10387.

Part IV
Human Development for Healthy Ageing

Chapter 13
Human Development Pathways for Empowering Older Adults: A Decade of Healthy Ageing Perspective

Md. Emaj Uddin

Acronyms and Abbreviations

COVID-19	Coronavirus Disease 2019
HD	Human Development

13.1 Introduction

The UN Decade of Healthy Ageing (2021–2030) brings together diverse sectors and stakeholders to take collaborative actions to foster healthy ageing, which is defined as the maintenance of functional ability and intrinsic capacity needed for well-being in old age (Keating, 2022; WHO, 2020). One of the principles of the Decade of Healthy Ageing initiative is to empower older adults to remain engaged in their communities (Keating, 2022; Rudnicha et al., 2020). Empowerment in this context is aimed at giving older adults a sense of belonging and equipping them with the skills, knowledge, and experience needed to remain engaged with life. One of the ways to encourage and support older adults to remain engaged with life is to provide age-friendly neighbourhoods where there are opportunities for social participation. This idea underpins the interest of stakeholders to widen the global network of age-friendly cities and communities (Rudnicha et al., 2020). Older adults must be empowered to use such cities and communities.

Empowerment in this chapter refers to the person's ability to control familial and neighbourhood resources, make informed choices, influence others and decisions, take advantage of services, and contribute to the community and society. Among

M. E. Uddin (✉)
Department of Social Work, University of Rajshahi, Rajshahi, Bangladesh
e-mail: emaj691@yahoo.com

N. Asiamah et al. (eds.), *Sustainable Ageing*,
https://doi.org/10.1007/978-3-031-69475-2_13

older adults, this ability is limited by poverty, low socioeconomic status, social inequality, ageism, and physiological problems (Thursz et al., 1995). Research suggests that disempowered older people (i.e., individuals without the above ability), in comparison with empowered ones, are less able to utilise neighbourhoods to maintain health (Buffel et al., 2023; De Witte & Van Regenmortel, 2023; Halvorsen et al., 2020; Tsubouchi et al., 2021). Particularly, disempowered older women and minority older adults are less capable of using neighbourhoods to maintain health. This fact reveals inequities even in the older adult population. Human development (HD) interventions or programmes (i.e., training and formal education) are, therefore, necessary not only for equipping older adults with the foregoing ability but also for eliminating inequalities.

HD programmes promote well-being by enabling older adults to remain engaged in life in the way of social participation, physical activity, and healthcare utilisation (Asiamah et al., 2023b; Uddin, 2024). In effect, they contribute to healthy longevity, enabling the individual to maintain functional ability and independence in later life. Yet, few studies to date have analysed how HD pathways can enable older people to utilise neighbourhoods for healthy ageing during crises. In this chapter, HD pathways are principles, values, or motivations governing or inspiring the design of HD programmes. They include autonomy, self-efficacy, and resilience, all of which serve as crucial abilities during crises. However, their role in older adults' utilisation of neighbourhoods for healthy ageing has not been sufficiently discussed in the literature. Uddin (2024) explained the link between the pathways and the use of neighbourhood resources for healthy ageing but did not consider implications for flagship initiatives such as the Decade of Healthy Ageing 2021–2030. Asiamah et al. (2023b) delineated a framework showing how older adults can be empowered to use assistive technologies during crises but failed to explain the role of the pathways in the use of neighbourhoods. Thus, there is no theoretical analysis of the HD pathways for empowering older adults to utilise neighbourhoods, considering the Decade of Healthy Ageing 2021–2030.

This chapter, therefore, aims to provide an understanding of how the HD pathways can be used to empower older adults to sustainably use neighbourhoods during crises. The chapter utilises the Decade of Healthy Ageing 2021–2030 campaign as a lens to elucidate the role of the pathways in using neighbourhoods during crises to maintain health and remain engaged with life. It guides future research on HD pathways and delineates implications for policy and healthy ageing during crises. The first section of the chapter, the introduction, sets out the aim and rationale of the chapter. In the second section, a theoretical framework that explains the significance of the HD pathways is formulated. The third section analyses the HD pathways, setting a basis for discussing implications for policy and healthy ageing in the fourth section. Limitations and future research directions are provided in the fifth section, whereas the sixth section presents concluding remarks.

13.2 Theoretical Framework

Studies to date informed by person–environment fit models have clearly demonstrated the role of neighbourhoods or human ecosystems in healthy ageing (Lawton, 1998; Wahl et al., 2012; Wahl & Gerstorf, 2020). Person–environment fit models advocate the design of neighbourhoods not only to enable individuals to remain engaged with life but also to empower them to use resources within the neighbourhoods. The Decade of Healthy Ageing initiative seeks to extend the global network of age-friendly cities and communities, partly in recognition of person–environment fit models. This assertion explains why this section focuses on theoretical perspectives on the role of neighbourhoods in healthy ageing and how individuals can be enabled to utilise age-friendly resources within their communities, especially during crises.

Person–environment fit models agree that socio-physical environments provide a worth of resources (i.e., parks, services, streets, and buildings) needed to enjoy life and remain actively engaged with life (Wahl & Gerstorf, 2020). Older adults meet their basic human needs and maintain well-being and social functioning by utilising these resources in the way of social engagement and physical activity participation (Lawton & Simon, 1968; Wahl et al., 2012). Specifically, the docility-proactivity model by Lawton (1989) critically asserts that willful utilisation of scarce resources may enable older people to maintain functional ability and intrinsic capacity over the life course.

More recently, some person–environment fit models suggested that the ideal place to age in good health embodies more than physically built environment attributes (da Schio et al., 2021). The Context Dynamics in Ageing framework, for example, recognises psychosocial factors such as peace and safety as important components of age-friendly contexts (Wahl & Gerstorf, 2020). The Socially Active Neighbourhood framework by Asiamah et al. (2023a) adds that a neighbourhood with the best-built infrastructure cannot support healthy ageing in crises situations without these psychosocial factors. Thus, the ultimate place to age characterises a built environment and psychosocial factors that encourage maximum engagement with life. The Socially Active Neighbourhood model admits, nevertheless, that whether people can utilise neighbourhoods to age in good health depends on some personal characteristics, such as functional capacity. Functional ability is implicit in the individual's overall ability, which should support sustained utilisation of services and other resources in a community.

From an HD perspective, every human needs the ability to use neighbourhoods to achieve life goals. This ability can be seen as knowledge, skills, and experiences. The Critical Social Theory supports this view and asserts that humans' patterns of activities in their communities can be influenced by what they know (i.e., knowledge) about these communities. Making people aware of crises such as floods, heatwaves, and violence in the community can enable them to make good decisions about how to use resources in the neighbourhood (Shearer & Reed, 2004). As mentioned earlier, the HD postulates of Asiamah et al. (2023b) recognise experiences

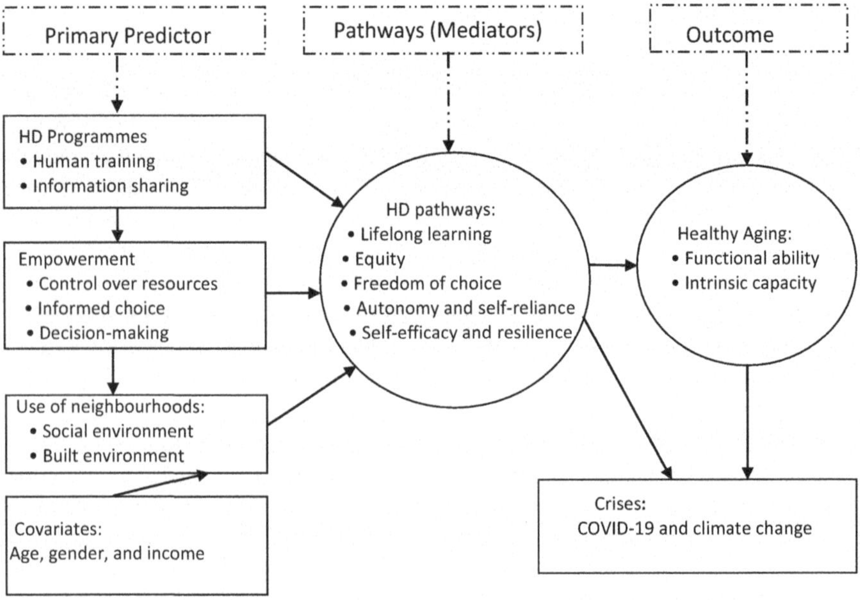

Fig. 13.1 The author's conceptualisation of the nexus between neighbourhood resources, HD pathways, healthy ageing, and crises. (Note: Not all potential covariates are in the fig. HD, human development; COVID-19, coronavirus disease 2019. Broken arrows and rectangles show the types of variables)

and skills as important enablers of social inclusion. The Activity Theory of Ageing similarly contends that sustained social participation over the life curse is influenced by how well the individual adapts previous experiences and skills (Asiamah et al., 2023b). Thus, the foregoing theories emphasise the importance of knowledge, skills, and experiences in well-informed action, especially in crises situations.

The HD postulates of Asiamah et al. (2023b) further elaborated the role of autonomy and resilience in the use of resources such as assistive technologies. While autonomy is needed by older adults to independently use resources, resilience is necessary for using such resources in crises situations. Based on these postulates and the literature (Anand & Sen, 2000; Blesh et al., 2019; Chowdhury et al., 2021), the integrated conceptual framework (see Fig. 13.1) is proposed as a model for understanding HD pathways, especially in contexts experiencing crises. The framework has three main parts: predictors, pathways or mechanisms, and outcomes. The primary predictor is any HD programme (i.e., training and information sharing) that gives older adults control over resources. Older adults should be able to choose the right resources for specific tasks and avoid any dangers associated with using these resources. During crises, it is crucial to keep safe while maintaining access to resources and support in neighbourhoods. If older adults can maintain control over resources, their use of resources will be sustained.

The HD pathways in the model are not necessarily traditional HD programmes but are rather the principles that should govern the implementation of these programmes. The principle of lifelong learning, for example, conveys a sense of continuous skills, knowledge, and experience acquisition. This idea implies that HD programmes must encourage lifelong learning in formal and informal ways. A formal way of learning is acquiring higher educational qualifications, whereas an informal route is learning from peers or social networks. Healthy ageing is the cardinal outcome of the pathways, suggesting that the predictors and pathways can positively contribute to the maintenance of functional ability and intrinsic capacity. If people age well, they can perform adaptive behaviour in response to crises such as climate change and disease outbreaks. Thus, healthy ageing during crises encompasses skills that foster the ability to adapt to adversity. Finally, the covariates in the model are other variables that can affect the pathways and where people live, as well as how they use the neighbourhood (Asiamah et al., 2023a).

As shown in Fig. 13.1, the predictors can be related to their influence on healthy ageing and the mediators. For instance, training and information sharing over the life course can improve older adults' ability to make informed decisions, exercise control over life situations, and make health-supporting choices (e.g., choosing walking as a mode of transportation over driving). This ability would, in turn, enhance the utilisation of social and built environment attributes. The mediators (e.g., lifelong learning) are direct outcomes of HD opportunities but a precursor for healthy ageing. According to Asiamah et al. (2023b), training and other HD opportunities (e.g., training) would have a maximum positive impact on healthy ageing if accessed over the life course. This is to say that individuals need HD opportunities sustained over the lifespan. Lifelong access to training would, thus, enable individuals to maintain their effective use of neighbourhood resources, thereby fostering healthy ageing through the mediators. Healthy ageing amidst crises is more likely if the HD programmes are designed to empower older adults to engage with life during adversities. This idea is depicted with the path linking the mediators and healthy ageing to 'crises'.

This integrated theoretical framework may help in understanding the relationship between neighbourhood resources, HD pathways, healthy ageing, and crises (Brown & Westaway, 2011; Wister et al., 2022). The model (Fig. 13.1) suggests that developing the HD principles or qualities such as lifelong learning, equity, freedom of choice, autonomy, self-reliance, and self-efficacy protects functional ability and intrinsic capacity amidst crises. It must be borne in mind, however, that the way this nexus would play out in practice may vary between contexts (e.g., poor vs. rich countries). This view unfolds the need for HD opportunities for older adults to be equitably distributed. Equity should be ensured in the support provided for older adults, their families, and communities through the Decade of Healthy Ageing 2021–2030 (Keating, 2022). To provide an understanding of how the proposed model applies to the Decade of Healthy Ageing initiative, the HD pathways are elaborated.

13.3 The HD Pathways

Crises such as climate change events (e.g., heatwaves and floods), natural disasters, and outbreaks of infectious diseases limit the potency of HD outcomes (e.g., health literacy) (UNDP, 2020, United Nations, 2022). Similarly, these crises hinder the implementation of HD interventions. For instance, climate change events and the outbreak of coronavirus disease 2019 (COVID-19) necessitated the closure of programmes providing continuous literacy to older people. This development meant that many older adults could not continue to acquire skills needed for daily living. This section analyses the role of the HD pathways in healthy ageing, with emphasis on how they may influence the implementation of the Decade of Healthy Ageing Campaign 2021–2030.

13.3.1 Lifelong Learning

Lifelong learning is one of the most fundamental HD processes through which older people acquire or protect abilities for utilising neighbourhood resources for healthy ageing amidst crises (Bastani et al., 2021; Cusack, 1999; Kump & KraŠovec, 2007). Lifelong learning refers to the process by which people acquire knowledge, skills, and abilities that empower them to overcome problems and achieve quality of life (Mirowsky & Ross, 2003; Merriam & Kee, 2013). The process helps individuals to succeed in their occupation, sustain or boost income, improve relationships, and protect health. It is assumed that the longer years of education people have, the greater knowledge, skills, and abilities they acquire and apply in making daily decisions (Mirowsky & Ross, 2003; Merriam & Kee, 2013). Skills acquired in lifelong learning are up-to-date and useful resources for remaining engaged with life since people continue to replenish their skills over time based on changing circumstances. Research has found that educated older adults or individuals who are successful lifelong learners make good decisions and informed choices and better engage with social networks to utilise neighbourhoods (Bastani et al., 2021; Merriam & Kee, 2013; Xia et al., 2014; Veloso & Guimarãs, 2014). Successful learners protect their cognitive abilities and are, therefore, able to make good decisions in social and physical activities.

Although lifelong learning is a process by which people can acquire and maintain abilities, this chapter treats it as a principle and value. As a personal value, lifelong learning can foster abilities that older adults need to use age-friendly neighbourhoods, identify and report ageist discrimination and abuse, and utilise health services. The Decade of Healthy Ageing 2021–2030 aims to combat ageism and give older adults access to age-friendly neighbourhoods as well as long-term and integrated health services. Hence, this campaign is more realistic in a context where lifelong learning is encouraged in older adults. Even so, learning should be aimed at acquiring skills that may help older adults to communicate with service providers and peers, identify dangers in the neighbourhood, and report their abusers. From another viewpoint, stakeholders can see lifelong learning as a principle, enabling them to invest in activities (i.e., formal and informal educational programmes) intended to equip older adults with skills. If lifelong learning is seen as a value and principle, governments are more likely to adopt policies to support and invest in it. Yet, there should be equity in the way opportunities for lifelong learning are discharged.

13.3.2 Equity

Equity in health, resources, and abilities among individuals is necessary for healthy ageing, especially from the perspective of the Decade of Healthy Ageing 2021–2030. As an HD principle, equity can encourage older adults to use neighbourhoods through social participation, including volunteering (Leach et al., 2018). It refers to giving people access to what they need, based on their circumstances, to be successful in daily routines and tasks (Alkire & Deneulin, 2009; Glover et al., 2020). When there is equity in the distribution of resources, people are happy and are willing to engage in life or support the economy. Evidence suggests that equitable distribution of resources or what people need to live a normal life encourages community engagement (Haase, 2020; Honey-Roses et al., 2020).

This chapter recognises equity as an HD principle for two main reasons. First, equitable distribution of resources (e.g., resources within age-friendly neighbourhoods) is the ideal way to empower older adults to succeed equally. Second, the aim of the Decade of Healthy Ageing campaign is to widen the network of age-friendly cities (Rudnicha et al., 2020) in the interest of fostering equity in the use of neighbourhood resources. If only a segment of people has access to age-friendly neighbourhoods, healthy ageing can only be a luxury for a minor segment of the population. Moreover, the recognition of equity as a necessary HD principle for providing access to resources is supported in research. Studies (Adger et al., 2006; Glover et al., 2020; da Schio et al., 2021) have found that older adults sufficiently used resources in their cities or neighbourhoods where equity is upheld as a principle. Therefore, it is necessary for stakeholders to achieve equity in their efforts to provide resources, services, and opportunities for lifelong learning.

13.3.3 Freedom of Choice

The Decade of Healthy Ageing initiative values freedom of choice and sees it as a factor influencing healthy ageing. Freedom of choice enables people to weigh options and utilise what best works for their situation. Given that globalisation continues to increase diversity in the older adult population, needs and wants can be expected to differ significantly in this population. If so, old adults are better empowered if they are allowed to make choices consistent with their backgrounds, health status, and goals. Research suggests older people who have freedom of choice are better able to use available neighbourhood resources in ways that support their longevity (UNDP, 2020). Nuhu et al. (2022) as well as Sheth and Bettencourt (2023) in the USA found that older people with higher levels of freedom of choice more frequently utilised neighbourhoods through social and physical activities.

Freedom of choice from this perspective includes having different routes (streets) to a supermarket, a variety of healthcare providers in one's neighbourhood, and multiple sources of social and financial support. It includes enabling individuals to identify and relish the best choice available. From the standpoint of the Decade of Healthy Ageing initiative, freedom of choice could be about having multiple channels where one can access long-term and integrated care, a variety of resources within age-friendly communities, and multiple avenues where older adults can report issues about ageism and abuse. As mentioned earlier, the ability to make the right decision and choice should be an outcome of HD programmes since it underscores autonomy.

13.3.4 Autonomy and Self-Reliance

Autonomy refers to the freedom to act independently as one deems appropriate (Heathcote, 2000). It is analogous to self-reliance, which refers to the ability to perform tasks or achieve goals without depending on others. The Decade of Healthy Ageing as a global campaign advocates autonomy for older adults (Rudnicha et al., 2020). Autonomy is a skill but can be viewed as a principle from the perspective of the Decade of Healthy Ageing campaign. Seeking autonomy as a principle would encourage stakeholders to develop HD programmes for equipping older adults with skills that give them independence from others. If older adults cannot have control over their lives and the way they use resources, their ageing may be fraught with health challenges. In contexts experiencing crises, autonomy is needed as a complement to resilience (Asiamah et al., 2023b). Given how widespread the crises have become, the recognition of autonomy as a value is necessary and would enable stakeholders to foster autonomy in the older adult population through HD programmes such as lifelong learning, Ad-hoc training, and informal education.

Autonomy does more for the individual in crises situations. It drives self-governance, self-esteem, a sense of responsibility, self-reliance, and self-determination, which are essential qualities needed by people to make decisions and engage with life without overly depending on others during adversities (Downie et al., 1990; Heathcote, 2000). Asiamah et al. (2023b) observed that autonomy is a source of happiness and a trait for healthy ageing. Research shows that more autonomous older adults, compared to less autonomous ones, better use the neighbourhoods and their resources to meet needs and successfully cope with adversities, including climate change events and diseases (Fotoukian et al., 2014; Greer &

Moore, 2023; McWilliam et al., 1994). This evidence signifies the importance of investment in interventions enhancing or preserving the autonomy of older adults.

13.3.5 Self-Efficacy and Resilience

The self-efficacy deteriorates over the life course, so older adults generally have less self-efficacy. This condition of older adults is problematic since self-efficacy is needed for utilising neighbourhood resources, including services. Self-efficacy refers to belief and confidence in one's ability and skills to effectively perform tasks (Bandura, 1986). Self-efficacy is an important life skill because people are unable to achieve goals without it. Studies (Kim & Kim, 2020; Meyer et al., 2022) have found that older adults with perceived self-efficacy better cope with stress and burnout during disasters (e.g., war, cyclone, flood, COVID-19). Dryhurst et al. (2020) also found that individuals with higher perceived self-efficacy believed they were more likely to survive COVID-19. Kim and Kim (2020) similarly found that individuals who were less vulnerable to COVID-19 had higher self-efficacy. A study by Cheng et al. (2018) has shown that self-efficacy minimises depressive symptoms among older adults experiencing crises.

Given the above pieces of evidence, self-efficacy can be seen as a value in HD programmes aimed at empowering older adults to use neighbourhoods during crises. HD programmes may not be effective if they do not equip people with self-efficacy since people cannot take certain actions if they do not believe in their ability to successfully perform these actions. The WHO and its partners may be successful in providing access to age-friendly neighbourhoods, but older adults may not utilise resources in these spaces without self-efficacy. This point suggests that efforts to support older adults, their families, and communities may not yield the expected outcomes if older adults do not believe in their ability to make effective use of available support and resources.

Self-efficacy can complement resilience in times of crises, enabling people to overcome challenges in their engagement with life. Resilience is suited for crises situations because it represents the ability to adapt easily despite adversities faced. Resilience is not only needed to remain calm and productive during crises but also allows individuals to support others. It is, thus, understandable why resilience is seen as a topmost trait necessary for healthy ageing (Leung et al., 2022). Emerging theories recognise it as a potential antidote to fear and burnout in settings experiencing humanitarian events (Wister et al., 2022). No doubt, the institutionalisation of HD programmes through key healthy ageing campaigns to enhance resilience among older adults is imperative. This assertion has implications for the implementation of the Decade of Healthy Ageing 2021–2030 campaign.

13.4 Implications for the Decade of Healthy Ageing

As illustrated in Fig. 13.1, the HD pathways can mediate between neighbourhood resources and healthy ageing as values, principles, or methods for equipping individuals with the ability to remain engaged with life in their neighbourhoods. This influence in the model depends on how well HD programmes targeted at older adults within organisations are governed by the aforesaid values and principles. For instance, lifelong learning needs to be treated as a value or principle in HD interventions to ensure that investment in them is sufficient and policy-driven. Similarly, autonomy, self-efficacy, equity, and freedom of choice should be viewed as valued outcomes of HD interventions rolled out by governments and organisations. If these values are treated as antecedents of HD programmes, they can facilitate life engagement and healthy ageing in the way individuals utilise them to access services, social networks, and social support, as well as the built environment.

The fact that the Decade of Healthy Ageing 2021–2030 aims to foster some of these values sets a worthwhile foundation for institutionalising the empowerment of older adults. The institutionalisation of empowerment in this context refers to adopting policies at the national and organisational levels to guide and regulate HD interventions for older adults. These policies ought to aim at the development of autonomy and self-efficacy with HD programmes. They should also provide opportunities for lifelong learning in social networks, employment activities, and community involvement opportunities. HD interventions are also expected to enable older adults to identify and rightly choose from multiple resources of support, services, and built environment attributes. This effort would not only give them freedom of choice but would also increase the enjoyability of service utilisation through social and physical activities. Older adults are more likely to remain engaged with life if they have different options to explore in their neighbourhoods. Finally, stakeholders may use the Decade of Healthy Ageing initiative as a tool to foster equity in the way HD programmes are implemented to equip older adults with autonomy and self-efficacy.

The HD pathways discussed have always been essential skills of life, but they are more useful in crises situations. Given that crises such as climate change events and violence are being globally felt (Asiamah et al., 2023b), these pathways are necessary values in emerging HD interventions. As such, concerted efforts must be made to design HD programmes to foster sufficient self-efficacy, resilience, autonomy, and freedom of choice for overcoming adversities. This view uncovers the need for policies to emphasise and value resilience over crises as a necessary skill for healthy ageing. Policies that emphasise resilience in times of crises would complement efforts to institutionalise HD programmes for encouraging lifelong learning through which individuals can acquire autonomy and self-efficacy. The Decade of Healthy Ageing 2021–2030 is an opportunity for WHO to work with governments and organisations to develop and implement these policies.

13.5 Limitations and Future Research

This chapter does not discuss the specific HD programmes (e.g., training) that can be employed to equip older adults with the abilities needed to utilise neighbourhoods during crises. Since such programmes have been extensively discussed in the literature (Asiamah et al., 2023b), this chapter focused only on principles and values that may be considered in empowering older adults to utilise neighbourhoods in contexts experiencing crises. The literature recognises traditional HD methods as HD pathways, but this chapter treats the above principles and values as HD pathways. This approach was adopted to emphasise the utmost significance of autonomy, resilience, and other related skills captured in the proposed model in healthy ageing in contexts experiencing crises. That is, lifelong learning and autonomy are not HD methods but should be valued as requirements for remaining engaged with life and ageing well in places experiencing crises. Moreover, this chapter was not based on a systematic review of the literature, so it may have missed vital complementary ideas in the literature. Finally, the proposed model (i.e., Fig. 13.1) has not been empirically tested; hence, future research aimed at testing it in whole or in part is necessary.

13.6 Conclusion

This chapter contributes to the literature through a narrative review of HD pathways, demonstrating how these pathways may contribute to healthy ageing in contexts experiencing crises. The pathways can be viewed as principles, values, and motivators of HD efforts aimed at empowering older adults to utilise neighbourhoods. Autonomy, resilience, and self-efficacy are necessary skills for remaining engaged with life over the life course during crises. Since lifelong engagement with life fosters healthy ageing, this chapter advocates human resources development interventions that equip older adults with these and other relevant skills. This chapter implies that investment in the HD pathways to empower and enable elderly people to sustainably use neighbourhood resources in promoting healthy ageing during crises is worthwhile. Investment aimed at improving skills captured in the proposed model may take place through the Decade of Healthy Ageing 2021–2030 campaign, which has become a standard for investment and policy development. Future researchers are encouraged to test the proposed model and provide empirical evidence that may encourage its adoption.

Review Questions

1. How important is HD in the realisation of the Decade of Healthy Ageing 2021–2030 campaign?
2. Why is it necessary for older adults to be equipped with the ability to utilise neighbourhood resources during crises?

3. Briefly explain how each of the HD pathways would contribute to healthy ageing during crises.
4. Why is the ability to adapt to adversity necessary for healthy ageing in crises situations?
5. Describe the role personal factors would play in the successful use of neighbourhood resources by older adults during crises.

References

Adger, W. N., Paavola, J., Huq, S., & Mace, M. J. (Eds.). (2006). *Fairness in adaptation to climate change*. The MIT Press.

Alkire, S., & Deneulin, S. (2009). Introducing the human development and capability approach. In S. Deneulin & L. Shahani (Eds.), *Introduction to the human development and capability approach: Freedom and agency*. Earthscan.

Anand, S., & Sen, A. (2000). Human development and economic sustainability. *World Development, 28*(12), 2029–2049.

Asiamah, N., Bateman, A., Hjorth, P., Khan, H. T. A., & Danquah, E. (2023a). Socially active neighborhoods: Construct operationalization for aging in place, health promotion and psychometric testing. *Health Promotion International, 38*(1), 1–10.

Asiamah, N., Danquah, E., Sghaier, S., Mensah, H. K., & Kouveliotis, K. (2023b). Assistive technologies for ageing in place: A theoretical proposition of human development postulates. In N. Asiamah, H. T. A. Khan, P. Villalobos Dintrans, M. J. Koohsari, E. Mogaji, E. R. Vieira, R. Lowry, & H. K. Mensah (Eds.), *Sustainable neighbourhoods for ageing in place* (pp. 161–178). Springer Nature Switzerland. https://doi.org/10.1007/978-3-031-41594-4_9

Bandura, A. (1986). *Social foundations of thought and action: A social cognitive theory*. Prentice Hall Inc.

Bastani, P., Mohammadpour, M., Samadbeik, M., Bastani, M., Rossi-Fedele, G., & Balasubramanian, M. (2021). Factors influencing access and utilization of health services among older people during the COVID-19 pandemic: A scoping review. *Archives of Public Health, 79*, 190. https://doi.org/10.1186/s13690-00719-9

Blesh, J., Hoey, L., Jones, A. D., Friedmann, H., & Perfecto, I. (2019). Development pathways toward “zero hunger”. *World Development, 118*, 1–14. https://doi.org/10.1016/j.worlddev.2019.02.004

Brown, K., & Westaway, E. (2011). Agency, capacity, and resilience to environmental change: Lessons for human development, well-being, and disasters. *Annual Review of Environment and Resources, 36*, 321–342.

Buffel, T., Yarker, S., Phillipson, C., Lang, L., Lewis, C., Doran, P., & Goff, M. (2023). Locked down by inequality: Older people and the COVID-19 pandemic. *Urban Studies, 60*(8), 1465–1482. https://doi.org/10.1177/00420980211041018

Cheng, S.-T., Leung, C. M. C., Chan, K. L., Chen, P. P., Chow, Y. F., et al. (2018). The relationship of self-efficacy to catastrophizing and depressive symptoms in community-dwelling older adults with chronic pain: A moderated mediation model. *PLoS One, 13*(9), e0203964. https://doi.org/10.1371/journal.pone.0203964

Chowdhury, J. R., Parida, Y., & Goel, P. A. (2021). Does inequality-adjusted human development reduce the impact of natural disasters? A gendered perspective. *World Development, 141*, 105394. https://doi.org/10.1016/j.worlddev.2021.105394

Cusack, S. A. (1999). Critical educational gerontology and the imperative to empower. *Education and Ageing, 1*, 21–37.

da Schio, N., Phillips, A., Fransen, K., Wolff, M., Haase, D., et al. (2021). The impact of the COVID-19 pandemic on the use and attitudes towards urban forests and green spaces: Exploring the instigators of change in Belgium. *Urban Forestry and Urban Greening, 65*, 127305. https://doi.org/10.1016/j.ufug.2021.127305

De Witte, J., & Van Regenmortel, T. (Eds.). (2023). *Silver empowerment: Fostering strengths and connections for an age-friendly society*. Leuven University Press.

Downie, R. S., Fife, C., & Tonnahill, A. (1990). *Health promotion: Models and values*. Oxford University Press.

Dryhurst, S., Schneider, C. R., Kerr, J., Freeman, A. L. J., Recchia, G., et al. (2020). Risk perceptions of COVID-19 around the world. *Journal of Risk Research, 23*(7–8), 994–1006. https://doi.org/10.1080/13669877.2020.1758193

Fotoukian, Z., Shahboulaghi, F. M., Hkoshknab, M. F., & Mohammadi, E. (2014). Concept analysis of empowerment in old people with chronic diseases using hybrid model. *Asian Nursing Research, 8*, 118–127.

Glover, R. E., van Schalkwyk, M. C., Akl, E. A., Kristjannson, E., Lotfi, T., Petkovic, J., et al. (2020). A framework for identifying and mitigating the equity harms of COVID-19 policy interventions. *Journal of Clinical Epidemiology, 128*, 35–48. https://doi.org/10.1016/j.jclinepi.2020.06.004

Greer, V., & Moore, K. D. (2023). Autonomy, identity, and design in the COVID-19 era. In F. Ferdous & E. Roberts (Eds.), *(re)designing the continuum of care for older adults: The future of long-term care settings* (pp. 263–281). Springer Nature Switzerland AG.

Haase, A. (2020). COVID-19 as a social crisis and justice challenge for cities. *Frontier in Sociology, 5*, 583638. https://doi.org/10.3389/fsoc.2020.583638

Halvorsen, K., Dihle, A., Hansen, C., Nordhaug, M., Jerpseth, H., et al. (2020). Empowerment in healthcare: A thematic synthesis and critical discussion of concept analyses of empowerment. *Patient Education and Counseling, 103*, 1263–1271.

Heathcote, G. (2000). Autonomy, health and ageing: Transnational perspectives. *Health Promotion Research, 15*(1), 13–24.

Honey-Roses, J., Anguelovski, I., Chireh, V. K., Daher, C., van den Bosch, C. K., et al. (2020). The impact of COVID-19 on public space: An early review of the emerging questions-design, perceptions and inequities. Cities and Health, 5, S263-S279

Keating, N. (2022). A research framework for the United Nations decade of healthy ageing (2021–2030). *European Journal of Ageing, 19*, 775–787.

Kim, S., & Kim, S. (2020). Analysis of the impact of health beliefs and resource factors on preventive behaviors against the COVID-19 pandemic. *International Journal of Environmental Research and Public Health, 17*, 8666. https://doi.org/10.3390/ijerph17228666

Kump, S., & KraŠovec, S. J. (2007). Education: A possibility for empowering older adults. *International Journal of Lifelong Education, 26*(6), 635–649.

Lawton, M. P. (1989). Environmental proactivity in older people. In V. L. Bengtson & K. W. Schaie (Eds.), *The course of later life* (pp. 15–23). Springer.

Lawton, M. P. (1998). Environment and ageing: Theory revisited. In R. J. Scheidt & P. G. Windley (Eds.), *Environment and ageing theory: A focus on housing* (pp. 1–31). Greenwood Press.

Lawton, M. P., & Simon, B. (1968). The ecology of social relationships in housing for the elderly. *The Gerontologist, 8*, 108–115.

Leach, M., Reyers, B., Bai, X., Brondizio, E. S., Cook, C., et al. (2018). Equity and sustainability in the Anthropocene: A social–ecological systems perspective on their intertwined futures. *Global Sustainability, 1*(e13), 1–13. https://doi.org/10.1017/sus.2018.12

Leung, D. Y. L., Chan, A. C. Y., & Ho, G. W. K. (2022). Resilience of emerging adults after adverse childhood experiences: A qualitative systematic review. *Trauma, Violence, Abuse, 23*(1), 163–181.

McWilliam, C. L., Brown, J. B., Carmichael, J. L., & Lehman, J. M. (1994). A new perspective on threatened autonomy in elderly persons: The disempowering process. *Social Science and Medicine, 38*(2), 327–338.

Merriam, S. B., & Kee, Y. (2013). Promoting community wellbeing: The case for lifelong learning for older adults. *Adult Education Quarterly, 20*(10), 1–17.

Meyer, N., Niemand, T., Davila, A., & Kraus, S. (2022). Biting the bullet: When self-efficacy mediates the stressful effects of COVID-19 beliefs. *PLoS One, 17*(1), e0263022.

Mirowsky, J., & Ross, C. E. (2003). *Education, social status, and health*. Aldine De Gruyter.

Nuhu, N. A., Baird, K., & Su, S. (2022). The association between the interactive and diagnostic use of financial and non-financial performance measures with individual creativity: The mediating role of perceived fairness. *Journal of Management Control, 33*(3), 371–402.

Rudnicha, E., Napierala, P., Podfigurna, A., Meczekalski, B., Smolarczyk, R., & Grymowicz, M. (2020). The World Health Organization approach to healthy ageing. *Maturitas, 139*, 6–11. https://doi.org/10.1016/j.maturitas.2020.05.018

Shearer, N. B. C., & Reed, P. D. (2004). Empowerment: Reformulation of a non-Rogerian concept. *Nursing Science Quarterly, 17*, 253–259.

Sheth, S., & Bettencourt, L. (2023). *The community human development index as a precision vulnerability metric and risk indicator*. Mansueto Institute for Urban Innovation Research Paper 35. Available at SSRN: https://ssrn.com/abstract=4328885 or https://doi.org/10.2139/ssrn.4328885

Thursz, D., Nusberg, C., & Prather, J. (1995). *Empowering older people: An international approach*. Auburn House.

Tsubouchi, Y., Yorozuya, K., Tainosyo, A., & Naito, Y. (2021). A conceptual analysis older adults' empowerment in contemporary Japanese culture. *BMC Geriatrics, 21*, 672. https://doi.org/10.1186/s12877-021-02631-x

Uddin, M. E. (2024). Human development pathways for understanding sustainable use of neighborhood resources and successful ageing in a world of crises. In R. Baikady et al. (Eds.), *The Palgrave handbook of global social problems* (pp. 1–21). Springer.

United Nations. (2022). *Climate change and population ageing in the Asia-Pacific region: Status, challenges and opportunities*. Economic and Social Commission for Asia and the Pacific (ESCAP). Available at: https://www.unescap.org/kp/2022/climate-change-and-population-ageing-asia-pacific-region-status-challenges-and

United Nations Development Programme (UNDP). (2020). *COVID-19 and human development: Assessing crisis, envisioning recovery*. UNDP.

Veloso, E., & Guimarãs, P. (2014). Education and empowerment in later life. In B. Schmidt-Hertha, S. J. Krašovec, & M. Formosa (Eds.), *Learning across generations in Europe: Contemporary issues in older adult education* (pp. 35–45). Sense Publishers.

Wahl, H.-W., & Gerstorf, D. (2020). Person-environment resources for ageing well: Environmental docility and life space as conceptual pillars for future contextual gerontology. *The Gerontologist, 60*(3), 368–375. https://doi.org/10.1093/geront/gnaa006

Wahl, H.-W., Iwarsson, S., & Oswald, F. (2012). Ageing well and the environment: Toward an integrative model and research agenda for the future. *The Gerontologist, 52*(3), 306–316. https://doi.org/10.1093/geront/gnr154

WHO. (2020). *Decade of healthy ageing: Baseline report*. World Health Organization.

Wister, A., Klasa, K., & Linkov, I. (2022). A unified model of resilience and ageing: Applications to COVID-19. *Frontiers in Public Health, 10*, 865459. https://doi.org/10.3389/fpubh.2022.865459

Xia, B., Skitmore, M., Buys, L., & Hu, X. (2014). Sustainability literacy of older people in retirement villages. *Journal of Ageing Research, 2014*, 919054. https://doi.org/10.1155/2014/919054

Chapter 14
Empowering Older Adults to Utilise Neighbourhoods: A Healthy Ageing Perspective

Simon Mawulorm Agyemang, Faith Hope Muhonja, Sarra Sghaier, Richmond Stephen Sorkpor, and Seyram Kafui Akude

Acronyms and Abbreviations

ATA	Activity Theory of Ageing
CTA	Continue Theory of Ageing
DHA	Decade of Healthy Ageing
DTA	Disengagement Theory of Ageing
ICT	Information, Communication, and Technology
SAN	Socially Active Neighbourhood
WHO	World Health Organization

S. M. Agyemang (✉)
Department of Science/Health, Physical Education, and Sports, Abetifi Presbyterian College of Education, Abetifi, Ghana
e-mail: smagyemang@abeticoe.edu.gh

F. H. Muhonja
Department of Community Health, School of Public Health, Amref International University, Nairobi, Kenya
e-mail: faith.muhonja@amref.ac.ke

S. Sghaier
Research Laboratory in Marketing (LRM), University of Sfax, Sfax, Tunisia

Department of Gerontology and Geriatrics, Africa Centre for Epidemiology, Accra, Ghana
e-mail: sarra.sgh@hotmail.com

R. S. Sorkpor
Department of Health Physical Education, Recreation, and Sports, University of Education Winneba, Winneba, Ghana
e-mail: rssorkpor@uew.edu.gh

S. K. Akude
Department of Science/Health Education, Peki College of Education, Peki, Volta Region, Ghana
e-mail: aseyramkafui@gmail.com

N. Asiamah et al. (eds.), *Sustainable Ageing*,
https://doi.org/10.1007/978-3-031-69475-2_14

14.1 Introduction

A prolonged and active lifespan represents a precious asset. It allows us to reevaluate the ageing experience and the unfolding trajectory of our lives (Beard & Bloom, 2015). However, the extent to which extended lifespans provide opportunities hinges significantly on a crucial variable: good health. Various circumstances have been identified as influencing mortality rates, the occurrence of illness, physical well-being, and mental health. These factors collectively contribute to population health disparities over time (Clarke & Nieuwenhuijsen, 2009). Among these disparities, older adults bear the most significant impact. The term "older adults" refers to individuals in the later stages of life, often characterised by retirement age and beyond (Rudnicka et al., 2020). While the specific age range of this demographic can vary, it generally encompasses people in their 60s and older. Some definitions also extend the category of older adults aged 65 and above (Asiamah et al., 2023e; Rudnicka et al., 2020).

Empirical evidence underscores the rapid increase in the ageing population compared to the recent past (Asiamah et al., 2023e; Boutros et al., 2019). For instance, in 2019, the global population of older adults (i.e., the aged population) reached 703 million (Barbaccia et al., 2022). Projections by the WHO suggest that by 2050, this figure will surge to 1.5 billion (Barbaccia et al., 2022). These findings aligned with existing literature (Barbaccia et al., 2022; WHO, 2020; Yeung et al., 2021), indicating that older adults now enjoy longer lifespans than previous generations (Boutros et al., 2019; Yeung et al., 2021).

This longevity can be attributed to significant advancements in medicine, public health, science and technology, education, self-awareness, self-esteem, and dietary practices (Boutros et al., 2019). Besides, many individuals within this demographic resist being labelled as "older people". Regardless, this cohort faces unique challenges related to physical health and lifestyle adjustments associated with ageing. The purpose of this chapter was to delineate specific strategies for empowering older adults to utilise their neighbourhoods to fulfil the goals of the healthy ageing agenda.

In pursuit of the United Nations (UN) 2030 Sustainable Development Agenda, which emphasises "Leave No One Behind," the WHO launched the iconic ageing initiative "Decade of Healthy Ageing" (DHA) (Andorra et al., 2020; Rudnicka et al., 2020; WHO, 2023). The central aim of this initiative is to enhance and safeguard the health of older adults (WHO, 2023). By prioritising the well-being of older populations, the UN seeks to improve the quality of life for older individuals, their families, and their communities (Keating, 2022; WHO, 2020).

Due to the rapid trajectory of the global older adult population, the overall global population is projected to increase by slightly over 60% between 2018 and 2050, reaching 7 billion inhabitants (Rugel et al., 2022). Concurrently, the number of older adults is expected to more than double, rising from 1 to 2.1 billion during this timeframe (Fallon & Karlawish, 2019). Research indicates that the proportion of individuals aged 60 and over is appreciating approximately three times faster in low- and middle-income countries than in income countries, significantly contributing to the overall population growth (WHO, 2018).

Sarkar et al. (2023) observed that global trends, including climate change events (e.g., extreme heat and flooding), adversely affect the civic rights of individuals, particularly older adults. Worse yet, global warming has increased the Earth's surface temperature over the past century, and the Earth's climate has fluctuated during this period (Meltzer, 2021). A critical examination of the data reveals that the average global temperature has increased by approximately 12 °F (1.18 °C) from the late nineteenth century to the present due to heightened carbon dioxide emissions and other human-induced factors (Wu et al., 2020).

Prolonged exposure to extremely high temperatures significantly impacts individuals with weakened or vulnerable health, such as older adults. Heart disease patients are particularly susceptible to elevated temperatures, as cardiac systems require extra effort to maintain an average body temperature. Moreover, in certain regions, older adults face the consequences of rising ozone levels (O_3), attributed to O_3 levels caused by climate change. Temperatures exceeding 90 °F can elevate ozone levels, adversely affecting lung health and leading to respiratory issues, including asthma.

Torrential rainfall frequently augments the risk of waterborne infections, particularly those associated with drinking water contaminated by sewage. As a significant driver of discomfort, climate change introduces weather fluctuations, elevated temperatures, altered precipitation patterns, and droughts. In regions lacking adequate drainage systems, heavy rains can lead to water stagnation, exacerbating the vulnerability to waterborne infections. Furthermore, climate change strains health systems, impacting disease dynamics through various consequences such as heightened temperatures and increased rainfall. Notably, global crises, including climate change, also reverberate through food security and hygiene (Brubacher et al., 2020).

Deductively, climate change events and other crises pose a threat to the population of older adults. Regardless of the support they may receive through the Decade of Healthy Ageing initiative, older adults are unlikely to live healthy and happy lives amidst climate crises. For this reason, an understanding of how to foster healthy ageing in contexts experiencing climate change events is imperative. This chapter, for the first time, provides ideas and postulates for empowering older adults to utilise neighbourhoods and their resources during climate crises. The ability to use contextual resources can be the difference between life and death for individuals experiencing crises. Thus, this book offers a unique opportunity to enable older adults to use neighbourhoods through the foregoing initiative.

This chapter is organised into eight sections, including the introductory section (Sect. 14.1) where the aim and significance of the chapter are elucidated. Section 14.2 defines healthy ageing and its associated factors, whereas a theoretical framework for understanding the role of the neighbourhood in healthy ageing is provided in Sect. 14.3. In Sect. 14.4, we proffer the importance of resilience and autonomy in the individual's effort to age well amidst crises. Section 14.5 provides insights into how the neighbourhood influences health and longevity, setting the foundation for Sect. 14.6, where strategies for utilising the neighbourhood from a human development perspective are analysed. Section 14.7 identifies the chapter's limitations and future research directions, whereas Sect. 14.8 offers concluding remarks.

14.2 The Concept of Healthy Ageing

Healthy ageing may be referred to as acquiring and sustaining functional capability. Specifically, it entails enabling older adults to engage in activities they enjoy, thereby promoting overall well-being in their later years (Michel & Sadana, 2017; WHO, 2020). This multidimensional concept encompasses physical, mental, and social aspects that contribute to an individual's quality of life as they age.

Healthy ageing revolves around maintaining functional capacity. This includes physical (such as mobility), cognitive functions (such as memory and decision-making), and sensory capacity (such as vision and hearing). By preserving and enhancing these capabilities, older adults can continue participating actively. Beyond the mere absence of disease or disability, healthy ageing emphasises holistic well-being. It encompasses physical health (e.g., managing chronic conditions), mental health (e.g., maintaining cognitive vitality), and social connectedness (e.g., building and maintaining relationships). These interconnected dimensions collectively contribute to a fulfilling life. In short, healthy ageing can be considered living well with multiple chronic conditions (Fallon & Karlawish, 2019). The right neighbourhood environment plays a pivotal role in health and ageing. Access to community resources, green spaces, social support networks, and age-friendly infrastructure empowers older adults to thrive. By harnessing these resources, they can lead vibrant lives and contribute meaningfully to their communities.

A neighbourhood is a geographically localised community within a larger city, town, suburb, or rural area. It encompasses the immediate geographical surroundings where people live, bounded by physical features such as streets, rivers, and train tracks (Asiamah et al., 2023b, d). Beyond physical boundaries, neighbourhoods possess an essential social element, representing the feeling of shared identity among residents (Bonaccorsi et al., 2020). It fosters social interaction, community cohesion, and a sense of belonging. Many older adults choose to age in place, residing in their neighbourhoods for extended periods of time. Consequently, the role of the neighbourhood is significant. It provides a familiar context where social ties, memories, and routines contribute to well-being.

As people age, functional capabilities may decline, particularly among older adults. *Functional capability* is the set of skills necessary to allow people of all ages to live their lives and do the things they cherish (Rudnicka et al., 2020; WHO, 2020). To promote healthy ageing, the WHO has identified five critical requirements for the maintenance of functional capability. These are the ability to fulfil fundamental requirements (our basic needs), learn, develop, and make decisions, freely move in the neighbourhood, build and maintain relationships (a social network), and give back to society in old age in the form of volunteering.

Notwithstanding, environmental influences can improve or hinder each critical functional capability. The secret to healthy ageing is living in a neighbourhood that upholds and enhances your inherent potential and functional capabilities. The degree of an individual's innate ability is determined by all their potential mental and physical abilities, which include their ability to move, think, see, hear, and recall. However, several factors can impact functional capability. These include the presence of illnesses, injuries, climate change, and age-related changes. Thus, healthy ageing can be made less realistic by prevailing "global crises," namely, climate change, radical industrialisation, extreme temperature, the outbreak of infectious diseases, flooding, and systemic violence (Asiamah et al., 2023c, d).

Successful empowerment of older adults to age healthily and utilise the neighbourhood largely depends on the built environment. This environment provides convenient access to essential services and other psychosocial features like peace and security. Walking within one's surroundings promotes health-seeking behaviours, underscoring the critical role of neighbourhood walkability in supporting ageing in place (Asiamah et al., 2023c, d, e, f). Walkability, as defined by Asiamah et al. (2023a, b), encompasses features promoting physical exercise and social interaction. These features include well-designed outdoor spaces and accessible services. Ageing in place is characterised by an individual's ability to remain physically capable, independent, and in good condition while growing older within their neighbourhood or residence. Three groups of factors interact to cause ageing in place: built environment features (i.e., streets, pavements, and traffic flow), social environment (e.g., social networks and support), and personal attributes (e.g., age and income). These factors jointly influence health and healthy longevity, as the following theoretical framework suggests.

14.3 Theoretical Framework

This work is grounded in several theories that shed light on the dynamics of ageing. One such theory is the Activity Theory of Ageing (ATA), which posits that older adults experience an improved quality of life when actively engaging with their social environment. Specifically, when older individuals maintain social connections, participate in community activities, and encourage mutual interaction among neighbours, their overall well-being is positively impacted (Asiamah et al., 2023e; Rudnicka et al., 2020). This implies that active lifestyles, social networking, and relationships are vital components positively associated with healthy ageing and ageing in place. This also implies that being actively involved in everyday activities in the neighbourhood is the path to achieving an awareness of healthy ageing. As a result, this engagement in neighbourhood activities helps to meet the basic needs of life, which are food and security. Again, the ATA suggests that if an enabler environment is created for older adults to be empowered to continue participating in neighbourhood activities, healthy ageing is made more realistic in crises situations.

The ATA adds that the healthy ageing process requires older adults to maintain a significant degree of functional ability, which encompasses a sense of independence and self-control, influenced by their ability to perform daily activities and make autonomous decisions. Engaging in fulfilling activities, such as employment, volunteerism, passions, or social responsibilities, contributes to the sense of fulfilment and direction that older adults experience. Maintaining consistency in responsibilities, habits, and relationships throughout life might help older adults feel more stable, which improves their general well-being. While ageing in place, older adults may experience changes in their social situations, cognitive capacities, and physical health as they get older. Their ability to navigate life's obstacles and persist with activities that hold meaning for them will determine whether they choose to continue engagement (as per the Continuity Theory of Ageing) or to disengage (as per the Disengagement Theory of Ageing (DTA)) (Asiamah et al., 2023b, c).

The DTA postulates that as individuals age, they progressively lose social connections, and their capacity for engagement with others diminishes over time (Asiamah, 2017; Nickerson, 2022; Ragini & Salwan, 2022). The DTA suggests that the ability for social interaction wanes with age, leading to a loss of connections with their social circles (Asiamah, 2017; Nickerson, 2022; Ragini & Salwan, 2022). As individuals commence the process of disengagement, they become exempt from societal norms that dictate social connections or neighbourhood engagement. The indifference towards societal conventions reinforces the syndrome of disengagement among older adults. Nickerson (2022) observes that, due to varying societal roles, the experience of disengagement differs between men and women. Nickerson (2022) further observes that fluctuations in ego associated with ageing punctuate an individual's life, resulting in a decline in cognitive and functional capabilities. Numerous studies have demonstrated that reliable technological advancements enable older adults with health concerns to maintain their independence at home, negating the need for permanent admission to a care facility for treatment (Dratsiou et al., 2022).

Ageing in place is associated with a fundamental physical transformation in older adults, characterised by decreased functional capability (Asiamah et al., 2023b, c, f). This transformation is precipitated by a lifelong, progressive reduction in bone and muscle strength, cardiorespiratory endurance, speed, and flexibility. Consequently, this leads to limited social and physical engagement, cognitive decline, and increased frailty. According to Sezgin et al. (2019), *frailty* is the deterioration and restrictions in bodily functionality in performing basic daily activities. These activities encompass grooming, dressing, toileting, eating, and ambulating. Furthermore, frailty also affects instrumental activities of daily living such as using a phone, preparing and serving one's meals, walking to the nearby supermarket or shops, managing finances, maintaining mobility, and administering medication.

Cognitive deficiencies in the context of frailty, which extend beyond mere bodily abnormalities, can be induced by memory impairment and other neurological disorders. As articulated by Asiamah et al. (2021) and Hoogendijk et al. (2018), ageing-induced functional declines encompass deficits related to physiology and cognition. As a result, the DTA claims that the scope of physical activities and social interactions that older adults can engage in will be limited because of these inevitable age-related changes. For instance, an individual's ability to walk 10 miles/day or ascend and descend 25 stairs repeatedly would be diminished or seized from doing so due to functional incapacity and frailty. Similarly, their social interaction and engagement—such as at funerals, weddings, festivals, church, or visits to friends or family members—will decrease. Due to their fragility, the individual might be incapable of persisting with walking and other related tasks. Therefore, empowering older adults to utilise neighbourhoods is imperative due to these age-related declines in functional ability (Asiamah, 2017).

The escalating prevalence of social disengagement among older adults is increasingly recognised as a significant public health concern. Research indicates that 43% of this group report feelings of loneliness, while 27% feel a sense of disconnection from others (Perissinotto et al., 2012; Solway et al., 2019). These findings highlight the significant impact that social disengagement and loneliness can exert on the lives of older adults. Disengagement or loneliness can precipitate a decline in quality of life, elevate the risk of health complications, impair mobility and self-care abilities, and potentially shorten life expectancy (Perissinotto et al., 2012). Furthermore, a correlation has been observed between reduced social interaction and an increased incidence of dementia. Fratiglioni et al. (2000) posit that elderly individuals who actively participate in their communities, harnessing their knowledge, skills, and expertise, can mitigate these adverse health effects. This active involvement not only enhances their health but also contributes positively to the health of their communities. Even so, the socially active neighbourhood (SAN) model posits that the ability to utilise skills to maintain health and functional capacity depends on whether the environment where one life is supportive.

The SAN model, originally developed by Asiamah and colleagues (2023b), serves as a theoretical framework that outlines strategies for fostering community engagement and social cohesion within residential areas. It argues that individual behaviours—such as social and physical interactions—are dependent on neighbourhood attributes or resources (Asiamah et al., 2023b). It further highlights the imperative of nurturing neighbourhood connectedness, social engagement, communal projects, and a feeling of inclusivity to foster healthier, more secure, and more dynamic neighbourhoods. As articulated by Asiamah et al. (2023b), according to Lawton and Simon's person-environment fit model, individuals and their respective neighbourhoods are interconnected through specific demands. An array of elements within the physical setting, such as resources, including social networks, technology, and transportation, characterises these demands. The needs of older adults can be met with the establishment of interpersonal relationships, neighbourhood engagement, and the utilisation of neighbourhood resources. This explains why social networks, technologies, and opportunities for volunteerism and social engagement promote healthy ageing in place.

The SAN concept generally offers a framework that enables families or neighbourhoods to maintain autonomy in their neighbourhoods and collaborate with peers to bring about constructive social transformation. This supports an action plan of the DHA initiative, which is to provide access to age-friendly neighbourhoods.

This campaign also aims to enable older adults to maintain resilience and autonomy for reasons discussed in the following section.

14.4 Importance of Autonomy and Resilience

Resilience and autonomy, both of which constitute essential requirements for healthy ageing, significantly enhance individuals' general health and quality of life. These attributes assist individuals in navigating the challenges and obstacles associated with later years. One of the key objectives of the DHA is to enhance the autonomy and resilience of older adults.

Autonomy is the capacity to exercise independent judgement and retain personal authority. According to Nietsche and Backes (2000), autonomy represents the ability to take charge of decisions for oneself and to act independently—that is, having the ability and willingness to take action on one's behalf. Autonomy can also be the ability to make decisions based on a conviction of our dependability as human beings (Lange et al., 2018). It becomes more robust as individuals modify their environment—initially with assistance and later independently—reproducing and disseminating the expertise to create innovative learning approaches. As a fundamental facilitator of longevity, autonomy contributes to understanding and establishing independence; thus, the significance of collaborative and participatory exploration becomes apparent. Supporting older adults' autonomy is crucial, allowing them to share responsibility for the variables that influence their physical and mental well-being (Lange et al., 2018). Autonomy is vital in fostering a sense of purpose, respect, self-esteem, and self-fulfilment during healthy ageing. Older adults experience greater satisfaction and well-being when empowered to make decisions about their daily activities, lifestyle, and health services. Additionally, autonomy promotes an appreciation for independence, enabling individuals to pursue their passions, form meaningful interpersonal connections, and uphold their self-identity and values. To be genuinely empowered, a person must have the ability to make choices, express their opinions, take initiative, and contribute autonomously to policy decisions across various dimensions of our existence as humans (Lancefield, 2023).

Resilience refers to the capacity to adapt and recover in global crises, including extreme temperatures, floods, pandemics (such as COVID-19), and other significant life events (e.g., fire outbreaks and challenging living conditions) (Merchant et al., 2022). In the context of healthy ageing, resilience enables individuals to navigate the mental, emotional, and social changes accompanying the ageing process. It involves establishing robust social support networks, maintaining an optimistic outlook, and developing effective coping strategies (Angevaare et al., 2020; Merchant et al., 2022). Older adults who possess resilience demonstrate excellent proficiency in managing life's fluctuations, such as declining health and its associated impacts, bereavement, and the challenges of ageing. Whether ageing healthily within their community or assuming caregiving responsibility, resilience plays a crucial role

(Angevaare et al., 2020; Athira et al., 2024; Gov.uk, 2022). They are able to find fresh meaning and fulfilment, keep a sense of purpose, and effectively handle stress. Resilience, as defined, is not just about adapting to life's demands within challenging or adverse social contexts. It is about finding fresh meaning and fulfilment, maintaining a sense of purpose, and effectively handling stress. It is about positive development that influences recovery rates following setbacks (Merchant et al., 2022).

Fundamentally, resilience connects risk factors, such as life-threatening conditions (e.g., disease, loss of social support, or financial hardships), to adaptive coping abilities (Angeler et al., 2018). The interplay of personal attributes (such as individuality, brainpower, and physiological health) and external resources (like a sense of community and socioeconomic security) significantly impacts psychological resilience (Laird et al., 2019). These factors can synergise with protective and promotive elements across physical, mental, social, and environmental domains, facilitating an individual's transition from adversity and disruption to adaptation, recovery, overall well-being, and even growth (Ungar et al., 2021). A critical societal intervention to enhance autonomy and resilience among older adults involves actively engaging them in their healthcare. This empowerment enables them to acquire self-care skills and make informed decisions throughout their lifespan (Lange et al., 2018). Notably, autonomy encompasses freedom of speech, inclusivity, interpersonal relationships, and neighbourhood connections, provided these actions do not harm others.

Arguably, the challenges to ageing in the twenty-first century are closely linked to maintaining autonomy and self-reliance while ageing in place (Lange et al., 2018). Consequently, developing strategies to promote autonomy among healthy older individuals presents valuable opportunities for improving their quality of life by leveraging neighbourhood resources. Neighbourhoods are crucial in empowering older adults' resilience, allowing them to lead fulfilling lives as they age within their community. This empowerment is achieved through supportive and health-promoting neighbourhood environments, accessible resources, and opportunities for meaningful participation.

14.5 Neighbourhood Resources and Healthy Ageing

To enhance healthy ageing in contexts experiencing climate change events, neighbourhood resources must be optimised and older adults empowered to use them to maintain engagement with life. Optimising neighbourhood resources involves leveraging community networks, which are an asset for improving older adults' social, emotional, and mental well-being. As such, the authors subsequently discuss approaches to empowering older adults to utilise neighbourhoods.

The first recommended step is the establishment of social or community centres for older adults. Establishing social centres for older adults and other intergenerational age groups is essential for education and training. These facilities often offer various programmes and events tailored to older adults, such as exercise regimens, educational seminars, creative arts gatherings, and volunteering opportunities. Empowering older adults to participate in these activities promotes cognitive well-being, encourages physical activity, and fosters social connections.

Neighbourhood centres offer a diverse range of educational programmes tailored to the preferences and needs of older adults (Krašovec & Kump, 2014). These initiatives encompass seminars, workshops, and talks covering nutrition, health, financial independence, and dietary choices. By providing opportunities for lifelong learning, neighbourhood centres empower older adults to acquire new skills, adopt positive behaviours, and access relevant information that contributes to their overall well-being. These centres can also serve as focal points for encouraging older individuals to lead active lives. They host wellness seminars, fitness programmes, and leisure activities that promote social interaction, physical exercise, and stress reduction. Additionally, community centres play a vital role in assisting senior citizens in establishing and maintaining healthy habits by creating environments that prioritise health and well-being (Age UK, 2024).

14.5.1 Maintaining Social Connectedness

Another approach to the empowerment of older adults is fostering social connectedness among older adults, not only with the creation of community centres but also with evidence-based interventions to social disengagement. Social connectedness refers to the personal experience of closely associated and fulfilling interactions with others (Seppala et al., 2013). According to Maslow's theory, compassionate and loving relationships with those around us are fundamental human requirements (Maslow, 1943). The lack of social network connections is a risk factor for early mortality comparable to several other major risk factors, such as obesity, flu shots, and physical inactivity (Holt-Lunstad et al., 2017). Individuals with strong social connections exhibit altered cognitive processing of stress by regulating emotions, which reduces anxiety-related inflammation and calms the nervous system (Detillion et al., 2004). The protective aspect of socialisation sensations is strongly associated with mental health (Holt-Lunstad et al., 2017; Seppala et al., 2013). Intergenerational programmes, including mentorship initiatives, volunteer opportunities, and intergenerational learning activities, foster mutual respect, understanding, and social relationships between older adults and younger generations. These programmes benefit both age groups. Moreover, promoting healthy eating habits among older adults can be achieved by empowering them to engage in neighbourhood or backyard gardening and by encouraging visits to neighbourhood farmer's markets, which offer fresh produce and opportunities for social interactions.

In coping with the global crises, older adults face the challenge of maintaining robust social ties (Asiamah et al., 2023a). The extent to which an individual achieves social connection is a multifaceted concept, encompassing both the quantity and quality of their interactions with others. The quality and quantity of one's social networks recall the role of security and peace in ageing in place, as explained by Asiamah et al. (2023a, b).

Healthy ageing is fundamentally linked to creating safe and secure neighbourhoods where older adults can reside, work, and socialise (Asiamah et al., 2023a, b). When older adults experience a sense of security and stability in tranquil neighbourhoods devoid of social upheaval, criminal incidents, and danger, their overall well-being is positively impacted. Establishing neighbourhoods that promote healthy ageing relies on fostering social unity and confidence, particularly among residents. These attributes are more readily nurtured in tranquil neighbourhoods. Older adults exhibit greater participation in social events, seek assistance proactively, and actively engage in local activities when they experience a sense of ease and attachment to their neighbours. Promoting opportunities for intergenerational interactions, organising neighbourhood gatherings, and implementing community initiatives can strengthen social bonds and foster a sense of inclusion among older adults.

According to Asiamah et al. (2023b), ageing in place becomes challenging within built environments characterised by traffic congestion, poor street connectivity, and a lack of psychosocial elements such as peace and security. Even if a neighbourhood offers essential psychosocial elements, successful ageing in place may be hindered if residents lack the physical capacity to utilise contextual features, such as available services. Neighbourhoods can create supportive environments that enable older adults to age in place, maintain autonomy, and lead fulfilling lives by leveraging local resources. Yes, crises from climate change and war or violence can erode a sense of community peace and security. For this reason, the goal of stakeholders and campaigns such as the Decade of Healthy Ageing 2021–2030 should be to foster community peace and security in a bid to provide age-friendly neighbourhoods. This goal will complement measures taken to preserve green spaces.

Access to green spaces, walking trails, and entertainment venues is crucial to encouraging outdoor activity and physical well-being. These elements are essential for maintaining cognitive function, heart health, and overall mobility, particularly among older adults. Additionally, targeted fitness programmes, health walks, and aerobic dance can motivate older individuals to prioritise their health. Research indicates that continuous exposure to vegetative environments can mitigate the adverse effects associated with ageing, leading to optimal psychological and physical outcomes (John et al., 2022).

Beyond their therapeutic benefits, green spaces actively contribute to healthy ageing. The Attention Restoration Theory posits that natural stimuli in ambient environments can mitigate attention fatigue during prolonged cognitive tasks (Joye & Dewitte, 2018; Kaplan, 1995; Stack & Shultis, 2013). In addition to facilitating social interaction and exercise, green spaces have been proven to reduce noise pollution, mitigate flood risks, improve air quality, provide shade and cooling, and enhance overall mental and physical well-being, especially in settings experiencing climate change events. Consequently, green spaces contribute to an improved quality of life within neighbourhoods by mitigating adverse environmental impacts (John et al., 2022). Parks with fitness facilities attract neighbours to their green surroundings, promoting social interactions and group exercise routines (Yi et al., 2022). They may also encourage the utilisation of neighbourhood services, including healthcare.

Collaboration among neighbourhood healthcare centres, pharmacies, over-the-counter drug sellers, and healthcare providers is essential to ensuring that older adults receive equitable access to medical attention, guidance on managing chronic conditions, and proactive health checkups. Informative resources and instructions related to medication management, injury prevention, first aid, and nutrition are also available at health expositions and wellness centres. The above-recommended measures unfold implications for the Decade of Healthy Ageing 2021–2030 initiative.

14.6 Implications for the Decade of Healthy Ageing Initiative

Empowering older adults to participate meaningfully in their neighbourhoods is essential for boosting good health, a sense of belonging, and promoting healthy ageing. The fact that the DHA campaign advocates the empowerment of older adults and the provision of age-friendly neighbourhoods provides an opportunity for healthy longevity in contexts experiencing crises.

The imperative to create age-friendly neighbourhoods underscores the need to consider the specific requirements of older adults. This involves deliberately planning and designing interventions that cater to the diverse needs of older adults. In this context, urban environments should be conducive to pedestrian traffic, offering well-designed walkways, strategically placed benches, easy ramps, and accessible public transportation. By fostering a walking-friendly and socially engaging physical environment, we empower older adults to actively participate in community life, including family gatherings, funerals, weddings, and other neighbourhood activities (Asiamah et al., 2023a, b, d). This measure is more crucial in poor countries where older adults are socioeconomically disadvantaged and, therefore, need support from governments to live happy and healthy lives. Such older adults need training in the use of technologies to utilise neighbourhood resources (Asiamah et al., 2023c).

Empowering older adults through exposure to digital tools—such as online courses, smartphone applications, and internet connectivity—can significantly enhance their functional capacity. These technological resources facilitate communication with family members, provide access to health-related information, and even offer recreational activities like computer games and videos (Asiamah et al., 2023c). By promoting access to these digital tools and services, we contribute to realising the Decade of Healthy Ageing initiative.

It is incumbent upon neighbourhoods to ensure the accessibility of age-appropriate internet sites, clear signage, and information, communication, and technology (ICT) training programmes and communication channels for older adults (Asiamah et al., 2023c). This provision may encompass the establishment of social media platforms such as WhatsApp, Telegram, Facebook, Twitter, or neighbourhood websites. Beyond enhancing the development of ICT usage, it is crucial to advocate for the utilisation of accessible technology.

Assistive technology, defined as any equipment, support, method, or instrument that aids older adults or those with disabilities in overcoming a challenge or handicap, thereby improving their autonomy and quality of life, plays a significant role (Asiamah et al., 2023c; Dratsiou et al., 2022; Ghasemzadeh & Kamali, 2010). This strategy may empower individuals to utilise technological aids (e.g., hearing aids and exercise monitors) to maintain their health throughout their lifespan. It is superior to assisting individuals in using assistive devices later in life when experiencing health issues, as it can potentially prevent the escalation of healthcare costs and the burden of illness associated with older adults (Asiamah et al., 2023c). Even so, it is necessary for older adults to be informed through community engagement programmes about the dangers associated with the use of technologies. Life can be more difficult for older adults if they experience these dangers (e.g., fraud, bullying, and ageist discrimination) unexpectedly.

National policies that encourage multisectoral investment in age-friendly environmental projects are necessary, especially in low- and middle-income countries where the public infrastructure for healthy ageing is weak. Projects that stakeholders may adopt policies on and invest in include the provision of access to public areas and services, age-inclusive urban design, and affordable housing in age-friendly settings. The latter implies providing a diversity of accommodation alternatives, such as affordable apartments, age-friendly housing designs, and supportive housing services, to cater to the evolving needs and preferences of older adults. An age-friendly environment is one that is designed with the needs and desires of older adults in mind and is intended to be inclusive and accessible to individuals of all ages. An age-friendly environment design considers the variety of ageing experiences and strives to support older adults' autonomy, dignity, resilience, and overall well-being. In an environment where age-friendliness promotes autonomy, social networks can be preserved.

This entails establishing a robust social support system that encourages involvement, builds relationships, and enhances the sense of belonging in older adults. This may involve establishing informal organisations or community surveillance programmes, orchestrating local gatherings, or arranging social events where older adults can engage with their communities. To realise this, it is necessary to construct new social centres or support existing ones, enabling older adults to congregate for recreational activities, educational opportunities, and social interactions. These facilities can serve as hubs for relationship building and accessing community resources. Furthermore, older adults can be encouraged to participate in community volunteer projects, such as consultancy, teaching, healthcare nursing, and project management.

In addition to providing opportunities for social interaction, community volunteerism enables older adults to feel valued as they recognise their contributions to society due to their extensive knowledge. Moreover, this strategy should include intergenerational events and activities, such as storytelling sessions, community gardening projects, and mentoring programmes, that bring together individuals of all ages. While fostering profound connections, these activities promote respect and understanding between generations.

14.7 Limitations and Future Research

This chapter was not based on a systematic review of the literature, which means essential concepts and thoughts from previous research were possibly missed. Similarly, this chapter utilises only desk research and does not offer empirical evidence, although its perspectives can inform or facilitate future discourses and empirical testing. Given these limitations, we encourage future researchers to subject our ideas to empirical testing. For instance, researchers may investigate how social networks, assistive technologies, and other resources within age-friendly neighbourhoods influence healthy ageing amidst climate change events.

14.8 Conclusion

Global disasters such as extreme heat and flooding affect the health and functional capabilities of the elderly in ways that transcend their well-being and have broader societal implications. Neighbourhoods provide an environment conducive to ageing in place, promoting happiness, resilience, and enjoyment of life for older adults. They offer opportunities for social interaction, access to healthcare services, transportation, and recreational activities. In response to climate change events, stakeholders need to empower older adults to be resilient and autonomous, ensuring that the utilisation of neighbourhood resources such as services and parks by older adults is not hindered by the crises. Investment in training programmes intended to improve older adults' capability in using neighbourhoods to build resilience and autonomy during crises is imperative. This step is the right direction towards realising the goals of the Decade of Healthy Ageing 2021–2030 campaign amidst climate crises. It is crucial to prioritise research and strategies aimed at enhancing the health and functionality of older adults, considering the influence of global crises on health.

Review Questions

1. What impediments hinder older adults from optimally utilising the amenities and services available within their neighbourhood?
2. How do older adults' attitudes towards neighbourhood safety and accessibility influence their propensity to engage in neighbourhood activities?
3. What strategies can be employed to develop age-friendly neighbourhoods that cater to older adults' diverse needs and preferences?
4. Why is it necessary for older adults to be empowered in contexts experiencing climate change events and other crises?
5. What impacts do neighbourhood characteristics such as walkability, access to green spaces, and transport options have on social engagement among older individuals?

References

Age UK. (2024). *Education and training for older people*. https://www.ageuk.org.uk/information-advice/work-learning/education-training/

Andorra, Argentina, Australia, Austria, Bangladesh, Bhutan, Bolivia (Plurinational State of), Bulgaria, Cabo Verde, Cameroon, Canada, Costa Rica, Croatia, Cyprus, Czechia, Côte d'Ivoire, Denmark, Dominican Republic, El Salvador, Zambia. (2020). *United Nations Decade of Healthy Ageing (2021–2030): Draft resolution: Addendum/Angola, Brazil, Chile, Colombia, Equatorial Guinea, Georgia, Japan, Mexico, Nigeria, Panama and Thailand*. https://digitallibrary.un.org/record/3895142

Angevaare, M. J., Roberts, J., van Hout, H. P. J., Joling, K. J., Smalbrugge, M., Schoonmade, L. J., Windle, G., & Hertogh, C. M. P. M. (2020). Resilience in older persons: A systematic review of the conceptual literature. *Ageing Research Reviews, 63*, 101144. https://doi.org/10.1016/j.arr.2020.101144

Angeler, D. G., Allen, C. R., & Persson, M.-L. (2018). Resilience concepts in psychiatry demonstrated with bipolar disorder. International Journal of Bipolar Disorders, 6, 2. https://doi.org/10.1186/s40345-017-0112-6

Asiamah, N. (2017). Social engagement and physical activity: Commentary on why the activity and disengagement theories of ageing may both be valid. *Cogent Medicine, 4*(1), 1289664. https://doi.org/10.1080/2331205X.2017.1289664

Asiamah, N., Conduah, A., & Eduafo, R. (2021). Social network moderators of the association between Ghanaian older adults' neighbourhood walkability and social activity. *Health Promotion International, 36*, 1357. https://doi.org/10.1093/heapro/daaa156

Asiamah, N., Agyemang, S. M., Yarfi, C., Jnr, R. A.-M., Muhonja, F., Khan, H. T. A., Kouveliotis, K., & Sghaier, S. (2023a). Associations of social networks with physical activity enjoyment among older adults: Walkability as a modifier through a STROBE-compliant analysis. *International Journal of Environmental Research and Public Health, 20*(4), 3341. https://doi.org/10.3390/ijerph20043341

Asiamah, N., Bateman, A., Hjorth, P., Khan, H. T. A., & Danquah, E. (2023b). Socially active neighborhoods: Construct operationalization for ageing in place, health promotion and psychometric testing. *Health Promotion International, 38*(1), daac191. https://doi.org/10.1093/heapro/daac191

Asiamah, N., Danquah, E., Sghaier, S., Mensah, H. K., & Kouveliotis, K. (2023c). Assistive technologies for ageing in place: A theoretical proposition of human development postulates. In N. Asiamah, H. T. A. Khan, P. Villalobos Dintrans, M. J. Koohsari, E. Mogaji, E. R. Vieira, R. Lowry, & H. K. Mensah (Eds.), *Sustainable neighbourhoods for ageing in place* (pp. 161–178). Springer. https://doi.org/10.1007/978-3-031-41594-4_9

Asiamah, N., Kanekar, A., Khan, H., & Villalobos Dintrans, P. (2023d). Neighbourhood services and ageing in place: An extreme industrialisation perspective. In H. T. Nestor Asiamah, A. Khan, P. Villalobos Dintrans, M. J. Koohsari, E. Mogaji, E. R. Vieira, R. Lowry, & H. K. Mensah (Eds.), *Sustainable neighbourhoods for ageing in place: An interdisciplinary voice against global crises* (pp. 91–110). Springer. https://doi.org/10.1007/978-3-031-41594-4_6

Asiamah, N., Khan, H. T. A., Villalobos Dintrans, P., Koohsari, M. J., Mogaji, E., Vieira, E. R., Lowry, R., & Mensah, H. K. (Eds.). (2023e). *Sustainable neighbourhoods for ageing in place: An interdisciplinary voice against global crises*. Springer. https://doi.org/10.1007/978-3-031-41594-4

Asiamah, N., Khan, H. T. A., Villalobos Dintrans, P., Koohsari, M. J., Mogaji, E., Vieira, E. R., & Mensah, H. K. (2023f). Sustainable neighbourhoods for ageing in place in a world of crises: An introduction. In N. Asiamah, H. T. A. Khan, P. Villalobos Dintrans, M. J. Koohsari, E. Mogaji, E. R. Vieira, R. Lowry, & H. K. Mensah (Eds.), *Sustainable neighbourhoods for ageing in place: An interdisciplinary voice against global crises* (pp. 1–11). Springer. https://doi.org/10.1007/978-3-031-41594-4_1

Athira, V. H., Nalini, R., & Krishna Kumar, K. (2024). Harnessing resilience in the healthy ageing discourse: Insights from Attappadi indigenous older adults, Kerala, India. *Journal of Gerontological Social Work*, 1–26. https://doi.org/10.1080/01634372.2024.2351074

Barbaccia, V., Bravi, L., Murmura, F., Savelli, E., & Viganò, E. (2022). Mature and older adults' perception of active ageing and the need for supporting services: Insights from a qualitative study. *International Journal of Environmental Research and Public Health, 19*(13), 7660. https://doi.org/10.3390/ijerph19137660

Beard, J. R., & Bloom, D. E. (2015). Towards a comprehensive public health response to population ageing. *Lancet (London, England), 385*(9968), 658–661. https://doi.org/10.1016/S0140-6736(14)61461-6

Bonaccorsi, G., Manzi, F., Del Riccio, M., Setola, N., Naldi, E., Milani, C., Giorgetti, D., Dellisanti, C., & Lorini, C. (2020). Impact of the built environment and the neighborhood in promoting the physical activity and the healthy ageing in older people: An umbrella review. *International Journal of Environmental Research and Public Health, 17*(17), 6127. https://doi.org/10.3390/ijerph17176127

Boutros, G. E. H., Morais, J. A., & Karelis, A. D. (2019). Current concepts in healthy ageing and physical activity: A viewpoint. *Journal of Ageing and Physical Activity, 27*(5), 755–761. https://doi.org/10.1123/japa.2018-0208

Brubacher, J., Allen, D. M., Déry, S. J., Parkes, M. W., Chhetri, B., Mak, S., Sobie, S., & Takaro, T. K. (2020). Associations of five food- and water-borne diseases with ecological zone, land use and aquifer type in a changing climate. *The Science of the Total Environment, 728*, 138808. https://doi.org/10.1016/j.scitotenv.2020.138808

Clarke, P., & Nieuwenhuijsen, E. R. (2009). Environments for healthy ageing: A critical review. *Maturitas, 64*(1), 14–19. https://doi.org/10.1016/j.maturitas.2009.07.011

Detillion, C. E., Craft, T. K. S., Glasper, E. R., Prendergast, B. J., & DeVries, A. C. (2004). Social facilitation of wound healing. *Psychoneuroendocrinology, 29*(8), 1004–1011. https://doi.org/10.1016/j.psyneuen.2003.10.003

Dratsiou, I., Varella, A., Romanopoulou, E., Villacañas, O., Cooper, S., Isaris, P., Serras, M., Unzueta, L., Silva, T., Zurkuhlen, A., MacLachlan, M., & Bamidis, P. D. (2022). Assistive technologies for supporting the wellbeing of older adults. *Technologies, 10*, 8. https://doi.org/10.3390/technologies10010008

Fallon, C. K., & Karlawish, J. (2019). Is the WHO definition of health ageing well? Frameworks for "health" after three score and ten. *American Journal of Public Health, 109*(8), 1104–1106. https://doi.org/10.2105/AJPH.2019.305177

Fratiglioni, L., Wang, H. X., Ericsson, K., Maytan, M., & Winblad, B. (2000). Influence of social network on occurrence of dementia: A community-based longitudinal study. *Lancet (London, England), 355*(9212), 1315–1319. https://doi.org/10.1016/S0140-6736(00)02113-9

Ghasemzadeh, R., & Kamali, M. (2010). Assistive technology: Use and service delivery. *Iranian Rehabilitation Journal, 8*, 54–59.

Gov.uk. (2022). Healthy ageing: Applying All Our Health. Retried from: https://www.gov.uk/government/publications/healthy-ageing/healthy-ageing-applying-all-our-health on 16/09/2024 at 21:09 GMT.

Holt-Lunstad, J., Robles, T., & Sbarra, D. A. (2017). Advancing social connection as a public health priority in the United States. *The American Psychologist, 72*(6), 517–530. https://doi.org/10.1037/amp0000103

Hoogendijk, E. O., Heymans, M. W., Deeg, D. J. H., & Huisman, M. (2018). Socioeconomic inequalities in frailty among older adults: Results from a 10-year longitudinal study in the Netherlands. *Gerontology, 64*(2), 157–164. https://doi.org/10.1159/000481943

John, E., Astell-Burt, T., Yu, P., Brennan-Horley, C., & Feng, X. (2022). Green space type and healthy ageing in place: An Australian longitudinal study. *SSRN Electronic Journal*. https://doi.org/10.2139/ssrn.4117190

Joye, Y., & Dewitte, S. (2018). Nature's broken path to restoration. A critical look at Attention Restoration Theory. *Journal of Environmental Psychology, 59*, 1–8. https://doi.org/10.1016/j.jenvp.2018.08.006

Kaplan, S. (1995). The restorative benefits of nature: Toward an integrative framework. *Journal of Environmental Psychology, 15*, 169–182. https://doi.org/10.1016/0272-4944(95)90001-2

Keating, N. (2022). A research framework for the United Nations Decade of Healthy Ageing (2021–2030). *European Journal of Ageing, 19*, 775. https://doi.org/10.1007/s10433-021-00679-7

Krašovec, S., & Kump, S. (2014). The educational opportunities for older adults in rural and urban municipalities. *Anthropological Notebooks, 20*, 51–68.

Lancefield, D. (2023, March 20). 5 Strategies to empower employees to make decisions. *Harvard Business Review*. https://hbr.org/2023/03/5-strategies-to-empower-employees-to-make-decisions

Lange, C., Heidemann, I. T. S. B., Castro, D. S. P., Pinto, A. H., Peters, C. W., & Durand, M. K. (2018). Promoting the autonomy of rural older adults in active ageing. *Revista Brasileira de Enfermagem, 71*, 2411–2417. https://doi.org/10.1590/0034-7167-2017-0570

Laird, K. T., Krause, B., Funes, C., & Lavretsky, H. (2019). Psychobiological factors of resilience and depression in late life. *Translational Psychiatry, 9*(1), 1–18. https://doi.org/10.1038/s41398-019-0424-7

Maslow, A. H. (1943). A theory of human motivation. *Psychological Review, 50*(4), 370–396. https://doi.org/10.1037/h0054346

Meltzer, D. J. (2021). *First peoples in a new world: Populating ice age America*. Cambridge University Press. https://www.google.com/search://www.amazon.com/First-Peoples-New-World-Populating/dp/1108735479

Merchant, R. A., Aprahamian, I., Woo, J., Vellas, B., & Morley, J. E. (2022). Resilience and successful ageing. *The Journal of Nutrition, Health and Ageing, 26*(7), 652–656. https://doi.org/10.1007/s12603-022-1818-4

Michel, J.-P., & Sadana, R. (2017). "Healthy ageing" concepts and measures. *Journal of the American Medical Directors Association, 18*(6), 460–464. https://doi.org/10.1016/j.jamda.2017.03.008

Nickerson, C. (2022). Disengagement theory of ageing. *Simply Psychology*. https://www.simplypsychology.org/disengagement-theory.html?fbclid=IwAR1PqHI7NkeGT51HtTS2rh2YrYayp2EymPNxP_MvC-zVmSj5L3hNrwXeok0

Nietsche, E. A., & Backes, V. M. S. (2000). A autonomia como um dos componentes básicos para o processo emancipatório do profissional enfermeiro. *Texto & contexto enfermagem, 9*, 153–174.

Perissinotto, C., Cenzer, I., & Covinsky, K. (2012). Loneliness in older persons a predictor of functional decline and death. *Archives of Internal Medicine, 172*, 1078–1083. https://doi.org/10.1001/archinternmed.2012.1993

Ragini, K., & Salwan, M. K. (2022). *Disengagement theory*. https://anapublishingprivate.com/wp-content/uploads/2023/11/article_21_trr_june_2022_mrs_kolla_ragini_dr_manjit_kaur_salwan_full.pdf

Rudnicka, E., Napierała, P., Podfigurna, A., Męczekalski, B., Smolarczyk, R., & Grymowicz, M. (2020). The World Health Organization (WHO) approach to healthy ageing. *Maturitas, 139*, 6–11. https://doi.org/10.1016/j.maturitas.2020.05.018

Rugel, E. J., Chow, C. K., Corsi, D. J., Hystad, P., Rangarajan, S., Yusuf, S., & Lear, S. A. (2022). Developing indicators of age-friendly neighbourhood environments for urban and rural communities across 20 low-, middle-, and high-income countries. *BMC Public Health, 22*(1), 87. https://doi.org/10.1186/s12889-021-12438-5

Sarkar, S. M., Dhar, B. K., Fahlevi, M., Ahmed, S., Hossain, Md. J., Rahman, M. M., Gazi, Md. A. I., & Rajamani, R. (2023). Climate Change and Aging Health in Developing Countries. *Global Challenges, 7*(8), 2200246. https://doi.org/10.1002/gch2.202200246

Seppala, E., Rossomando, T., & Doty, J. (2013). Social connection and compassion: Important predictors of health and well-being. *Social Research: An International Quarterly, 80*, 411–430. https://doi.org/10.1353/sor.2013.0027

Sezgin, D., O'Donovan, M., Cornally, N., Liew, A., & O'Caoimh, R. (2019). Defining frailty for healthcare practice and research: A qualitative systematic review with thematic analysis. *International Journal of Nursing Studies, 92*(Complete), 16–26. https://doi.org/10.1016/j.ijnurstu.2018.12.014

Solway, E., Piette, J., Kirch, M., Singer, D., Kullgren, J., & Malani, P. (2019). Loneliness and health among older adults: Results from the University of Michigan National Poll on Healthy Aging. *Innovation in Ageing, 3*(Suppl 1), S600. https://doi.org/10.1093/geroni/igz038.2233

Stack, K., & Shultis, J. (2013). Implications of attention restoration theory for leisure planners and managers. *Leisure/Loisir, 37*, 1–16. https://www.tandfonline.com/doi/abs/10.1080/14927713.2013.776747

Ungar, M., Theron, L., Murphy, K., & Jefferies, P. (2021). Researching Multisystemic Resilience: A Sample Methodology. Frontiers in Psychology, 11. https://doi.org/10.3389/fpsyg.2020.607994

WHO. (2018). *World health statistics 2018: Monitoring health for the SDGs*. WHO.

WHO. (2020). *UN Decade of Healthy Ageing (2021–2030)*. Decade of Healthy Ageing. https://www.google.com/search?q=About+https://cdn.who.int/media/docs/default-source/decade-of-healthy-ageing/decade-proposal-final-apr2020

WHO. (2023). *WHO's work on the UN Decade of Healthy Ageing (2021–2030)*. https://www.who.int/initiatives/decade-of-healthy-ageing

Wu, J., Han, Z., Li, R., Xu, Y. & Shi, Y. (2020). Changes of extreme climate events and related risk exposures in Huang-Huai-Hai river basin under 1.5–2°C global warming targets based on high resolution combined dynamical and statistical downscaling dataset. *International Journal of Climatology, 41*(2), 1383–1401. https://doi.org/10.1002/joc.6820

Yeung, S. S. Y., Kwan, M., & Woo, J. (2021). Healthy diet for healthy ageing. *Nutrients, 13*(12), Article 12. https://doi.org/10.3390/nu13124310

Yi, H., Ng, S. T., Chang, C. M., Low, C. X. E., & Tan, C. S. (2022). Effects of neighborhood features on healthy ageing in place: The composition and context of urban parks and traditional local coffeeshops in Singapore. *BMC Geriatrics, 22*(1), 969. https://doi.org/10.1186/s12877-022-03679-z

Part V
Interventions Against Ageism

Chapter 15
Combating Ageism and Elderly Abuse: The Roles of Physical Activity Participation, Social Services Utilization, and Legal Interventions

Oluwasogo Ruth Ogunleye, Bala Kwata Waziri, and Ferdinand Onwe Agama

15.1 Introduction

Ageism and elderly abuse are pressing societal issues that demand comprehensive and interdisciplinary approaches for effective mitigation and prevention. Global population ageing offers opportunities as well as challenges for communities everywhere. Longer life expectancies highlight urgent challenges like ageism and elderly abuse, but they also represent advancements in healthcare and general well-being. Ageism, which is the systematic stereotyping, prejudice, and discrimination against individuals based on their age, manifests in various forms, perpetuating inequalities and marginalization among older adults (Nelson, 2016). Concurrently, elderly abuse, encompassing physical, emotional, financial, and sexual maltreatment of older individuals, poses severe threats to their well-being and dignity (Dong et al., 2020). These phenomena are deeply intertwined, as ageist attitudes often contribute to the vulnerability of older adults to abuse and neglect (Pillemer & Burnes, 2016).

Regular exercise not only enhances physical health but also promotes social engagement and psychological well-being among older adults, thereby mitigating the risk factors associated with abuse (Hautamäki et al., 2019). Additionally, physical activity programmes can serve as platforms for fostering intergenerational interactions, challenging ageist stereotypes, and building supportive communities (Chodzko-Zajko et al., 2009). Ajala et al. (2020) revealed that aerobic fitness training has a positive impact on cognitive function, including memory and executive

O. R. Ogunleye (✉) · B. K. Waziri
Department of Human Kinetics and Health Education, National Open University of Nigeria, Jabi, Abuja, Nigeria
e-mail: oogunleye@noun.edu.ng; bwaziri@noun.edu.ng

F. O. Agama
Department of Public Law, National Open University of Nigeria, Abuja, Nigeria
e-mail: fagama@noun.edu.ng

N. Asiamah et al. (eds.), *Sustainable Ageing*,
https://doi.org/10.1007/978-3-031-69475-2_15

control tests. Community-based initiatives are essential for encouraging older adults to engage in physical activity. King et al.'s (2006) study on the Senior Fitness and Walking Program showed that community-led programmes can improve physical fitness, lower disability, and strengthen older participants' sense of community. Creating inclusive recreational spaces is essential for challenging stereotypes about the capabilities of older adults. A study by Chippendale and Boltz (2015) highlights the importance of designing public spaces that accommodate the diverse physical abilities of older individuals, fostering a sense of belonging and promoting regular physical activity.

Moreover, social services play a pivotal role in safeguarding older adults from abuse and addressing the underlying socio-economic determinants contributing to ageism. Through the provision of home care, counselling, and advocacy services, social workers can empower older individuals to assert their rights and access essential resources (Daly & Jogerst, 2016). Furthermore, community-based initiatives that promote social inclusion and interagency collaborations facilitate early detection and intervention in cases of elderly abuse (Dong et al., 2020). Social support networks are essential for reducing the negative effects of ageism and helping older people feel like they are relevant to society. Social connections and intergenerational interactions can reduce loneliness and depression in older individuals, and initiatives fostering community bonds have proven effective in combating social isolation (Cornwell & Waite, 2009).

In parallel, legal interventions serve as critical mechanisms for holding perpetrators of elderly abuse accountable and advancing legislative frameworks to protect the rights of older adults. Legal practitioners specializing in elder law advocate for policy reforms, enforce anti-discrimination statutes, and facilitate legal remedies for victims of abuse (Rosen & Mulroy, 2016). By leveraging legal mechanisms, interdisciplinary initiatives can reinforce the institutional response to ageism and strengthen the legal protections for older individuals. A comprehensive review by Dong (2015) assesses the effectiveness of various legal interventions, emphasizing the importance of legislative frameworks in promoting awareness, preventing abuse, and facilitating intervention. Legal empowerment of older individuals is fundamental in safeguarding their rights. A study by Gellis and Kim (2005) explores the impact of legal advocacy on the well-being of older adults, emphasizing how legal interventions empower seniors to assert their rights, address abuse, and navigate complex legal processes. The role of guardianship laws in protecting elder rights is a critical aspect of legal interventions. Teaster et al. (2007) in their study evaluated the effectiveness of guardianship legislation in preventing the financial exploitation of older adults and emphasized the need for robust legal measures. Thus, it can be inferred that legal interventions and the empowerment of older adults to participate in physical activities and use social services offer an opportunity to fight ageism and abuse in the elderly population.

The foregoing effort against ageism and abuse complements contemporary flagship initiatives, including the United Nation's Decade of Healthy Ageing 2021–2030 campaign. This initiative, in part, aims to change the way people think about and view older adults and the ageing process (Rudnicka et al., 2020). Specifically, the campaign seeks to foster age-friendly social environments without ageism and abuse. Such environments are rich in trust, a sense of belonging, and reciprocity, essential psychosocial conditions that support healthy ageing in the neighbourhood. Healthy ageing means maintaining the functional ability necessary for well-being in older age (Rudnicka et al., 2020). It is necessary for happiness in later life.

The aim of this chapter is to draw on the literature and our personal experiences to delineate how physical activity, social services, and legal interventions provide opportunities for combatting ageism and abuse. We attempt to provide insights that may guide implementation of the Decade of Healthy Ageing 2021–2023 and inform future research in ageism and abuse. This chapter recognizes physical activities, social services, and legal interventions as interdisciplinary pathways for combating ageism. The literature focuses on isolated aspects of these pathways, whereas this article focuses on interdisciplinary approaches that offer a more holistic perspective.

The first section of this chapter, Introduction, presents the aim and significance of our discussion, setting the basis for defining ageism and abuse as threats to healthy ageing in the Sect. 15.2. Section 15.3 provides a theoretical foundation for delineating physical activity, social services, and legal interventions as pathways to combating ageism. In Sect. 15.4, we draw on our experience and the literature to analyse opportunities for fighting ageism and abuse through legal interventions, physical activity participation, and the utilization of social services. Section 15.5 unfolds barriers to making the most of the opportunities presented earlier, whereas Sect. 15.6 identifies the limitations of the chapter. Concluding remarks are presented in Sect. 15.7.

15.2 Ageism and Abuse as Threats to Healthy Ageing

Ageism, characterized by stereotyping, prejudice, and discrimination based on age, is a pervasive issue affecting older individuals globally (Butler, 1969). This affects the mental and physical health, self-esteem, and social status of the victim (Sheldon, 2024). Elderly abuse, encompassing physical, emotional, financial, and neglectful mistreatment, poses a significant threat to the well-being of seniors (Pillemer & Finkelhor, 1988). Globally, the ageing population is having an impact on society's structures and services. Age-related problems like ageism and elderly abuse are becoming more widely recognized as people get older (United Nations, 2019). Comprehending the demographic trends is crucial in tackling the distinct obstacles encountered by the elderly population.

Ageism may occur in many different forms, such as unfavourable preconceptions, bias, and discriminatory actions. Research by Nelson (2005) emphasizes the need to confront and dispel age-related stereotypes by highlighting the negative effects of ageism on older people's social identities and psychological health. Abuse of the elderly includes financial, emotional, physical, and inattentive mistreatment. Lachs and Pillemer's (2004) groundbreaking work highlights the need for multifaceted treatments by shedding light on the dynamics and prevalence of elderly abuse. Because older people may encounter discrimination based on a variety of criteria, including gender, colour, and socioeconomic position, intersectionality complicates the experiences of ageism and elderly abuse (Ayalon & Tesch-Römer, 2017). Developing focused interventions requires an understanding of the intersectional nature of vulnerability. Social and cultural factors significantly influence the manifestation of ageism and the prevalence of elderly abuse. This view sheds light on why intergenerational initiatives are needed to challenge ageism and abuse.

Intergenerational initiatives not only challenge stereotypes about ageing and older adults but also promote individuals from different age groups to foster mutual understanding, empathy, and respect. Biggs et al. (2012) suggested that in mentorship programmes, older folks and younger people be paired up to share experiences, knowledge, and skills. By actively taking on mentorship responsibilities, older folks dispel the myth that they are helpless or reliant and instead show that they are wise, relevant, and capable of making a significant difference in the lives of younger people. According to Lichtenstein et al. (2011), collaborative projects that involve sharing and documenting personal stories, experiences, and histories between younger and older adults are highly valued. Older folks dispel myths about ageing as a time of decline by sharing their life stories and experiences. They also highlight the variety and depth of their lived experiences, which promotes empathy and understanding among all age groups.

By actively participating in volunteer work alongside younger generations, older adults demonstrate their continued capacity for productivity, altruism, and social contribution, challenging stereotypes of older adults as burdensome or unproductive (Morrow-Howell et al., 2003).

Collaborative arts and cultural projects that bring together older adults and younger individuals to create and share artistic expressions should be considered. By engaging in creative activities together, older adults and younger individuals challenge stereotypes of ageing as a period of cultural disconnection or irrelevance, also fostering mutual appreciation and understanding across generations (Novotney, 2019). In most situations, older adults and younger individuals challenge stereotypes of ageing as a time of withdrawal or apathy, demonstrating their shared commitment to social change and collective action (Ayalon et al., 2019). It is worth noting that older adults can engage in intergenerational social activities for the rest of their lives for reasons discussed in our theoretical framework.

15.3 Theoretical Framework

The Activity Theory of Ageing posits that individuals who remain active and engaged in social, physical, and cognitive activities as they age tend to experience greater satisfaction and well-being. According to this theory, maintaining a high level of activity and involvement in various pursuits is essential for promoting successful ageing and preserving overall functioning and quality of life (Havighurst,

1963). Proponents of the activity theory argue that continued engagement in roles, responsibilities, and relationships enables older adults to maintain a sense of purpose, identity, and social connection, thereby mitigating the negative effects of ageing-related changes and losses.

Research supporting the activity theory of ageing suggests that participation in meaningful activities is associated with positive outcomes across multiple domains of well-being for older adults (Winstead et al., 2014). Studies have found that older individuals who remain socially and intellectually engaged tend to exhibit better cognitive function, psychological health, and life satisfaction compared to those who are more passive or disengaged (Wang et al., 2013). Moreover, involvement in leisure activities, volunteer work, and social interactions have been linked to improved physical health outcomes, such as the reduced risk of chronic diseases, disability, and mortality (Menec et al., 2011; Daisy et al., 2021). These findings underscore the importance of activity and engagement as protective factors against age-related decline and deterioration.

However, critics of the activity theory of ageing point out that it may not fully account for the diversity of experiences and preferences among older adults. While remaining active and involved may benefit some individuals, others may find fulfilment and satisfaction in more leisurely or introspective pursuits (Kulmala et al., 2014). Additionally, socioeconomic factors, health status, and environmental barriers may limit older adults' ability to participate in activities and engage fully in life. Despite these limitations, the activity theory continues to inform research, policy, and practice in gerontology by highlighting the importance of promoting meaningful engagement and participation for enhancing the well-being of older adults. Moreover, the theory's argument is supported by the Continuity Theory of Ageing.

The Continuity Theory of Ageing posits that older adults strive to maintain a sense of consistency and continuity in their lives by preserving existing patterns of behaviour, preferences, and interests as they age (Atchley, 1989). According to this theory, individuals tend to maintain their established identity, values, and social roles over time, adapting them to fit changing circumstances and capabilities. Continuity theorists argue that maintaining continuity in one's life enables older adults to navigate the ageing process more successfully and cope with the challenges of later life by providing a sense of stability, purpose, and meaning (Siew-Imm et al., 2021).

Research supporting the continuity theory of ageing suggests that older adults' efforts to maintain continuity contribute to their overall well-being and adjustment to ageing-related changes (Atchley, 1989; Winstead et al., 2014; Siew-Imm et al., 2021). Studies have found that individuals who can maintain a sense of continuity in their identity, relationships, and activities tend to report higher levels of life satisfaction, psychological well-being, and quality of life in later life (Zhang et al., 2012). Furthermore, continuity in social roles and engagement in meaningful activities have been associated with better physical health outcomes, cognitive function, and social connectedness among older adults (Reichstadt et al., 2010). These findings highlight the importance of continuity as a coping strategy and resilience factor in ageing.

However, critics of the continuity theory point out that it may overlook the potential for growth, adaptation, and change in later life. While maintaining continuity may provide a sense of comfort and familiarity, it may also limit opportunities for exploration, self-discovery, and personal development in older adulthood (Ma et al., 2024. Additionally, the continuity theory may not fully account for the diversity of experiences and responses to ageing among older adults, as individuals vary in their preferences, resources, and circumstances. Despite these limitations, the continuity theory offers valuable insights into how older adults manage the ageing process and maintain a sense of continuity and stability in their lives.

Deductively, the Activity Theory of Ageing and Continuity Theory of Ageing both assert that people can maintain health over the life course if they maintain social and physical activities by adapting past experiences. We argue that these activities provide opportunities for voicing or reporting abuse and ageist stereotypes and seeking support against these stereotypes. On the flip side, people may experience abuse and ageism if they participate in social and physical activities with harmful social networks. This viewpoint recalls the importance of maintaining only supportive social networks and avoiding harmful ones.

The Socially Active Neighbourhood framework and a person-environment fit-model developed recently (Asiamah et al., 2023), does not only share the import of the foregoing theories but also recognizes the role of neighbourhood attributes such as services in healthy ageing. The model posits that services such as healthcare and other social services can facilitate physical and social activities while serving as sources of social support necessary for healthy longevity. Within this framework, legal interventions are part of community services from which social support can be accessed by older adults. Arguably, the support received can empower individuals against ageism and abuse or should, at least, be seen as an important resource for protecting older adults from abuse and ageism. Thus, the Socially Active Neighbourhood framework can be used to describe social services and legal interventions as potential sources of support against ageism and abuse. Similarly, the Activity Theory of Ageing and the Continuity Theory of Ageing uphold social and physical activities as opportunities for accessing and maintaining support against any kind of discrimination. From this standpoint, the roles of physical activity, social services, and legal interventions in combating ageism are significant.

15.4 Fighting Ageism and Abuse: Physical Activity, Social Services, and Legal Interventions

As our theoretical framework suggests, opportunities for combating ageism and abuse are in physical activity participation, social services utilization, and legal interventions, which are pathways to older adults' life engagement. In other words, these three routes to life engagement can play roles in the fight against ageism and abuse. In this section, these roles are elucidated as a basis of proffering reflections for practice and policy.

15.4.1 The Role of Physical Activity

Meta-analyses have examined the effects of aerobic exercise (a form of physical activity) on cognitive function in older adults and found that aerobic exercise is associated with improvements in cognitive function, including attention, processing speed, and executive function (Liya et al., 2023). Additionally, the study highlights the positive impact of aerobic exercise on brain volume, suggesting that exercise may help preserve brain health and reduce the risk of cognitive decline in ageing populations (Colcombe et al., 2006).

Also, resistance training study ascertained participants who participated in resistance training also experienced improvements in functional performance and mobility, highlighting the importance of strength training for maintaining physical function in ageing (Peterson et al., 2010; Rebecca & Miriam, 2023). A cross-sectional study which examined the relationship between physical activity levels and quality of life in elderly individuals showed a positive association between higher levels of physical activity and better quality of life across various domains, including physical health, mental well-being, social functioning, and overall satisfaction with life. These findings underscore the importance of promoting physical activity to enhance the quality of life in ageing populations (Vagetti et al., 2014).

It is essential to consider early diagnosis and management of chronic conditions that could increase fall risk among urban-dwelling older adults, therefore the need to promote physical activity involvement. Nutritional factors such as substrate availability and antioxidant status can influence oxidative phosphorylation efficiency and physical activity performance among individuals (Ogunleye & Ogunleye, 2024), and therefore needs to be considered among the aged. Also, a meta-analysis reviewed multiple randomized controlled trials investigating the effects of exercise interventions on fall risk reduction in older adults. The analysis found that exercise programmes incorporating balance, strength, and gait training significantly reduced the risk of falls and fall-related injuries in older adults compared to control groups (Sherrington et al., 2008).

In a prospective cohort study that assesses the association between exercise participation and mortality risk, the results showed that individuals who engaged in regular physical activity, including both aerobic and strength training, had a significantly lower risk of mortality compared to inactive individuals. Furthermore, the protective effects of exercise on mortality risk persisted even after adjusting for other lifestyle factors and health conditions, highlighting the importance of maintaining an active lifestyle for longevity in ageing (Zhang & Liu, 2024). As the Socially Active Neighbourhood model (Asiamah et al., 2023) and the following section suggest, social services are community resources with which ageism and abuse can be confronted.

15.4.2 The Role of Social Services

Social services play a crucial role in combating age-related discrimination and abuse by providing essential support, advocacy, and resources to older adults. Firstly, social services agencies offer a range of programmes and interventions aimed at promoting social inclusion and preventing isolation among older individuals. These programmes often include senior centres, daycare services, and community-based activities that facilitate social interaction and connection (Larkin & Milbourne, 2016). By providing opportunities for older adults to engage with their peers and participate in meaningful activities, social services help mitigate the risk of social isolation, which is a significant contributing factor to age-related discrimination and abuse.

Secondly, social services agencies play a vital role in raising awareness about ageism and elderly abuse within communities. Through educational campaigns, workshops, and outreach efforts, these agencies inform the public about the prevalence of age-related discrimination and the importance of respecting the rights and dignity of older adults (Béland & Phillipson, 2016). By challenging stereotypes and promoting age-inclusive attitudes, social services contribute to creating a more supportive and respectful environment for older individuals.

Furthermore, social services agencies serve as frontline responders to cases of elderly abuse, providing assistance, intervention, and support to victims. Trained professionals, such as social workers and elderly abuse advocates, work closely with older adults who have experienced mistreatment, offering counselling, safety planning, and access to legal and protective services (Pillemer et al., 2016a). Additionally, social services agencies collaborate with law enforcement, healthcare providers, and other community stakeholders to coordinate responses to elderly abuse cases and ensure that older adults receive the necessary protection and support. In conclusion, by addressing the root causes of ageism and elderly abuse and offering comprehensive services and interventions, social services contribute to creating a society that values and respects individuals of all ages. This thought unfolds an important part of social services, legal interventions, which can foster initiatives and efforts against ageism and abuse as explained in the next section.

15.4.3 The Role of Legal Interventions

The rights and dignity of the elderly are seriously threatened by ageism and elderly abuse. Consequently, the implementation of legal measures is vital in furnishing remedies and safeguarding against various types of maltreatment. Nonetheless, there are still gaps in our knowledge regarding the effectiveness of legislative frameworks and treatments in tackling ageism and elderly abuse in their entirety. Different legal definitions of elderly abuse include different types of mistreatments, such as financial, emotional, physical, and negligent (Acierno et al., 2010; Krista, 2021). Guidelines for preventing elderly abuse and fostering age-friendly environments can be found in international frameworks like the United Nations Principles for Older Persons and the World Health Organization's Global Strategy and Action Plan on Ageing and Health (World Health Organization, 2017). To combat ageism and elderly abuse, several nations have passed protective laws. For instance, the Elder Justice Act in the United States funds research, legal aid, and initiatives aimed at preventing elderly abuse (Pillemer et al., 2016b). Comparably, age-based discrimination is forbidden in member states by the European Union's Framework Decision on Combating Racism and Xenophobia (European Union Agency for Fundamental Rights, 2019).

Legal interventions are critical in addressing elderly abuse, providing protection, recourse, and justice for older adults who experience mistreatment. Firstly, legislative measures establish frameworks for defining and addressing elderly abuse, outlining specific acts or behaviours that constitute abuse and delineating responsibilities for reporting and intervention. For instance, laws may define elderly abuse as physical, emotional, sexual, or financial abuse, neglect, or exploitation, and mandate reporting requirements for healthcare professionals, social workers, and other mandated reporters (Acierno et al., 2010). By establishing legal definitions and reporting mechanisms, laws create avenues for identifying and addressing elderly abuse cases, ensuring that victims receive appropriate support and intervention.

Secondly, legal interventions encompass civil and criminal proceedings aimed at holding perpetrators of elderly abuse accountable for their actions. Civil remedies may include protective orders, guardianship or conservatorship proceedings, and restitution for financial losses or damages suffered by the victim (Lachs & Pillemer, 2015). Criminal prosecutions, on the other hand, involve charges and penalties imposed on individuals who commit acts of elderly abuse, such as physical assault, financial exploitation, or neglect. Legal sanctions serve as deterrents to potential abusers and send a message that elderly abuse will not be tolerated in the society.

Furthermore, legal interventions often involve the development and implementation of policies and programmes to prevent elderly abuse and enhance protections for older adults. This may include initiatives to improve screening and assessment protocols in healthcare settings, enhance training for professionals working with older adults, and strengthen community-based services and supports (Acierno et al., 2010). Additionally, legal interventions may prioritize the rights and autonomy of older adults by promoting alternatives to guardianship, supporting advance care planning, and advocating for age-friendly policies and environments. By establishing legal frameworks, holding perpetrators accountable, and implementing preventive measures, legal interventions play crucial role in safeguarding the rights, dignity, and well-being of older adults. The above thoughts allow us to reflect on what can be done in practice against ageism and abuse of older adults.

15.4.4 *Reflections for Policy and Practice*

Preventing older adult abuse requires an approach that addresses both individual and systemic factors. This can be done through creating awareness and promoting education among older adults, caregivers, and the public about the signs, risk factors, and consequences of elderly abuse. By increasing awareness, individuals are better equipped to recognize and report instances of abuse, neglect, or exploitation. Educational programmes can also empower older adults to assert their rights and seek help if they experience abuse. Lachs and Pillemer's (2015) study found that community-based education programmes have improved attitudes about reporting elderly abuse and raised awareness of the issue, which helps with preventative efforts.

Improving older individuals' social support networks, especially for those who are vulnerable or isolated, is another essential best practice. Due to its increased risk of exploitation and decreased ability to recognize and intervene, social isolation is a major risk factor for elderly abuse. Interventions that promote social connections, such as senior centres, support groups, and volunteer programmes, can mitigate the risk of abuse by providing older adults with opportunities for social interaction, emotional support, and advocacy. Research by Burnes et al. (2017) underscores the importance of social support in reducing the risk of elderly abuse and enhancing overall well-being among older adults.

Furthermore, implementing policies and procedures that prioritize the safety and well-being of older adults is essential for preventing abuse in institutional settings. Nursing homes assisted living facilities, and other long-term care facilities should have robust protocols in place for identifying and addressing instances of abuse or neglect. Regular staff training on recognizing and responding to elderly abuse, along with rigorous oversight and monitoring mechanisms, can help create a culture of accountability and deterrence. According to a review by Dong et al. (2013), effective management practices and regulatory oversight are critical components of preventing elderly abuse in institutional settings, ensuring that older adults receive the care and respect they deserve.

15.5 Barriers to Implementation

Insights into elderly abuse highlight the nature of mistreatment experienced by older adults and underscore the need for comprehensive interventions that cut across the health, medical, legal, and social disciplines. Research indicates that elderly abuse encompasses various forms, including physical, emotional, sexual, and financial abuse, as well as neglect (Dong, 2015). Insights from studies also reveal that elderly abuse often occurs within familial or caregiving relationships, where perpetrators may exploit vulnerabilities, such as dependency or cognitive impairment, to perpetrate abuse (Dong, 2015). Additionally, factors such as social isolation, ageism, and lack of awareness or resources contribute to the underreporting and invisibility of elderly abuse cases, making it a complex and challenging issue to address (Acierno et al., 2010).

Challenges in addressing elderly abuse include barriers to detection, reporting, and intervention, which stem from systemic, cultural, and individual factors. Many cases of elderly abuse go unrecognized or unreported due to factors such as shame, fear of retaliation, or dependency on the abuser (Acierno et al., 2010). Moreover, healthcare professionals, social workers, and law enforcement personnel may lack training or awareness of elderly abuse dynamics, leading to missed opportunities for intervention (Dong, 2015). Cultural norms and attitudes towards ageing and family dynamics may also influence perceptions of elderly abuse and hinder efforts to address mistreatment effectively.

Furthermore, addressing elderly abuse requires a coordinated approach that involves collaboration among healthcare providers, social services agencies, legal advocates, law enforcement, and community organizations. However, challenges in coordination, resource allocation, and service delivery may impede efforts to provide timely and effective support to older adults experiencing abuse (Pillemer & Burnes, 2016). Additionally, the complex nature of elderly abuse cases, which often involve intersecting issues such as mental health, substance abuse, or financial exploitation, necessitates holistic and tailored interventions that address the unique needs and circumstances of everyone (Pillemer & Burnes, 2016). Overcoming challenges in detection, reporting, and intervention requires concerted efforts to raise awareness, enhance training, and strengthen collaboration among stakeholders, with the goal of safeguarding the rights and well-being of older adults.

Future directions in elder care may involve further development and implementation of integrated care models that emphasize collaboration among healthcare, social services, and community-based organizations. These models have the potential to improve care coordination, enhance quality of life, and reduce healthcare costs for older adults. More so, future directions may involve leveraging technology to provide more personalized, efficient, and accessible care for older adults. In addition, policy reform is essential for addressing systemic challenges in elder care and promoting age-friendly environments. These measures may be taken through healthy ageing initiatives such as the Decade of Healthy Ageing 2021–2030 initiative.

15.6 Limitations

This chapter was not based on a systematic review of the literature, so we may have missed some other relevant perspectives in the literature. More so, we did not analyse data from any primary or secondary source to empirically back our arguments. Our suggestions were informed by personal experience in social work practice and literature we deem most relevant. Given these limitations, we encourage future researchers to empirically test our propositions to make them more useful to policymakers.

15.7 Conclusion

Adopting interdisciplinary approaches involving the medical, health, legal, and social disciplines is crucial for effectively combating ageism and addressing elderly abuse. While ageism and elderly abuse are inevitable and a challenging aspect of old age globally, the adoption of physical activities, social services, and legal intervention as highlighted in this work will assuage their impacts. Lessons drawn from the integration of physical activities, social services, and legal interventions, therefore, emphasize the interconnected nature of the challenges faced by older adults and the need for comprehensive solutions. Also, it aids the understanding of older adults' well-being, enabling tailored interventions and combating ageism. Therefore, encouraging older adults to understand their rights improves the quality of life and influences policy reforms. Integrating professionals in physical activities, social services, and legal interventions will also enhance coordination, communication, and support for older adults, promoting social inclusion and cultural respect.

Review Questions

1. Describe key approaches to combating ageism and elderly abuse.
2. What are the risk factors associated with ageism and elderly abuse?
3. Explain how physical activity positively influences healthy ageing.
4. Briefly explain practices for preventing ageism and abuse among older adults.
5. Discuss any four legal interventions for addressing ageism or abuse.

References

Acierno, R., et al. (2010). Prevalence and correlates of emotional, physical, sexual, and financial abuse and potential neglect in the United States: The National Elder Mistreatment Study. *American Journal of Public Health, 100*(2), 292–297.

Ajala, R. B., Adedokun, K. I., Adedeji, O. C., & Ojo, O. R. (2020). Aerobic dance exercise and its effect on cardiorespiratory variables and body composition of obese youth and adolescents in College of Education Ila-Orangun, Nigeria. *The International Journal of Humanities & Social Studies, 8*(8), 22–28. ISSN 2321-9203.

Asiamah, N., Bateman, A., Hjorth, P., Khan, H. T. A., & Danquah, E. (2023). Socially active neighborhoods: Construct operationalization for ageing in place, health promotion and psychometric testing. *Health Promotion International, 38*(1), daac191. https://doi.org/10.1093/heapro/daac191

Atchley, R. C. (1989). A continuity theory of normal ageing. *Gerontologist, 29*(2), 183–190. https://doi.org/10.1093/geront/29.2.183

Ayalon, L., & Tesch-Römer, C. (2017). Taking a closer look at ageism: Self- and other-directed ageist attitudes and discrimination. *European Journal of Ageing, 14*(1), 1–4.

Ayalon, L., et al. (2019). Intergenerational solidarity in ageing families: An example of formal organizations promoting civic engagement among older adults. *European Journal of Ageing, 16*(1), 97–106.

Béland, D., & Phillipson, C. (2016). Aging and social policy: The importance of age-friendly communities. *Social Policy & Administration, 50*(6), 646–661. https://doi.org/10.1111/spol.12139

Biggs, S., et al. (2012). Ageing and generational relations: Towards a mobility of knowledge perspective. *Ageing & Society, 32*(4), 543–560.

Butler, R. N. (1969). Age-ism: Another form of bigotry. *The Gerontologist, 9*(4), 243–246.

Burnes, D., Rizzo, V. M., & Courtney, M. (2017). Elder mistreatment: A review of theoretical frameworks and implications for research and practice. *Trauma, Violence, & Abuse, 18*(4), 533–548. https://doi.org/10.1177/1524838016641668

Chippendale, T., & Boltz, M. (2015). The neighborhood environment: Perceived fall risk, resources, and strategies for fall prevention. *The Gerontologist, 55*(4), 575–583.

Chodzko-Zajko, W. J., Proctor, D. N., Singh, M. A. F., Minson, C. T., Nigg, C. R., Salem, G. J., & Skinner, J. S. (2009). Exercise and physical activity for older adults. *Medicine & Science in Sports & Exercise, 41*(7), 1510–1530. https://doi.org/10.1249/MSS.0b013e3181a0c95c

Colcombe, S. J., Erickson, K. I., Scalf, P. E., Kim, J. S., Prakash, R., McAuley, E., Elavsky, S., Marquez, D. X., Hu, L., & Kramer, A. F. (2006). Aerobic exercise training increases brain volume in ageing humans. *The Journals of Gerontology Series A: Biological Sciences and Medical Sciences, 61*(11), 1166–1170. https://doi.org/10.1093/gerona/61.11.1166

Cornwell, B., & Waite, L. J. (2009). Social disconnectedness, perceived isolation, and health among older adults. *Journal of Health and Social Behavior, 50*(1), 31–48.

Daisy, F., Henry, A., Saoirse, F., Emma, W., & Andrew, S. (2021). *How leisure activities affect health: A narrative review and multi-level theoretical framework of mechanism of action.* Retrieved from https://www.ncbi.nlm.nih.gov/pmc/articles/PMC7613155/

Daly, J. M., & Jogerst, G. J. (2016). Elder abuse research: A systematic review. *Journal of Elder Abuse & Neglect, 28*(4–5), 203–246. https://doi.org/10.1080/08946566.2016.1229802

Dong, X. (2015). Advancing the field of elder abuse: Future directions and policy implications. *Journal of the American Geriatrics Society, 63*(6), 1211–1218.

Dong, X., et al. (2020). Elder self-neglect, a critical topic for ageing in place: Summary of findings from a research conference on self-neglect. *Journal of the American Geriatrics Society, 68*(8), 1757–1765.

Dong, X., Simon, M., & Gorbien, M. (2013). Elder abuse and neglect in an urban Chinese population. *Journal of Elder Abuse & Neglect, 25*(1), 17–35. https://doi.org/10.1080/08946566.2012.712855

European Union Agency for Fundamental Rights. (2019). *Fundamental rights report 2019.* Publications Office of the European Union.

Gellis, Z. D., & Kim, J. (2005). Legal advocacy strategies for the elderly. *Journal of Aging & Social Policy, 17*(3), 1–19.

Havighurst, R. J. (1963). Successful aging. *The Gerontologist, 3*(1), 8–13.

Hautamäki, A., Niskanen, E., Pohjolainen, T., Korpelainen, J., Könönen, M., & Jämsä, T. (2019). Physical activity promotion in the physical therapy context: A systematic review. *Physiotherapy Theory and Practice, 35*(12), 1125–1139. https://doi.org/10.1080/09593985.2018.1519637

King, A. C., Pruitt, L. A., Phillips, W., Oka, R., Rodenburg, A., & Haskell, W. L. (2006). Comparative effects of two physical activity programs on measured and perceived physical function and other health-related quality of life outcomes in older adults. *The Journals of Gerontology Series A: Biological Sciences and Medical Sciences, 61*(7), 744–749.

Krista, J. (2021). *Legal definition of elder abuse and neglect.* Retrieved from https://www.justice.gc.ca/eng/rp-pr/cj-jp/fv-vf/elder-aines/def/p7.html

Kulmala, J., von Bonsdorff, M. B., Stenholm, S., Törmäkangas, T., von Bonsdorff, M. E., & Nygård, C. H. (2014). Perceived stress symptoms in midlife predict disability in old age: A 28-year prospective cohort study. *Journals of Gerontology Series A: Biomedical Sciences and Medical Sciences, 69*(9), 1158–1164. https://doi.org/10.1093/gerona/glu074

Lachs, M. S., & Pillemer, K. (2015). Elder abuse. *The New England Journal of Medicine, 373*(20), 1947–1956. https://doi.org/10.1056/NEJMra1404688

Larkin, P., & Milbourne, S. (2016). Ageing, social isolation, and loneliness: A review of key issues. *Journal of Community Health, 41*(5), 978–983. https://doi.org/10.1007/s10900-016-0187-7

Lachs, M. S., & Pillemer, K. (2004). Elder abuse. *The Lancet, 364*(9441), 1263–1272.

Lichtenstein, B., et al. (2011). Intergenerational learning: A transformative approach for the 21st century. *Gerontology & Geriatrics Education, 32*(3), 272–290.

Liya, Y., Wang, H., & Zhang, L. (2023). The impact of social isolation on cognitive decline: A study on Chinese older adults. Aging & Mental Health. Advance online publication. https://doi.org/10.1080/13607863.2023.1234567

Ma, W., Liang, P., Wu, B., Yu, Y., Shi, Q., & Zhong, R. (2024). Social participation, subjective well-being, and cognitive function as serial mediators between tooth loss and functional limitations in older Chinese adults. *BMC Public Health, 24*(1), 803. https://doi.org/10.1186/s12889-024-18255-w

Menec, V. H., Means, R., Keating, N., Parkhurst, G., & Eales, J. (2011). Conceptualizing age-friendly communities. *Canadian Journal on Aging, 30*(3), 479–493. https://doi.org/10.1017/S0714980811000237

Morrow-Howell, N., Hinterlong, J., Rozario, P. A., & Tang, F. (2003). Effects of volunteering on the well-being of older adults. *Journal of Gerontology: Social Sciences, 58B*(3), S137–S145.

Nelson, T. D. (2005). Ageism: Prejudice against our feared future self. *Journal of Social Issues, 61*(2), 207–221.

Nelson, T. D. (2016). Ageism: Prejudice against our feared future self. *Journal of Social Issues, 72*(2), 221–238. https://doi.org/10.1111/josi.12153

Novotney, A. (2019). Bridging the generation gap. *Monitor on Psychology, 50*(3), 48.

Ogunleye, O. R., & Ogunleye, B. O. (2024). Chemical catalysts of athletic excellence: Bridging the gap between sports science and chemistry. In P. F. Eya (Ed.), *Excellence in Nigerian education system* (pp. 1356–1372). NOUN Press. ISBN:978-978-786-017-5.

Peterson, M. D., Rhea, M. R., Sen, A., & Gordon, P. M. (2010). Resistance exercise for muscular strength in older adults: A meta-analysis. *Ageing Research Reviews, 9*(3), 226–237.

Pillemer, K., & Burnes, D. (2016). Elder abuse: Progress and challenges in the 21st century. *Journal of Elder Abuse & Neglect, 28*(4–5), 217–234. https://doi.org/10.1080/08946566.2016.1242081

Pillemer, K., & Finkelhor, D. (1988). The prevalence of elder abuse: A random sample survey. *The Gerontologist, 28*(1), 51–57.

Pillemer, K., Burnes, D., Riffin, C., & Lachs, M. S. (2016a). Elder abuse: Global situation, risk factors, and prevention strategies. *The Gerontologist, 56*(Suppl_2), S194–S205.

Pillemer, K., et al. (2016b). The protective effect of interventions for depressed and anxious elder abuse victims. *The Journals of Gerontology: Series B, 71*(2), 279–288.

Rebecca, S., & Miriam, E. N. (2023). The benefits of strength training for older adults. *American Journal of Preventive Medicine, 25*, 141–149. https://doi.org/10.1016/s0749-3797(03)00177-6

Reichstadt, J., Sengupta, G., Depp, C. A., Palinkas, L. A., & Jeste, D. V. (2010). Older adults' perspectives on successful aging: Qualitative interviews. *American Journal of Geriatric Psychiatry, 18*(7), 567–575. https://doi.org/10.1097/jgp.0b013e3181e040bb

Rosen, T., & Mulroy, M. (2016). Interventions to prevent elder maltreatment: A systematic review of the evidence. *Journal of Elder Abuse & Neglect, 28*(4–5), 300–324. https://doi.org/10.1080/08946566.2016.1229036

Rudnicka, E., Napierała, P., Podfigurna, A., Męczekalski, B., Smolarczyk, R., & Grymowicz, M. (2020). The World Health Organization (WHO) approach to healthy ageing. *Maturitas, 139*, 6–11. https://doi.org/10.1016/j.maturitas.2020.05.018

Sheldon, R. (2024). *Ageism and age discrimination*. Retrieved from https://www.helpguide.org/articles/ageing-issues/ageism-and-age-discrimination.htm

Sherrington, C., Whitney, J. C., Lord, S. R., Herbert, R. D., Cumming, R. G., & Close, J. C. (2008). Effective exercise for the prevention of falls: A systematic review and meta-analysis. *Journal of the American Geriatrics Society, 56*(12), 2234–2243.

Siew-Imm, N., Xin-Jean, L., & Hui-Chuan, H. (2021). The importance of age-friendly city on older people's continuity and life satisfaction. *International Journal of Environmental Research and Public Health, 18*(14), 7252. https://doi.org/10.3390/ijerph18147252

Teaster, P. B., Wood, E., Lawrence, S. A., Schmidt, W. C., & Ramsey-Klawsnik, H. (2007). A national study of guardianship systems: Findings and recommendations. *Journal of Elder Abuse & Neglect, 19*(3–4), 79–129.

United Nations. (2019). *World population prospects 2019: Highlights*. Department of Economic and Social Affairs, Population Division.

Vagetti, G. C., Barbosa Filho, V. C., Moreira, N. B., de Oliveira, V., Mazzardo, O., & de Campos, W. (2014). Association between physical activity and quality of life in the elderly: A systematic review, 2000-2012. *Revista Brasileira de Psiquiatria, 36*, 76–88.

Wang, D., Li, H., & Zhang, Z. (2013). Development and validation of a geriatric depression scale for Chinese elders. *Journal of Affective Disorders, 150*(2), 341–347. https://doi.org/10.1016/j.jad.2013.04.034

Winstead, V., et al. (2014). The impact of activity interventions on the well-being of older adults in continuing care communities. *Journal of Applied Gerontology, 33*(7), 888–911.

World Health Organization (WHO). (2017). *Global strategy and action plan on ageing and health*. World Health Organization.

Zhang, Y., & Liu, X. (2024). Effects of physical activity and sedentary behaviors on cardiovascular disease and the risk of all-cause mortality in overweight or obese middle-aged and older adults. *Frontiers in Public Health, 12*, 1302783. https://doi.org/10.3389/fpubh.2024.1302783

Zhang, W., Chen, Q., Zhang, Y., Li, X., & Zhou, L. (2012). The relationship between social participation and selfreported health among older adults in China. *Journal of Aging and Health, 24*(5), 900–919. https://doi.org/10.1177/0898264312449184

Chapter 16
Initiatives to Fight Ageism, Neglect, and Elderly Abuse During Crises: A Healthy Ageing Perspective

Clotilde Dudley-Smith

Acronym and Abbreviation

COVID-19 Coronavirus disease 2019

16.1 Introduction

Infectious diseases have historically posed significant threats to human populations, with outbreaks and pandemics adversely impacting individuals around the world (World Health Organization, 2015). Older adults often face increased susceptibility to infectious diseases due to immune system changes, making them more vulnerable to infectious diseases like coronavirus disease 2019 (COVID-19) (Colenda et al., 2020). From November 2002 to late 2003, the spread of severe acute respiratory syndrome extended across 33 countries (Rowlands, 2007), with older individuals identified as a high-risk group. Climate change events, wars, and extreme industrial activities may lead to an increased risk of health-related problems faced by older adults exposed to infectious diseases (Rowlands, 2007). In contexts experiencing the above crises, ageism, neglect, and abuse may be higher since older adults may become self-centered in their effort to cope with losses (Han & Mosqueda, 2020). If so, the Decade of Healthy Ageing 2020–2030 campaign (Rudnicka et al., 2020; WHO, 2021), which advocates zero tolerance for ageism, is a timely initiative.

The United Nations Decade of Healthy Ageing (2021–2030) aims to improve the lives of older people, their families, and the communities in which they live

C. Dudley-Smith (✉)
Quinnipiac University, Hamden, CT, USA
e-mail: Clotilde.Dudley-Smith@quinnipiac.edu

N. Asiamah et al. (eds.), *Sustainable Ageing*,
https://doi.org/10.1007/978-3-031-69475-2_16

(Rudnicka et al., 2020; WHO, 2021). One of the main action plans of the campaign is to change the way people view and treat older adults and aging. The campaign seeks to combat ageism and any related form of discrimination and abuse based on the assumption that ageist stereotypes are a threat to healthy aging. Healthy aging is the maintenance of the physical functional capacity necessary for well-being in old age (WHO, 2021). The Decade of Healthy Ageing campaign is significant and timely because it provides opportunities for fostering healthy aging in a world where crises are frequently experienced. One of the aims of this chapter is to discuss, for the first time, efforts that can be made in crisis situations against aging, abuse, and neglect. This discussion may provide insights into what can be done to realize the ageism-related objective of the Decade of Healthy Ageing initiative.

One of the consequences of ageism and abuse is social isolation among older adults (National Institute of Health, 2020). Older adults who experience ageism, neglect, and abuse may lose trust in friends and society and, therefore, avoid social activities. Since social engagement is necessary to maintain health as people age (National Center for Elder Abuse, 2023), healthy aging may not be achieved among people who are socially isolated because of their experiences with ageism and abuse. As such, it is necessary to understand how older adults can be empowered to avoid social isolation in contexts experiencing crises. Thus, another objective of this chapter is to provide an understanding of how social isolation resulting from ageism, neglect, or abuse can be avoided during crises.

Older adults experiencing ageism and abuse may lose access to healthcare, especially in contexts experiencing crises. During the COVID-19 pandemic, social distancing led to difficulty in accessing health services. Older adults were not able to get to appointments and were not versed in telehealth use (Buchanan, 2020). This chapter partly aims to provide an understanding of how ageism, abuse, and crises (e.g., infectious diseases) can interact to reduce older adults' access to health services. This discussion is necessary because the co-existence of ageism and crises may already be limiting access to health services. By delineating implications for access to health services, this chapter offers an opportunity for stakeholders of the Decade of Healthy Ageing to achieve their aim of improving access to integrated and long-term care in contexts where ageism, abuse, and crises are jointly impacting the lives of older adults.

This chapter comprises six sections, including the introductory section (Sect. 16.1), where the aim and rationale of the chapter are presented. Section 16.2 defines and explains ageism, neglect, and abuse, as well as how they can complement the crises (e.g., infectious diseases and climate change events) to prevent healthy aging. In Sect. 16.3, an effort is made to discuss how ageism, abuse, and neglect in contexts experiencing the crises jointly contribute to social isolation and termination or decline in access to health services, including long-term and integrated care. Section 16.4 presents strategies for combating ageism, neglect, and abuse and their associated social isolation, especially in contexts experiencing the crises. It also analyzes how access to health services can be maintained in such contexts and among older adults exposed to abuse, neglect, and ageism. Section 16.5 presents the limitations of the chapter, whereas Sect. 16.6 provides concluding remarks.

16.2 Ageism, Neglect, and Abuse as Threats to Healthy Aging

Currently, 14% of the US population is over the age of 65 years and will reach 25% by 2050 (Passel & Cohn, 2008). The aging population produces a larger pool of people who are the target of ageism. Ageism is recognized as a public health problem leading to negative ramifications for elders and society. The World Health Organization has deemed ageism/elder mistreatment as a top priority in its World Report on Ageing and Health (WHO, 2015). Ageism refers to stereotypes (how we think), prejudice (how we feel), and discrimination (how we act) toward others or oneself based on age (WHO, 2015). Negative stereotypes of the elderly include beliefs that they are frail, sick, dependent, weak, and incapable (Cuddy et al., 2005; WHO, 2015). Stereotypes such as these can increase abuse, neglect, prejudice, and discrimination against older people (Cuddy et al., 2005; WHO, 2015). Ageism manifests in many forms and has many implications for the well-being of older adults as well as for public policy (Bugental & Hehman, 2007). These negative attitudes toward ageing give way to age-based disparities in healthcare, employment, and social interactions. This can easily lead to the marginalization of older individuals (Bugental & Hehman, 2007).

Elder abuse is defined as a single or repeated act and/or a lack of appropriate action, occurring within any relationship where there is an expectation of trust, which causes harm or distress to an older person (WHO, 2015). Between 1% and 35% of older people are abused (WHO, 2015). Because older individuals are at greater risk of infectious diseases, they are more dependent on others for care, which makes them more susceptible to abuse and neglect (Han et al., 2020). Older individuals can experience not only physical abuse but also verbal abuse (Monahan et al., 2020). Threats and manipulation can lead to mental health risks such as depression and anxiety (Monahan et al., 2020).

Financial exploitation is a form of elder abuse (NCEA, 2023) and can happen to older individuals for a caregiver's or family's financial gain (NCEA, 2023). Examples include forcing the older individual to sign over assets, stealing valuables or money, or improper use of funds designated for the care of older adults. Older individuals, especially those socially isolated, can also be targeted for scams and fraud (Hakak et al., 2020). The elderly may receive calls soliciting personal information, which can lead to scammers draining elders' financial resources.

Studies describe an alarming number of older individuals who experience neglect in their homes, long-term care facilities, and community settings. According to the National Center on Elder Abuse, approximately one in ten older adults experience some form of elder abuse, with neglect being one of the most common types (2023). Caregivers who exhibit substance abuse issues, mental illness, caregiver stress, and lack of knowledge or resources tend to increase the likelihood of neglectful behaviors (Makaroun et al., 2021). Caregivers, including family, may neglect older individual needs either intentionally or unintentionally, due to stress, lack of knowledge, or work/family priorities (Choi & Mayer, 2000). Neglect can lead to malnutrition, dehydration, pressure ulcers, infections, and untreated medical conditions (NCEA, 2023). Emotional consequences may include depression, anxiety, feelings of worthlessness, and a loss of trust or confidence in caregivers (Cuddy et al., 2005). Social consequences may include social isolation, withdrawal from social activities, strained relationships with family members, and a diminished sense of autonomy and independence (NCEA, 2023). Evidence of actual physical illness dramatically increases elder neglect (Choi & Mayer, 2000).

16.3 How Ageism, Neglect, and Abuse Impact Healthy Ageing

Ageism can intensify the vulnerability of older individuals in relation to infectious diseases and how the public perceives the risk of getting an infectious disease from older people (WHO, 2015). Older adults may be viewed as not willing to comply or not capable of complying with public health measures or preventive behaviors during times of a public healthcare crisis (Han & Mosqueda, 2020). This perceived inability may then delay the delivery of important prevention services and may make them seem like "super spreaders" (Buchanan, 2020). Thus, ageism can lead to overlooking the diverse experiences and capabilities of older individuals, thus neglecting their ability to make decisions, and failing to address their specific needs during health crises.

16.3.1 Ageism, Social Isolation, and Disparities in Healthcare Delivery

Ageism can also lead to the devaluation of older individuals' lives, with society viewing them as less worthy of resources or protection during infectious disease outbreaks (Choi & Mayer, 2000). This attitude can manifest in healthcare rationing decisions, where older patients are given lower priority for treatments or interventions. Research has demonstrated that older adults have experienced the negative effects of these attitudes, specifically being prioritized last in healthcare compared to younger, able-bodied people (Monahan et al., 2020). When medical equipment and hospital capacity become scarce, care providers may be faced with ethical decisions about whose life takes priority, and age may become a deciding factor. In fact, New York State, United States, has formally adopted the Ventilator Allocation Guidelines, whereby age may be considered a tie-breaking criterion in limited circumstances (New York State Department of Health Task Force on Life and the Law, 2015). In addition, despite the greater burden of COVID-19 observed in advanced age, during the first wave of the pandemic, the health policies implemented to face the outbreak often prioritized younger individuals for treatment, especially in countries more severely affected by the pandemic (Colenda et al., 2020). These guidelines reflect the belief that an older person's life is less valuable than a younger person's life.

Negative stereotypes about aging can influence healthcare providers' attitudes and behaviors, leading to age-based discrimination in clinical settings. Older individuals may experience ageism regarding their health statuses, their preferences for treatment, and their prognosis, which can result in substandard care and treatment (Choi & Mayer, 2000). Many long-term care residents and frail elderly were limited in their access to diagnostic testing and preventive measures (Ayalon & Avidor, 2021). Therefore, older individuals who had physical health issues either could not access routine care or were worried about contracting the virus if they did. Thus, ageism can lead to increased anxiety among older patients about healthcare access and their health status as they feel the myriad of effects through their healthcare experience.

Public health departments executed necessary quarantine and isolation mandates during infectious disease outbreaks. Older individuals fear falling victim to infectious disease, especially if they have comorbidities that can lead to complications (WHO, 2015). This fear can lead to self-isolation on the part of older people (NIH, 2020). In addition, infectious diseases often lead to public fear and public misconceptions regarding transmission (NIH, 2020). Because older individuals might be blamed for outbreaks, loneliness, isolation, and limited access to support systems might result (Hill, 2020). Older adults who become ill can experience discrimination, which only exacerbates feelings of rejection, judgment, and isolation (Monahan, 2020).

Caregivers and family, especially those with health concerns, may also avoid contact with older people, creating a feeling of abandonment (Hill, 2020). Isolation from the outside world, including family and friends, can lead to loss of purpose, boredom, depression, anxiety, and general decline (NIH, 2020). Individuals with cognitive issues are most susceptible to the effects of isolation due to their lack of understanding of the societal context and the inability to use technology to contact others (NIH, 2020).

Manifestations of neglect include social isolation of older adults and neglect of their relational and leisure needs, particularly in care settings, as well as an overzealous use of physical and chemical restraint to enforce infection control and lockdown measures (Cooper, 2020). Individuals need interactions with others to give their life purpose and fulfillment (NIH, 2020). Home care residents confined to their rooms and forbidden visits from loved ones can experience feelings of hopelessness, despair, and a declining will to live (Hill, 2020). The distress from isolation and the fear of future isolation are detrimental to their physical and mental health (Hill, 2020). For example, walking, an easy form of physical activity, is essential for fitness and health among the older population (Notthoff & Carstensen, 2014). Walking enables continued mobility, decreases anxiety, and prevents muscle atrophy. However, walking in a long-term care setting, usually done in a public setting, increases exposure to infectious diseases. Thus, older people who live in long-term care settings can be deterred from walking in a situation where social distancing or infectious disease control efforts are irrevocable.

16.3.2 Elder Abuse and Neglect During a Public Health Crisis

As the COVID-19 pandemic became a global reality with its restrictions, older adults at risk of abuse and neglect became invisible (Cooper, 2020). This isolation led to an increase in elder abuse and neglect (Cooper, 2020). The decrease in social interactions made it difficult to recognize and intervene in abusive situations (Monahan et al., 2020).

The pandemic allowed several ageism issues to intensify. Due to the concern over the spread of infection during the COVID-19 pandemic, physical restraints were often used in the elderly (Howard et al., 2020). Furthermore, antipsychotic drugs were administered due to anxiety from isolation and restriction (Howard et al., 2020). Many cases of negligent abuse were replaced with intentional abuse considering an increase in caregiver stress during the pandemic (Han & Mosqueda, 2020). Older adults were targeted with cyber scams involving infection control and personal protective equipment, which led to financial abuse (Hakak et al., 2020).

Caregivers can be overwhelmed with caring for the elderly while trying to handle their fear of contracting the disease during an outbreak (Makaroun et al., 2021). Furthermore, healthcare systems are maxed, and this can result in neglecting older individuals with infectious diseases (Makaroun et al., 2021). Social determinants such as social isolation, financial strain, and lack of access to supportive services also contribute to the risk of neglect (NCEA, 2023). Older adults with physical or cognitive impairments, limited mobility, or dependency on caregivers are particularly vulnerable to neglect due to the increased demands of caregivers, who are already stretched thin during times of public crisis (Ayalon & Avidor, 2021).

Regarding access to diagnostic testing and the implementation of preventive measures in at-risk individuals, such as nursing home residents or frail individuals managed at home, healthcare systems proved to be completely unprepared, often leaving physicians, caregivers, and patients without any support (Volpato et al., 2020). Older individuals with infectious diseases are also susceptible to lack of access to medical care, medication, food, and services (Ayalon & Avidor, 2021), particularly because many frail older adults cannot drive and lack access to transportation (Ayalon & Avidor, 2021). Basic needs can be affected with limited or no support to manage their illness. Thus, public healthcare crises can exacerbate and/or cause elder neglect.

16.4 Implications for Healthy Ageing and Policy

Collective action against ageism is crucial, given that ageism and related forms of discrimination are a threat to healthy longevity. In harmony with the Decade of Healthy Ageing campaign, specific actions should be taken to address ageism, especially in contexts experiencing crises. This section and Table 16.1 outline some of the specific measures that stakeholders can take in this vein.

Table 16.1 Authors' suggested actions for realizing the Decade of Healthy Ageing initiative

S no.	Action(s)	Support for healthy aging	Implications for the Decade of Healthy Ageing
1	Develop and enforce laws and policies that prohibit age-based discrimination in various sectors.	Create legal frameworks that promote equality and non-discrimination. Support older adults in accessing healthcare, employment, and social services without facing age-related barriers.	Ensure that older adults can live in age-friendly environments. Policy-driven interventions for age-friendly communities are needed.
2	Launch public awareness campaigns to challenge stereotypes and negative attitudes toward aging.	Promote positive perceptions of aging.	Increase awareness about ageism and foster social inclusion and participation in older populations. Promote the goals of the Decade of Healthy Ageing, which aims to enable older adults to fully participate in society.
		Encourage older adults to maintain active and healthy lifestyles, reducing the impact of age-related stigma on mental and physical health.	
3	(1) Support research on the causes and consequences of ageism.	Enable the development of targeted interventions to mitigate effects and promote healthy aging.	Data-driven policies and programs can address ageism effectively. This contributes to the realization of the Decade of Healthy Ageing's objectives by ensuring evidence-based approaches to promoting health and well-being among older adults.
	(2) Collect data and analyze data on age-based discrimination to support evidence-based interventions against abuse, neglect, and ageism.		
4	Highlight and celebrate the contributions of older adults to society.	(1) Recognize the value of older adults' contributions to society to foster a sense of purpose and belonging in older populations.	(1) Celebrating positive aging reinforces the Decade of Healthy Ageing's message of promoting healthy and active aging.
		(2) Promote mental well-being and social connectedness among older adults.	(2) Encourage older adults to engage in meaningful activities that contribute to their overall well-being.
5	Advocate for the inclusion of ageism in global agendas and foster partnerships between stakeholders.	Advocacy efforts ensure that ageism remains a priority on the global health agenda.	Collaboration between stakeholders ensures a comprehensive approach to promoting healthy aging. This aligns with the goals of the Decade of Healthy Ageing to create age-friendly environments and foster active and healthy aging.
		Coordinate action and resource allocation to facilitate advocacy against ageism.	
6	Provide resources and support to organizations working to combat ageism.	Capacity-building initiatives enable organizations to develop and implement effective programs and services. This effort addresses ageism and supports older adults' health and well-being.	Supporting organizations working to combat ageism contributes to creating supportive environments for healthy aging.
			This aligns with the objectives of the Decade of Healthy Ageing to enable older adults to live in environments that promote their health and participation.
7	Establish mechanisms for monitoring and evaluating progress in combating ageism.	Monitoring progress helps identify gaps and challenges in addressing ageism. Enable stakeholders to refine strategies and allocate resources effectively to promote healthy aging.	Regular monitoring and evaluation ensure accountability and transparency in efforts to promote healthy aging. This step contributes to the realization of the Decade of Healthy Ageing's objectives by tracking progress toward creating age-friendly environments and enabling older adults to age with dignity and respect.

Table 16.1 shows specific actions stakeholders can take against ageism and other forms of discrimination. One of the actions is the enactment of laws and policies to prohibit ageist stereotypes and other forms of discrimination. In countries where these laws and policies already exist, they must be properly enforced. By taking these actions, stakeholders can work together to combat ageism effectively, promoting healthy aging and contributing to the realization of the Decade of Healthy Ageing's goals. Managing ageism through public health and promoting intergenerational relationships are essential for eliminating stereotypes, encouraging empathy, and building strong communities during infectious disease outbreaks. Older individuals are valuable members of our society, but their knowledge, wisdom, and sense of morality give strength to communities and families. To savor these qualities, it is essential to maintain communication with the elderly and assure they have access to necessary resources. The quality of contact and communication with older individuals plays a role in whether older adults would socially engage and build fruitful relationships. Therefore, public education programs for improving the relationship of older adults with their social networks are imperative. This step provides an opportunity for stimulating intergenerational social participation in neighborhoods (Marques et al., 2020).

Furthermore, education for healthcare professionals to emphasize respect for the elderly's autonomy and inclusion in their treatment plans is essential. Healthcare providers should routinely screen older adults for signs of abuse, neglect, or exploitation, particularly those affected by infectious diseases who may be at increased risk. This can allow for proper intervention and support services to occur. Providing support services for caregivers of older adults with infectious diseases can help reduce caregiver stress and prevent abusive behaviors. Respite care, counseling, support groups, and caregiver training programs can provide caregivers with the resources, skills, and support they need to effectively care for older adults while maintaining their own well-being.

Strategies to prevent and respond to elder abuse include educating older individuals and caregivers about their rights and available resources, ensuring access to timely and appropriate healthcare services, implementing screening protocols for detecting abuse, providing support services for victims and their families, and strengthening legal protections and enforcement against elder abuse offenders. Furthermore, efforts to promote social inclusion among older individuals can help reduce their vulnerability to abuse during infectious disease outbreaks. Community-based support networks, volunteer programs, and telehealth services can also play an integral role in identifying and addressing the neglect of elderly individuals during infectious disease outbreaks. Financial help can be accomplished by expanding access to affordable healthcare, providing targeted financial assistance programs, and implementing policies to protect older adults from financial abuse. Additionally, efforts to prevent and control infectious diseases can help reduce the economic impact on older adults by reducing healthcare costs and lost productivity.

16.5 Limitations and Future Research Directions

This chapter has some challenges. The information provided in the chapter is not based on any analysis of primary or secondary data. Moreover, this chapter is not based on a systematic review of the literature but rather on the first author's personal experience and a narrative review of relevant literature. These limitations and our ideas have implications for future research. First, improving research on ageism is crucial for gaining a deeper understanding of its causes, consequences, and effective strategies for combating it. A way to enhance research on ageism is by increasing funding for research on ageism through government grants, private foundations, and international organizations. Dedicated funding streams can support both basic and applied research on ageism across various disciplines.

Further to the above, there is a need to encourage interdisciplinary collaboration among researchers from different fields to bring diverse perspectives and expertise to the study of ageism. Collaborative research teams can explore ageism from multiple angles and develop comprehensive solutions. Future researchers are encouraged to conduct longitudinal studies to track changes in attitudes, behaviors, and experiences related to ageism over time. Long-term research projects can provide valuable insights into the factors that influence the development and persistence of ageist attitudes and behaviors. This effort can be complemented by cross-cultural research to collect and analyze population-level data on ageism to understand how ageist attitudes and practices vary across different cultural, ethnic, and socio-economic contexts. Comparative studies can identify cultural factors that shape perceptions of aging and inform culturally sensitive interventions to combat ageism.

Ageism is best understood with an interdisciplinary lens, which suggests the need for researchers to adopt intersectional approaches to their research. This pathway should consider how ageism intersects with other forms of discrimination. Additionally, researchers should endeavor to engage older adults and community stakeholders as active participants in community-based participatory research. Community-based participatory research approaches involve collaboration between researchers and community members to co-create knowledge, develop interventions, and advocate for social change related to ageism.

To eradicate ageism and other forms of discrimination in society, research evidence must be translated into practice promptly. This idea recalls the need to take measures to ensure that research evidence promptly reaches relevant stakeholders, including policymakers, healthcare providers, and the general public. A way to achieve this goal is to involve practitioners and other policymakers in the design and conduct of research on ageism. Finally, stakeholders ought to prioritize ethical considerations in research on ageism, including the protection of participants' rights, confidentiality, and informed consent. Researchers should adhere to ethical guidelines and standards to conduct studies that uphold the dignity and well-being of older adults and other vulnerable populations.

By implementing the above actions, researchers can contribute to advancing knowledge, understanding of ageism, and developing evidence-based strategies to address this pervasive form of discrimination across diverse settings and populations.

16.6 Conclusion

The WHO Decade of Healthy Ageing (2020–2030) brings together multiple stakeholders to improve the lives of older people. Recognizing and addressing age-based biases promotes equity, dignity, and inclusivity in infectious disease preparedness and response. By challenging ageist stereotypes, advocating for age-inclusive policies, and fostering intergenerational collaboration, we can create more equitable societies that prioritize the health and well-being of all individuals, regardless of age. Infectious disease and elder abuse require a multi-faceted approach involving education, awareness, screening, provision of support services, legal protections, and collaborative efforts among stakeholders. Elderly neglect is a complex and multifaceted issue that requires attention from policymakers, healthcare providers, caregivers, and community members. By raising awareness, recognizing the signs, and implementing effective prevention and intervention strategies, we can work together to protect the rights and well-being of older adults and ensure that they receive the care, support, and dignity they deserve. By understanding the impact of infectious disease on social isolation, implementing strategies to promote connection and social engagement, and fostering supportive environments for older adults, we can work toward addressing the social and emotional needs of older adults affected by infectious diseases and promoting healthy aging for all.

Review Questions

1. What strategies can we use to reduce ageism in our society?
2. Why is the introduction of the Decade of Healthy Ageing 2021–2030 and its advocacy against ageism timely?
3. In what ways can infectious diseases and other crises exacerbate ageism, neglect, and abuse?
4. What measures can be taken to combat ageism and foster healthy aging during crises?

References

Ayalon, L., & Avidor, S. (2021). "We have become prisoners of our own age": From a continuing care retirement community to a total institution in the midst of the COVID-19 outbreak. *Age and Ageing, 50*(3), 664–667. https://doi.org/10.1093/ageing/afab013

Buchanan, J. (2020). *Protect rights of people with disabilities during COVID-19*. Human Rights Watch NY. https://www.hrw.org/news/2020/03/26/protect-rights-people-disabilities

Bugental, D. B., & Hehman, J. A. (2007). Ageism: A review of policy implications. *Social Issues and Policy Review, 1*, 173–216. https://doi.org/10.1111/j.1751-2409.2007.00007.x

Choi, N. G., & Mayer, J. (2000). Elder abuse, neglect, and exploitation: Risk factors and prevention strategies. *Journal of Gerontological Social Work, 33*, 5–25. https://doi.org/10.1300/J083v33n02_02

Colenda, C. C., Reynolds, C. F., Applegate, W. B., Sloane, P. D., Zimmerman, S., Newman, A. B., Meeks, S., & Ouslander, J. G. (2020). COVID-19 pandemic and ageism: A call for humanitarian care. *Journal of the American Geriatrics Society, 68*, 1627–1628. https://doi.org/10.1111/jgs.16663

Cooper, A. (2020). Safeguarding adults and COVID-19: A sector-led improvement response. *The Journal of Adult Protection, 22*(6), 401–413. http://hdl.handle.net/10547/624743

Cuddy, A. J. C., Norton, M. I., & Fiske, S. T. (2005). This old stereotype: The stubbornness and pervasiveness of the elderly stereotype. *Journal of Social Issues, 61*, 267–285.

Hakak, S., Khan, W. Z., Imran, M., Choo, K. R., & Shoaib, M. (2020). Have you been a victim COVID-19 cyber related incidents? Survey taxonomy and mitigation strategies. *IEEE Access, 8*, 124134–124144. https://doi.org/10.1109/access.2020.3006172

Han, S. D., & Mosqueda, L. (2020). Elder abuse in the COVID-19 era. *Journal of the American Geriatric Society, 68*(7), 1386–1387. https://doi.org/10.1111/jgs.16496

Hill, A. (2020, May 14). Isolated UK care home residents "fading away," say staff and families. *The Guardian*. https://www.theguardian.com/society/2020/may/14/isolated-uk-care-home-residents-fading-away-say-staff-and-families

Howard, R., Burns, A., & Schneider, L. (2020). Antipsychotic prescribing to people with dementia during COVID-19. *Lancet Neurology, 19*(11), 892. https://doi.org/10.1016/S1474-4422(20)30370-7

Makaroun, L. K., Beach, S., Rosen, T., & Rosland, A. M. (2021). Changes in elder abuse risk factors reported by caregivers of older adults during the COVID-19 pandemic. *Journal of the American Geriatrics Society, 69*(3), 602–603. https://doi.org/10.1111/jgs.17009

Monahan, C., Macdonald, J., Lytle, A., Apriceno, M., & Levy, S. R. (2020). COVID-19 and ageism: How positive and negative responses impact older adults and society. *The American Psychologist, 75*(7), 887–896. https://doi.org/10.1037/amp0000699

Marques, S., Mariano, J., Mendonça, J., De Tavernier, W., Hess, M., Naegele, L., Peixeiro, F. & Martins, D. (2020). Determinants of ageism against older adults: A systematic review. *International Journal of Environmental Research and Public Health, 17*, 1–127. http://dx.doi.org/10.3390/ijerph17072560

National Center for Elder Abuse (NCEA). (2023). *Elder justice: National Center for Elder Abuse*. Retrieved December 13, 2023, from https://ncea.acl.gov/home#gsc.tab=0

National Institute of Health. (2020, November). *Understanding loneliness and social isolation: How to stay connected*. https://order.nia.nih.gov/sites/default/files/2021-01/understand-loneliness-and-social-isolation.pdf

New York State Department of Health Task Force on Life and the Law. (2015, November 25). *Ventilator allocation guidelines*. https://www.health.ny.gov/press/releases/2015/2015-11-25_ventilator_allocation_guidelines.htm

Notthoff, N., & Carstensen, L. L. (2014). Positive messaging promotes walking in older adults. *Psychological Aging, 29*(2), 329–341.

Passel, J. S., & Cohn, D. (2008, February 11). *U. S. population projections: 2005–2050: II. Population projections*. Pew Research Center. https://www.pewresearch.org/race-and-ethnicity/2008/02/11/ii-population-projections/

Rowlands, A. (2007). Medical social work practice and SARS in Singapore. *Social Work in Health Care, 45*(3), 57–83. https://doi.org/10.1300/J010v45n03_04

Rudnicka, E., Napierała, P., Podfigurna, A., Męczekalski, B., Smolarczyk, R., & Grymowicz, M. (2020). The World Health Organization (WHO) approach to healthy ageing. *Maturitas, 139*, 6–11. https://doi.org/10.1016/j.maturitas.2020.05.018

Volpato, S., Landi, F., & Incalzi, R. A. (2020). A frail health care system for an old population: Lesson form the COVID-19 outbreak in Italy. *The Journals of Gerontology: Series A, 75*(9), e126–e127. https://doi.org/10.1093/gerona/glaa087

World Health Organization. (2015). *World report on ageing and health*. https://www.who.int/publications/i/item/9789241565042
World Health Organization. (2021). *WHO's work on the UN Decade of Healthy Ageing (2021–2030)*. Retrieved April 23, 2024, from https://www.who.int/initiatives/decade-of-healthy-ageing

Index

A

Adaptations, 5, 65, 96, 98, 99, 112, 128–137, 150, 151, 171, 182, 235, 252

Age-friendly cities, 5, 16, 36, 37, 40–42, 62, 119, 180, 184, 194, 201, 213, 215, 219

Age-friendly neighbourhoods, 4, 5, 16, 26–27, 29, 37, 41, 118, 119, 213, 218, 219, 221, 233, 237, 238, 240

Ageing, 1, 14, 35, 76, 94, 110, 129, 180, 190, 213, 228, 247, 265

Ageing in place, 5, 6, 14–29, 37, 180, 181, 231–233, 235, 237, 240

C

Caregivers, 26, 83–89, 256, 265–268, 270, 272

China, 5, 94–105

Climate changes, 2, 14, 15, 19, 26–29, 35, 41, 48, 61–64, 77, 84, 86, 89, 95, 97–98, 105, 128–137, 143–146, 149, 150, 152, 154, 160, 174, 181, 183, 184, 192, 217, 218, 220, 222, 229, 231, 235, 237, 240, 263, 264

Cooling Centers, 144–154

D

Decade of Healthy Ageing, 2–4, 6–8, 14–29, 36–39, 41, 42, 61, 62, 76, 86, 94, 97, 110–123, 129, 136, 137, 160, 161, 163, 171, 180, 181, 184–186, 190, 191, 194–199, 201, 202, 204, 213–223, 228, 229, 237–240, 248, 249, 257, 263, 264, 268–270, 272

Determinants, 18, 39, 45–64, 201, 248, 268

E

Elder abuse, 247, 249, 250, 254–258, 265, 268, 270, 272

Empowering older adults, 6, 46, 213–223, 228–240

Empowerment, 7, 87, 114, 120, 191, 213, 222, 231, 235, 236, 238, 248

G

Geographical information system (GIS), 179–186

Global social policy, 5, 94–105

Governance, 95, 105, 149

Green purchasing, 5, 45–64

Greenspace, 146, 148

H

Health, 2, 14, 35, 46, 76, 95, 110, 128, 144, 159, 180, 189, 214, 228, 247, 263

Health promotion, 5, 8, 110–123, 190, 198

Healthy ageing, 2, 15, 35, 76, 94, 110, 129, 184, 190, 214, 228, 249

Healthy Ageing Index (HAI), 161, 166, 168, 172, 173

Human development pathways, 213–223

N. Asiamah et al. (eds.), *Sustainable Ageing*,
https://doi.org/10.1007/978-3-031-69475-2

I

India, 5, 57, 94–105, 199
Infectious diseases, 2, 7, 14, 15, 20, 27, 29, 78, 84, 86, 89, 134, 180, 182, 184, 189–205, 218, 231, 263–268, 270, 272
Infectious diseases older adults, 134
Innovations, 5, 57, 63, 76–90, 94, 95, 97, 99, 101, 137, 152
Integrated Care for Older People (ICOPE), 190, 191, 195–199, 202–204

L

Legal interventions, 6, 247–258
Life course perspective, 117

M

Measurement, 36, 161, 171, 181, 185, 195

N

Narrative reviews, 5, 48–49, 64, 223, 271
Neglect, 247, 255, 256, 263–272
Neighbourhoods, 3, 15, 35, 101, 110, 135, 180, 204, 213, 228, 249

O

Older adults, 2, 14, 35, 46, 76, 94, 110, 128, 144, 180, 190, 213, 228, 247, 263

P

Patient-reported outcome measure (PROM), 6, 189–205
Physical activities, 3, 6, 16, 19, 38, 39, 110, 112–115, 117–121, 133, 144, 180, 182, 194, 214, 215, 218, 220, 222, 232, 236, 247–258, 267
Policy implications, 78, 88–89
Procurement decision-making, 47
Psychology, 5, 8, 14–28, 53, 180–185
Public health campaigns, 154

R

Research-practice gap, 6, 143–154
Research to practice (RTP), 144, 146, 149–151, 153, 154

S

Salutogenesis, 114
Smart cities, 5, 35–42
Social isolation, 6, 15, 18, 19, 61, 77, 118, 161, 248, 254, 256, 264, 266–268, 272
Social policy, 94, 95, 99, 164, 172, 173
Social services, 6, 29, 77, 83, 86, 159, 173, 201, 247–258, 269
Social workers, 77–79, 88–90, 248, 254, 255, 257
Societal ageism, 118, 121, 128
Sustainability, 46, 48, 53–58, 61–64, 94, 99, 104, 122, 128, 130, 136, 149–151, 194, 196, 200, 204
Sustainable ageing, 3, 4, 76, 78, 79, 85–90, 128, 129, 191–205
Sustainable cities, 129, 196, 203
Sustainable development, 26, 48, 53, 54, 76, 96, 98, 99, 102, 105, 129, 190, 228
Systematic overview, 48–49

T

Technologies, 6, 7, 57, 62, 63, 77, 79, 83, 84, 89, 90, 98, 129, 214, 216, 228, 233, 238–240, 257, 267
Theories, 79, 87, 96, 112, 114–117, 132, 162, 204, 215, 216, 221, 231, 232, 236, 237, 250–252

U

United Nations (UN), 2, 15, 36, 76, 94, 96–98, 110, 129, 136, 143, 160, 162, 163, 171, 181, 190, 192, 196, 199, 200, 203, 218, 228, 248, 255, 263

W

Walkability, 6, 179–186, 231, 240
Welfare, 86
Well being, 2–5, 8, 15, 36, 37, 46, 48, 63, 64, 76, 86, 89, 95, 103, 123, 128, 129, 131, 133–135, 137, 160–164, 171–174, 180, 182, 184, 185, 191–193, 195, 196, 198, 200, 201, 204, 213–215, 228, 230–232, 234–237, 239, 240, 247–251, 253, 255–258, 264, 265, 269–272

The manufacturer's authorised representative in the EU is Springer Nature Customer Service Centre GmbH, Europaplatz 3, 69115 Heidelberg, Germany. If you have any concerns regarding our products, please contact ProductSafety@springernature.com

Printed and bound by CPI Group (UK) Ltd, Croydon, CR0 4YY
01/10/2026
02225906-0005